The Art and Science of Health Care

The Art and Science of Health Care

Psychology and Human Factors for Practitioners

Bruce D. Kirkcaldy
(Editor)

International Centre for the Study of Occupational
and Mental Health, Düsseldorf, Germany

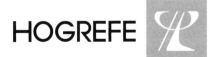

HOGREFE

Library of Congress Cataloging-in-Publication Data

is available via the Library of Congress Marc Database under the
LC Control Number 2011926764

Library and Archives Canada Cataloguing in Publication

The art and science of health care : psychology and human factors for practitioners / Bruce Kirkcaldy (editor).
Includes bibliographical references.

ISBN 978-0-88937-423-2

1. Medicine and psychology. 2. Medical personnel and patient. 3. Clinical medicine. 4. Integrative
medicine. I. Kirkcaldy, Bruce D. (Bruce David), 1952-

R726.5.A78 2011   610.1'9   C2011-902666-X

© 2011 by Hogrefe Publishing

PUBLISHING OFFICES
USA: Hogrefe Publishing, 875 Massachusetts Avenue, 7th Floor, Cambridge, MA 02139
          Phone (866) 823-4726, Fax (617) 354-6875; E-mail customerservice@hogrefe-publishing.com
EUROPE: Hogrefe Publishing, Rohnsweg 25, 37085 Göttingen, Germany
          Phone +49 551 49609-0, Fax +49 551 49609-88, E-mail publishing@hogrefe.com

SALES & DISTRIBUTION
USA: Hogrefe Publishing, Customer Services Department,
          30 Amberwood Parkway, Ashland, OH 44805
          Phone (800) 228-3749, Fax (419) 281-6883, E-mail customerservice@hogrefe.com
EUROPE: Hogrefe Publishing, Rohnsweg 25, 37085 Göttingen, Germany
          Phone +49 551 49609-0, Fax +49 551 49609-88, E-mail publishing@hogrefe.com

OTHER OFFICES
CANADA: Hogrefe Publishing, 660 Eglinton Ave. East, Suite 119 - 514, Toronto, Ontario M4G 2K2
SWITZERLAND: Hogrefe Publishing, Länggass-Strasse 76, CH-3000 Bern 9

Hogrefe Publishing
Incorporated and registered in the Commonwealth of Massachusetts, USA, and in Göttingen, Lower Saxony,
Germany

Cover image: "Das Grundprinzip der Medizin ist die Liebe" [The basic principle of medicine is love] (2004),
[acrylics and oil pastel on canvas], [200 x 150 cm], by Hubertus Salinger.
Reproduced by permission of Hubertus Salinger. Internet: www.lebenstaucher.de

Printed and bound in the USA
ISBN 978-0-88937-423-2

Table of Contents

Acknowledgments

I would like to express my sincere thanks to those persons and organizations that helped develop this book. Once again, it was an honor for me to draw on an international, multidisciplinary team, the 26 contributors who shared my enthusiasm and goals of producing a distinct series of essays which would depict the state-of-the-art in medicine and health care both in Europe and North America. Hogrefe, represented by Robert Dimbleby, a fellow British traveler who made his way to Germany, had the interest and courage to publish it and offered invaluable assistance on the structure, development, and presentation of the final "product," and for the help and effort of Lisa Bennett and her team in the production phase of the book. In the final stages of editing, when time pressures prevailed (one half of the manuscripts arrived in the month before submission!), I was extremely grateful for the support of some colleagues and friends: Terrence Martin (Ireland), Georg Siefen (Bochum), Claire Schulze (Cologne), and Richard Bogue (Florida) to act as "additional" readers for the final manuscripts and thus double proof some of my corrections and editorial comments. They responded to my urgent pleas irrespective of what time of day or night. I value not only their academic qualities, but their friendship and continued support in times of need! I was fortunate too in having reserved some time to visit my native Cheshire, relaxing during the day and being able to read through those manuscripts in the comfort of my "culture of origin," whilst being able to recuperate a bit from my daily clinical tasks in order to focus on editing the manuscripts. Finally, my thanks go to my wife, Elizabeth, and two daughters, Lisenka and Eliana, who in their own way provided me with the emotional support – in the form of discussions and midday walks through the forests – to motivate me in my research and writing endeavors.

Introduction

Introduction

Bruce D. Kirkcaldy

International Centre for the Study of Occupational and Mental Health Düsseldorf, Germany

This book aims to unite various fields of health sciences in a multidisciplinary venture drawing on academics and clinicians from medicine, psychology (clinical, organizational, and cognitive), nursing sciences, biochemistry, economics, and neurosurgery. In part it has grown out of my own professional career of 30 years, the first half of which focused primarily on research and the latter half on clinical practice. Throughout these three decades I am extremely fortunate to have met and collaborated with many colleagues in clinical, health, and organizational psychology who share my enthusiasm to unite clinical psychology, especially psychological health, with occupational and leisure psychology. Ironically, this quest for unity has taken place at a time when conventional authorities in psychology would have viewed such fusion as virtually impossible.

The interdisciplinary approach adopted here has assembled medical and health specialists – representing a rare ensemble of outstanding academics *and* clinicians, all experts in their fields. Collectively, their scholarly outputs reveal the interplay between medicine and psychology and social sciences from many different cultures and faculties, and share my vision of the nexus of psychology and human factors in healthcare.

Getting individuals to participate in such a publishing venture resembles the management of a sailing expedition across unexplored seas. It requires a competent and enduring crew, each an expert in their own field, and a willingness and motivation to endure the hardships whilst not rebelling or abandoning the journey underway. Hence, I value having completed this journey with them and seeing not a single person abandoned or thrown overboard from launch to completion – although the journey had some perilous moments and required the occasional around the clock watch (writing through the midnight hours to meet the deadlines!).

Each chapter addresses questions which will be central for social and policy makers in the public health field in the 21st century. This volume is intended as a creative and exploratory set of guidelines for a wide audience of medical and health professions, including general practitioners, psychiatrists, allied health personnel such as social workers, nurses and counselors and clinical psychologists, and hopefully prove to be of value for health professionals during their training and influence health policy makers. We have deliberately maintained a low level of mathematical or scientific expression to promote clarity of exposition which should ensure its popularity among professionals, researchers, and students alike.

The book is divided into five sections. The first focuses on culture, health, and medicine, the second on personality and health outcome determinants of the medical and healthcare profession. The third section addresses cultural and individual aspects of patient care. A fourth domain centers on cognitive psychology and medical/therapeutic treatment. The volume closes with a section on the barriers of economics and literacy in health care. To some extent this division is idiosyncratic. It could have easily been dichotomized into the more and less scientific/artistic categories. But that would have given a distorted impression that health sciences are an "either (science) or (art)" domain, when many of us in this crew feel that the health sciences require a fusion of both, a blend of art and science.

Again we all hope that the reader finds this collection of essays both up-to-date and practical. We have aimed to produce an innovative book offering creative guidance on the changing face of medicine. The book is also international, it assumes that there are common aspects in the experience of "being a health professional." It focuses on the physician's and health practitioner's experience, including the psychosocial environment in which she or he works and lives. It broadens common conceptions, and provides stimulation for physicians and others as they seek to understand more about their journeys across the unsettled seas of health and medicine.

Let me briefly provide a summary of the structure and content of the sections of the book.

Martin Brune begins from a biological perspective. Evolutionary medicine is a highly interdisciplinary field that draws from biology, psychology, anthropology, and diverse fields of medicine. One view argues that many contemporary social, psychological, and physical ills are the result of incompatibilities between the environments of human evolution and those in which most of us live today. This chapter provides an overview of the field of evolutionary medicine with selected examples and proposes that, by adopting an evolutionary perspective, medical researchers, and healthcare providers may be able to approach contemporary health challenges in ways that improve health and well-being. The chapter begins with an introduction to evolutionary medicine and goes on to examine selected health challenges from an evolutionary perspective, including: Medical consequences of bipedalism, evolved bodies and modern lifestyles, and evolution and reproduction. Martin then outlines further an evolutionary view of "normal" health and offers his ideas on what medicine can gain from an understanding of evolution.

In clinical practice, irrespective of medical or psychological ailment, health practitioners will observe sleeping disorders amongst their patients, although the effects of such problems are frequently overlooked. Indeed medical and allied personnel themselves are often "victims" of such disruptions in circadian rhythms. In Chapter 2, Timo Partonen, Finland Institute of Mental Health, examines the impact of biological rhythms of work and health among medical doctors and nursing personnel. His chapter defines the concept of circadian misalignment, followed by a brief introduction to the circadian and sleep processes in humans. Timo then summarizes relevant research results from simulated (Laboratory) and field (real situation) studies of shift work on performance in medical profession, and makes recommendations based on scientific trials regarding monitoring sleep-wake patterns and to improve adaptation to night-shift work in particular.

Over the last two decades, there has been a significant increase in the use of pharmaceuticals especially in the developed industrialized nations for the treatment of ill-health and psychological disorders. Some have labeled this an "Era of Medication." Chapter 3 by Bruce Kirkcaldy, Adrian Furnham, and Georg Siefen begins with a review of the literature on the relationship between well-being and medication. Drawing on various cross-cultural data bases from the World Health Organization, the UN and additional sources, the authors examine cross-cultural differences in psychopharmaceutical expenditure, highlighting specific psycho-pharmacological agents such as antidepressives, anxiolytic medication, and hypnotics/sedatives medication. They analyze the relationship between medication health costs and life satisfaction. Exploratory analyses are provided on the prevalence of psychological disorders and suicide rates across countries, as well as the relationships between psychotropic drug use and psychological well-being and physical health. Finally, the association between socioeconomic factors and psychopharmaceutical consumption are examined, and the implications of these findings for future healthcare research.

In an American contribution, Richard Bogue and colleagues from Florida provide an overview of the research and prominent lines of thought related to physician motivation, physician satisfaction, and what it means to be an excellent physician. The chapter begins by exploring why people choose to become physicians, and the factors influencing choice of medical speciality. They then review three general lines of physician satisfaction research: (1) the most prominent in hospitals and health systems asks doctors to provide feedback on their work environment, (2) a second area focuses on how features of work and organization affect physician satisfaction, often using the term "career satisfaction," and (3) a third line of work attempts to index and understand physician satisfaction from the standpoint of physicians, including their work environment, work tasks, work relationships, and personal lives. They conclude by focusing on the two dimensions of being an effective physician, the cure and the care of medicine, being a flawless technician and a complete person.

In the next chapter, Bruce Kirkcaldy and colleagues provide a comprehensive review of the literature in stress and health outcomes among the medical professions. They begin by examining the "changing face of medicine," resulting in part from statutory, legislative, and technological innovations that have shifted the traditional medical health care into a new "orbit." Different personalities seem to be gravitating towards the occupation of medicine, whilst others are being pushed away. The authors examine the magnitude of the problem of stress and specific sources of stress among health professionals. A review follows on the consequences of stress in terms of emotional and psychological distress, job burnout, self-destructive behavior, physical illness (and absenteeism), work satisfaction, and worker-related accidents. As in the chapter by Bogue and colleagues, they look at differences between generalists and specialists. Finally, sociodemographic factors are examined such as age, gender and parenthood. They include details of analyses derived from their German survey(s) of the medical profession, showing, among other findings, that medical practitioners' perception of occupational stress and work climate differed significantly between general practitioners and specialists. The implications of these findings are discussed and practical advice is given on how to tackle problems of stress-related ailments among the medical health profession.

Adrian Furnham's chapter reviews the literature on factors influencing our choice of medical practitioner. How do patients decide by which medical doctor they prefer to be treated? Adrian looks at the choices involved in selecting a general practitioner and those for a specialist. The chapter explores the medical consultation from the perspective of the patient and focuses on the academic literature on patient choice. It includes a section on communicative competence and subjective evaluation of clinical competence. He explores studies on demographic preferences, especially age and ethnicity, and their role in patient selection of medical treatments, and then examines why patients like what health professionals in alternative medicine do.

The practice of psychiatry and medicine does not occur in a vacuum. Society determines resources in training and salaries. The last chapter in the second section on medical health professionals is written by the British psychiatrist Dinesh Bhugra and his Indian colleague, Gurvinder Kalra, and they emphasize the methods of teaching the trainers and what works for medical professionals. Professionalism, they argue, is about primacy of patient welfare, managing resources effectively, ethical practice, and altruistic service. The medical and psychiatric professions would like to have autonomy, but recent medical scandals in the UK have changed the landscape of healthcare regulation. Consequently, instilling professionalism and leadership skills at an early stage is important. The authors explore the attributes of professionalism and leadership, the role of training and its components, and the various tools available to trainers. Finally, the implications of different approaches to training and instilling professionalism are explained.

The third section of this volume shifts towards patient care. A contribution from Rachel Davis and Charles Vincent, both from London, explores patient involvement in medical management. They describe what patient involvement is, introducing the terminology used in the literature and discussing discrepancies among definitions. They review why involvement is important and when the movement from paternalism to patient-centered care began, mentioning some of the key initiatives, such as the "expert patient program." They go on to explore ways in which patients can be involved, including self-management and patient safety. Rachel and Charles review the literature on whether and when patients want to be involved in their own care and discuss that patient involvement means different things for different patients: Being informed, for example, versus actually participating in health-related behaviors. Several relevant questions are raised: What the barriers are to patient involvement (health literacy, cultural factors, self-efficacy, power differentials)? How can these barriers be overcome? What interventions have been conducted? What works? Finally, they attempt to bring all the above ideas together in the form of key messages for this research for health policy makers.

Jutta Lindert from Germany provides an original contribution on "idioms of ill-health," first defining "idioms of distress" and then analyzing this construct in the context of the DSM IV and the DSM V. Jutta then offers an individual, familial, and cultural model associated with idioms of expression. The author examines diverse studies on idioms of distress of migrants, patterns of migration (phases of migration) and help-seeking behavior. Finally, the relationships between distress, help-seeking behavior, and social class are explored.

Drug and alcohol abuse are reportedly increasing quite dramatically in the European Community and elsewhere. Our contribution from Greece examines problems dealing with drug abuse especially among immigrant families. Alexander-Stamatios Antoniou and Marina Dalla present their study concentrating on immigration and drug abuse and models for professionals treating refugee and immigrant drug abusers. The main questions addressed are: How do immigrants deal with immigration and acculturation? What risk factors are related to drug abuse among immigrants and refugees? What are the differences in drug abuse among immigrants and natives in Greece? How can professionals become more culturally sensitive in servicing immigrant and refugee drug abusers and their families? Ultimately, immigrants are understood to differentiate their behavior in relation to drug abuse involvement and drug abuse treatment in ways that are instructive to the healing professions.

Over the years Lorraine Sherr has researched intensively in the area of health medicine, especially regarding difficult situations and patients in clinical settings. Together with Natasha Croome they introduce the concepts of difficult patients, difficult situations, and difficult topics. They offer psychological approaches that allow for enhanced abilities to prevent problems in the first place, particularly through doctor-patient communication. Clinicians and practitioners at various levels are offered methods for breaking bad news, and handling subsequent interactions. The chapter also examines mental health problems in nonmental health consultations: Picking up mental health cues, knowing how to handle them, and how they may affect consultations. After providing guidance on dealing with difficult patients they look at "difficult situations" – and handling difficult situations – such as abandoned babies, pregnancy as a result of rape, gender disappointment in childbirth, and mental health problems. Finally, the authors move on to difficult topics including HIV, sex-related issues, dealing with young children, and taking a detailed sexual history.

There has been a surge of interest over the last decade or two of introducing concepts of mindfulness in psychosomatic medicine. In the next chapter, American colleagues address the effect of mindfulness training on health outcome. Shauna Shapiro and her colleague Caitlin Burnham provide a chapter introducing the role of mindfulness in health care, focusing on the implications of mindfulness as it relates to: (1) the mindful therapist, (2) mindfulness-informed therapy, and (3) mindfulness-based therapy. Each of these topics is reviewed, drawing on current research and clinical anecdotes, pointing to the effectiveness of mindfulness training as a way of enhancing therapist effectiveness as well as therapist well being. They also address the issue of clinician stress and burnout, suggesting mindfulness as a self-care technique. And they offer advice on using mindfulness as a health intervention in our daily practices and in clinical training programs. Future directions include the further exploration of the relationship between mindfulness and clinical outcomes, and the incorporation of mindfulness training into education curricula.

Michael Eysenck, a cognitive psychologist by trade, looks in detail at the contribution cognitive psychology has made to medical health care. He first reviews the literature on cognitive functioning and its relevance to health care, particularly through the association of health literacy. He suggests convincingly that low health literacy is related to lower compliance to medical treatment plans, with subsequent inferior health outcomes. Such limitations in cognitive functioning are manifested in deficits in executive functioning, long-term memory, and language comprehension. Eysenck goes on to present compelling evidence that individual differences in various personality dimensions (e.g., neuroticism) play an important role in the development and maintenance of several medical conditions. He focuses in particular on emotion regulation (e.g., distraction, cognitive reappraisal) and the relationship between personality and medical condition, which is often mediated in part by cognitive biases. There has been a rapid increase in our understanding of the cognitive processes and mechanisms contributing to ill health. This research has proved very useful in terms of cognitive interventions designed to reduce the symptoms of diverse medical conditions, such as pain perception, fibromyalgia, and chronic fatigue syndrome, and some of the more successful interventions are discussed in detail.

Willi Ruch, Appletree Rodden, and Rene Pryor combine the expertise of a researcher, a medical practitioner, and a neurosurgeon/artist in their original contribution. For many years the Swiss-German team have explored key concepts in humor and laughter in psychology and medicine. They emphasize the value of implementing humor and laughter in medical and therapeutic scenarios in "appropriate dosages." Laughter "binds people together, leads to relaxation and enhances pain tolerance ... But humor and laughter also represent a double-edged sword." They introduce the field and the measurement of humor and humor-related moods and traits. They explore cognitive and motivational processes associated with humor. The chapter focuses on results from studies on the impact of humor on mental health, and on physical health. Moreover, the question is addressed as to whether humor can be learned/trained? They look at humor and the health movement and the various implementations of humor in hospitals and clinical settings, such as clinic clowns. Finally, the authors explore the potential of implementing humor and other positive oriented interventions in the health setting.

The volume's next chapter looks more intensively at economic factors that relate to health care, centering on the UK model. Douglas McCullough begins with "scarcity and choice" – simple questions, but complex value-laden answers. He discusses in detail the incorporate information costs and economy in health care, the importance of budget definitions, the impacts of patient travel to distant large-scale hospitals, how to ensure adequate numbers of rare cases in physician training, and other economic factors in health care. Douglas then examines and explains prioritizing mechanisms, such as the quality adjusted life year, cost-utility analysis, lattice analysis, and programmed budgeting and marginal analysis (PBMA). He then turns his attention to the scarcity of researchers' time and the resulting conservative bias of research. As the number of researchers increases, so does the degree of competition and the conservative bias of new work, also making support staff harder to get. The author attempts to resolve the question as to who's the "perfect agent" for the public interest. In this context, he reviews the economic relevance of patient lifestyle choices, sanctions, and the roles of the state, the doctor, and the voter.

Finally, John Skelton from Birmingham Medical School in the UK provides a novel chapter on narrative and literature in health care. His chapter looks at the development over the years of the significance of story-telling for the clinical professions, and suggests how it may develop in the future. The concept of narrative medicine has thrived in recent years in the context of a shifting emphasis, since the 1970s, on the holistic nature of medicine. Skelton makes clear that neither holism nor the idea that the clinician should be a well-rounded individual are new ideas. The pages of *Academic Medicine* from the 1920s frequently reflect on the need for doctors to have an understanding of the Humanities. He demonstrates, however, that in recent years the sophistication of the debate has increased.

There is a nexus of ideas which are generally held to be part and parcel of "holism": Patient-centeredness, empathy and so on. At worst, these are interpreted as a kind of intellectual laziness, the replacement of knowledge and logic by a kind of unfocussed sense of caring and sharing. But in fact, what is at stake is a different understanding of the nature of our world and its people, one which goes beyond the concept of "evidence" defined as the conclusions from experiment. An evidence-based understanding seeks to improve our understanding (and our grasp of how to help patients) by reducing uncertainty. A narrative approach recognizes, in a tradition that goes back to Empson (1930), that this kind of reductionist approach is not the only way of making sense of life. Sometimes to represent the world truly is to represent it as inherently ambiguous.

Let me return to the primary intention of the book. Our goal in inviting contributors to participate in writing these 16 chapters was to reach a target readership of academics and practitioners in the health professions. We are also hopeful this book will meet the needs of pre-med programs and their students, medical schools, medical school students, and the counselors or behaviorists in residency programs, or working for or with health systems. Many of us, in addition to our research and clinical tasks, do some form of teaching and certainly are familiar with the literature in our respective fields. Hence we want to offer not only scientific information relevant for students and professionals alike, but to share some of the more creative and artistic aspects of our work which may be difficult to find in a single authored volume. We hope this book provides diverse strategies and techniques for health practitioners, by interweaving ideas from art and science, hopefully filling a niche in the health literature, and at the very least maybe stimulating new areas for clinical research and practice.

Bruce David Kirkcaldy[1,2]
[1]International Centre for the Study of Occupational and Mental Health, Düsseldorf, Germany
[2]Visiting Professor in Psychology, Jagiellonian University, Cracow, Poland

Culture, Health, and Medicine

Evolutionary Aspects in Medicine

Martin Brüne

Research Department of Cognitive Neuropsychiatry and Psychiatric Preventive Medicine,
LWL University Hospital Bochum, Department of Psychiatry, Ruhr University, Bochum, Germany

What Is Evolutionary Medicine and Why Do We Need It?

Clinicians usually take for granted that any body function can go wrong at some point in life and they do not waste time thinking about why this is so. This is a somewhat distorted view of human nature, because it suggests that the human body is a defective gadget that is poorly adapted to the burden of life (Schiefenhövel, 2000). Starting with Morel's (1857) thesis some 150 years ago, physicians believed that the most plausible explanation of disease was that humans escaped the forces of evolution, and consequently succumbed to increasing "degeneration" (Brüne, 2007). Disease was thus seen as something that did not affect individuals, but entire populations – Social Darwinism was born (Roehlke, 1997). The fundamental flaws of this pseudo-evolutionary view on human nature have been dealt with elsewhere (e.g., Brüne, 2001). To this end, I shall argue that the opposite approach is actually more substantiated by evolutionary theory: Body functions can go wrong, in spite of their superb design. Put differently, from an evolutionary point of view it is all but straightforward to assume that body dysfunction is so widespread, especially when acknowledging that selection has shaped the functional properties of organs over eons close to optimum, albeit sometimes constrained by opposing adaptive mechanisms. Conversely, pathologies – regardless whether physical, cognitive, emotional, or behavioral – convey fitness disadvantages in terms of survival and reproduction, and, therefore, should have been eliminated by selection. So, the most pertinent questions in medicine are why disease exists in such frequencies at all, what can be done to deal with dysfunction, and how illness can be prevented.

Evolutionary medicine offers a couple of important answers to these questions – in fact, I contend that these questions cannot be answered without an evolutionary approach. To begin with, a common misconception of evolution by natural selection is to assume that adaptations are always optimal by design. When looking at individual traits, however, it becomes quite obvious that design failures are inevitable, because selection may have shaped a trait in the attempt to "reconcile" diametrical demands posed by evolution on that trait – just remember the oft-cited example of the peacock's tail, which makes peacocks sexually attractive to peahens the more "eyes" the tail contains, but also puts the peacock at risk of being devoured, because escape from predators is obstructed by the mere size of the tail and because its conspicuous colors may even attract predators (Darwin, 1871). Another example is human bipedalism, which putatively evolved to travel long distances at relatively low energy consumption (Fleagle, 1992), but renders humans vulnerable to develop instability of the vertebral column, including slipping disks, and also forced our ancestors to deliver birth to immature babies (Day, 1992) – a compromise that radically changed the way we care for our children. This latter issue will be discussed in greater detail later in this chapter. At this point, these examples may illustrate that the human body (like all other living organisms) comprises a set of design compromises, and that individual adaptations cannot be seen in isolation from other, sometimes counter-running, adaptive mechanisms (Nesse & Williams, 1994).

Another (in evolutionary standards) recent – human-specific – problem has occurred due to the divergent speed at which cultural and biological changes take place. The "mismatch" between the two reflects the fact that biological evolution cannot keep pace with cultural evolution, another crucial aspect with fundamental consequences for vulnerability to disease (Nesse & Williams, 1994). The evolutionary mismatch becomes evident in almost every health-related issue, ranging from problems caused by "modern" diet (Eaton, Konner, & Shostak, 1988), to changes in exposure to microbiotic environments (Torrey & Yolken, 2005), and physical exercise (Cordain, Gotshall, & Eaton, 1997). All "classic" diseases of civilization including hypertension, diabetes, substance abuse, obesity, autoimmune disorders, cancer, and mental disorders are perhaps mainly caused by mismatch-related problems. That is, adaptations that were shaped by selection in the past are no longer suitable for many problems encountered in the present (Nesse & Williams, 1994). This does not mean that genetic variation between individuals is not important in this regard; individuals differ, of course, with regard to vulnerability to disease. However, many genetic polymorphisms may have been selectively neutral in the past, or were even advantageous, and only in recent days may some variants have become "susceptibility alleles" due to mismatch with recent adaptive problems (Belsky et al., 2009; Keller & Miller, 2006). For instance, there is good evidence to suggest that our contemporary high-caloric diet, which contains large amounts of unsaturated fatty acids and sugar, contributes to atherosclerosis (Omenn, 2010). Finally, pathogens such as bacteria and viruses evolve so fast that immune systems struggle to cope; our modern environment may not only foster the emergence of new and resistant strains of germs, it may also help spread infections in populations. A well-known example from the recent past is the plague that killed a large proportion of the European population.

So, the claim that clinicians can learn a lot more about disease when taking into account evolutionary aspects of human nature is clearly supported, yet hardly put into practice with regard to the curricula of medical faculties around the world (Nesse et al., 2010).

In highlighting selected examples from evolutionary medicine, pertaining to diverse domains such as internal medicine, obstetrics and gynecology, and psychiatry, this chapter aims at illustrating that insights from evolutionary theory not only improve our understanding of disease, but may also help to find new ways to deal with human ailments in terms of prevention and treatment. Before doing so, however, I shall try to briefly summarize the ancestral conditions under which our species evolved.

Human Ancestral Environments and Genetic Issues

Environments of Evolutionary Adaptedness

Research into the life of extant hunter-gatherer tribes suggests that ancestral humans lived in small, kin-based and mostly patrilocal tribal groups that were relatively egalitarian in social structure, with accumulation of material goods largely absent (Ehrlich, 2000). Estimates of group size propose that ancestral communities comprised perhaps not more than 30–40 individuals, which together with neighboring groups or extended kin made up to 150 people who personally knew each other (Dunbar, 2003). Trade, but also warfare with adjacent groups was probably prevalent throughout human history. Data from recent horticultural societies under intense pressure to compete for scarce resources suggest that about one in four men dies a violent death, mainly in between-group battle (Schiefenhövel, 1995), and similar figures may be assumed for ancestral hunter-gatherers (Radcliffe-Brown, 1948). This model probably prevailed for most of human history. Cooperation was critical within groups to secure food from game hunting and foraging. Moreover, cooperative behaviors included mutual aid of women who raised children (thereby probably shortening between-birth intervals from 5 to 6 years down to 3 to 4 years; Hrdy, 2000), and between men to protect the group from large predators and competing human groups.

The smallest functional unit within ancestral human societies was the nuclear family consisting of father, mother, and children. Anatomical features including testes size and sexual dimorphism (differences in body size between the sexes) suggest that mild polygyny was perhaps common in ancestral humans, yet critically depending on whether or not a male could "afford" more than one spouse in terms of provision of sufficient resources, including offspring he fathered (Buss, 1999). From a human infant's perspective, the most crucial task was to manage survival. Compared with other newborn apes, human babies are physiologically preterm by about 13 months. Put differently, if human babies were at birth as mature as chimpanzee babies the human gestation period would last approximately 22 months. As indicated above, human preterm parturition represents an evolved design compromise, which is ultimately linked to the evolution of bipedalism. Upright walking was accompanied by a change of the human pelvis anatomy, which consequently led to a narrowing of the birth canal. This was not a problem as long as ancestral hominoid species had relatively small chimpanzee-like brains of approximately 350 cm^3. However, as the brain started to grow larger over evolutionary time, the problem of a narrow birth canal became more vital. The increase in brain size – according to the "Social Brain" hypothesis (Brothers, 1990; Dunbar, 2003), which was most likely spurred by a progressively more complex social environment that selected for larger brains – selected for antedating parturition. The reason for this was that a brain (and skull) larger than that of contemporary human newborns would not have been able to pass the birth canal. In turn, the evolution of bigger brains came at the expense of greater immaturity of offspring at birth.

This special situation of human newborns implied that the formation of a dyad between mother and offspring became one of the most crucial psychological adaptations in early humans (Bowlby, 1969). Successful attachment on the baby's side and bonding on the mother's side have remained vital for psychological well-being throughout human evolution to the present day in every known culture. In addition, the dependence of the mother on helpers increased proportionally, such that close cooperation between women, between mother and father of the child, and kinship alliances were positively selected. For example, women with young children were often supported by their mothers, who contributed a substantial amount of resources to the survival of young offspring (Hrdy, 2000). This so-called "grandmother model" may explain why selection has increased the postmenopausal lifespan of human women to more than 20 years. It is also conceivable that diminishing sexual dimorphism, a trend towards monogamy or mild polygyny, and concealed ovulation, that is, the loss of visible signs of ovulation such as genital swellings, which are typical for our closest extant relatives, are (secondary) adaptive consequences of walking on two legs. All these aspects, presented here in a nutshell, are core features of human ancestral conditions, or the human "Environments of Evolutionary Adaptedness" (EEA; Bowlby, 1969).

Genetic Make-Up

Humans differ from each other regarding their genetic make-up. However, interindividual differences are rather small, because ancestral human populations were genetically shaped by several evolutionary "bottlenecks." Genes are represented in DNA, a highly conservative biological structure. The DNA of two randomly picked humans is more than 99% identical. Differences or variation may occur at any part of the DNA and is mainly brought about by mutation through replacement of a single base or nucleotide. If the frequency of at least two alleles at a given locus is greater than 1% of the population, these variants are called polymorphisms. Single nucleotide polymorphisms (SNP) are common and believed to occur on average once every 1,500 bases. Since most SNPs lie in noncoding regions, they are phenotypically silent. However, SNPs can have dramatic effects if they are located in coding regions, promoter regions, enhancer or silencer regions of the genome that may affect gene expression. Similarly, the insertion or deletion (loss) of one or more bases can have profound consequences for the functioning of the respective stretch of the genome. Insertions, deletions, duplications, and complex multi-site variants have recently been subsumed under the term copy number variations (CNV) or copy number polymorphisms (CNP). Such variations are much more frequent in the human genome than previously assumed. An estimated 1,400+ regions comprising CNVs have been identified so far, covering approximately 12% of the human genome (Cardno & McGuffin,

2005). The functional significance of CNVs is poorly understood, as are their evolutionary origins. It can be expected, however, that research into CNV loci will ultimately have implications for psychiatry in the near future. In any event, from an evolutionary point of view it is crucial to note that a variant producing a mere 1% fitness advantage would increase in population frequency from 0.1% to 99.9% in roughly 4,000 generations, hence, in humans within 100,000–120,000 years.

There is little doubt that an individual's genetic make-up may be associated with vulnerability to dysfunction, disorder or disease. However, despite increasing knowledge about genetic susceptibility for human disease, the situation is still complex, because genes interact with environmental conditions in manifold ways. Only a few human diseases follow a Mendelian pattern of inheritance with simple dominance recessivity relationships. Also, genes may differ in expression and penetrance, that is, the probability of a specific phenotype as a function of a certain genotype. Likewise, many medical conditions differ from "normalcy" by degree, not kind, that is, traits are quantitatively or continuously distributed in populations.

For organisms to grow, both nature (genes) and nurture (environment) are necessary ingredients. Some disorders are more, others less under genetic control. The emergence of some disorders depends more on certain environmental conditions, for example, stress, malnutrition, hypercaloric diet, lack of exercise, etc., others less so. In the context of human disease, it is important to emphasize that an evolutionary perspective does not necessarily imply that a given trait or genotype "determines" the phenotype. Instead, knowing the complex interaction between genes and environment will be vital to improve health care and prevention of illness.

Selected Contemporary Health Challenges From an Evolutionary Perspective

Internal Medicine

Atherosclerosis, Myocardial Infarction, and Stroke
Atherosclerotic-associated diseases such as coronary heart disease and stroke account for some 40% of annual deaths in developed countries. Hypertension, dyslipidemia, overweight, lack of physical exercise, tobacco smoking, and diabetes are among the most common risk factors for atherosclerotic diseases. According to estimates from the Center for Disease Control and Prevention (2005), mortality could be reduced by a quarter through treatment of hypertension and hypercholesterinemia. Most, if not all, of the risk factors mentioned clearly belong to the category "evolutionary mismatch." In Western cultures, people are exposed to a variety of chronic stressors that induce activation of the HPA axis. This may be one of the leading mechanisms that cause hypertension. In traditional societies, including hunter-gatherers, blood pressure is usually much lower, and this seems to be more specific to the diastolic pressure (Lindeberg, Nilsson-Ehle, Terént, Vessby, & Scherstén, 1994; Trowell & Burkitt, 1981). Conversely, elevated blood pressure is a disease of modern civilization, and blood pressure does not rise in traditional populations

before middle age. Regarding blood lipids, findings are more diverse. In some traditional populations, the prevalence of ischemic diseases such as myocardial infarction and stroke is low despite blood lipid levels that resemble those seen in Western societies (Lindeberg et al., 1994). Lindeberg (2010), for example, reports that hypercholesterolemia can occur in the indigenous people of Kitava (Trobriand Islands), which is most likely due to a high intake of saturated fat from coconuts. Overweight is very rare among hunter-gatherers (Lindeberg et al., 1994; Trowell & Burkitt, 1981). In traditional societies, the average Body Mass Index (BMI) at age 40 was found to hover around 20 kg/m^2 for men and 19 kg/m^2 for women, and waist circumference larger than hip circumference is absent in most traditional societies (Lindeberg, 2010).

Type -II diabetes seems to be absent in most traditional societies, as long as they stick to their traditional diets (Joffe et al., 1971; Spielman et al., 1982). This seems to change dramatically in some populations, when exposed to a Western diet, which is rich in saturated fatty acids. One plausible explanation is that in many places around the world episodic food shortages were prevalent throughout human evolutionary history, such that selection favored individuals who were carriers of "thrifty genes" (Neel, 1962). The "thrifty gene hypothesis" suggests that in ancestral conditions genes were selected for maximum calorie extraction, which nowadays, in times of oversupply and abundance of high-caloric diet, causes harm. Thrifty genes may also account for our preference of sweets and food rich in cholesterol. Contemporary human populations such as the indigenous peoples of North and South America, which until recently lived under environmental restrictions to the availability of such foods, now suffer from enormous prevalence rates of type-II diabetes and atherosclerotic diseases causing premature death (Zhang et al., 2008).

In fact, myocardial infarction is conspicuously absent in populations that have not transitioned to a Western lifestyle, as recorded in a number of clinical investigations and autopsy studies across the globe (summarized in Lindeberg, 2010). Conversely, the emergence of ischemic heart disease has been well-documented in several populations after they switched to a Western lifestyle. Accordingly, individual cases of myocardial infarction have been observed in these societies with increasing incidence rates since the 1950s (INTERHEALTH Steering Committee, 1991).

In a similar vein, ECG examinations in traditional populations have shown no indication of left ventricular hypertrophy (Lindeberg & Lundh, 1993) or a shift toward leftward deviation of the heart's electrical axis with increasing age. Heart failure is also not observed in traditional societies (Lindeberg, 2010).

A similar case can be made for the incidence of stroke in traditional societies. Lindeberg and Lundh (1993) did not detect a single incidence of paralysis on one side of the body (hemiplegia), inability to speak (aphasia), or sudden loss of balance, as indicating cerebellar infarction (Lindeberg & Lundh 1993). Moreover, clinical examinations of Kitava inhabitants revealed no manifestations of stroke. Since a substantial number of people are 60 years or older, the absence of cerebral ischemia could not be accounted for by age-related factors alone. Similarly, (noninfectious) stroke was not reported in indigenous populations of Papua New Guinea before transition to a more Western lifestyle (Breinl, 1915) or East African countries (Trowell & Burkitt, 1981).

This sheds some light on the evolutionary history of atherosclerosis-associated diseases. The clear relationship of increasing incidence rates in traditional societies of myocardial infarction, stroke, and heart failure with lifestyle changes in an extremely short period of time (in evolutionary standards) suggests that differences in genetic make-up between traditional and Western populations are negligible in this regard, but probably play a role in within-group variation in terms of vulnerability.

Cancer

Malignant diseases – as a group – are the second leading cause of mortality in the developed countries. In addition to age, which constitutes a risk factor alone, infections, tobacco smoking, alcohol consumption, other nutritional factors, and exposure to cancerogenic material figure among the most important nongenetic causes for cancer. Genetic factors, by comparison, account for only 4% of cancers (Trevathan, Smith, & McKenna, 2008).

Tobacco smoking increases the risk for lung, esophagus, larynx, pharynx, urinary bladder, kidney, pancreas, breast, and colon cancer. Although inhalation of psychoactive substances has been known for thousands of years, tobacco smoking has dramatically increased since the 16th century, when tobacco plants were introduced to Europe (Greaves, 2000). Therefore, malignant diseases associated with tobacco smoking are another example of an "evolutionary mismatch." It seems likely that humans were not exposed to regular inhalation of toxic fumes for the most part of their evolutionary history. A similar case can be made for alcohol consumption. Although small quantities of ethanol can be found in ripe fruits, the commercial production of alcoholic beverages is a quite recent development. This does not preclude the assumption that early humans regularly ingested psychotropic substances for various purposes, particularly as stimulants or sedatives. For example, betel nut (*Areca catechu*) chewing increases brain acetylcholine levels; cocaine, the active alkaloid in *Erythroxylum coca*, is a powerful reuptake inhibitor of norepinephrine and dopamine. Betel quid chewing is known to be an important risk factor for oral cancer, due to the strongly alkaline environment that develops in the mouth by adding slacked lime (from heated coral) to the betel quid (Boyle et al., 1990; MacLennan, Paissat, Ring, & Thomas, 1985). Thus, in those parts of the world where betel nut is regularly consumed, oral cancer is quite common (Atkinson, Chester, Smyth, & ten Seldam, 1964; Wallington, 1986). However, other types of cancers seem to be remarkably less prevalent in traditional societies compared to developed countries.

Cancers caused by regular consumption of psychotropic substances could be reduced in number by preventing consumption; however, this is much easier said than done, because these substances, consumed regularly and excessively, not only exceed the organism's detoxification potential, they also usurp the phylogenetically ancient "reward system" in the brain by signaling the prospect of getting a reward. This mainly dopaminergic reward system has no built-in stopping device, which in the past was not selected for, because in natural conditions the exhaustion of resources terminated the activation of the reward system, and the appetitive or seeking behavior ceased automatically. This is presumably one cause of the excessive intake of psychotropic substances such as tobacco or alcohol by some individuals, which renders them more vulnerable to develop cancer through oxidative stress and damage to the DNA (Lende & Smith, 2002).

Compared to lung cancer and other malignant disorders that are clearly linked with tobacco smoking or alcohol consumption, the origins of prostate cancer may be different. Prostate cancer is increasing in prevalence, mainly due to aging of Western societies. From an evolutionary perspective, the prostate is interesting, because it has increased in size such that the human prostate is larger compared to other mammals. The large human prostate gland could be the result of the prevailing mating system in ancestral human populations, that is, mild polygyny. The production of viable sperm depends on testosterone, and retaining male fertility to an advanced age could have been a selective advantage. If such a scenario came close to reality, prostate cancer could be seen as an evolutionary "cost" or trade-off for the ability to retain sperm production in older men (Greaves, 2000). Since prostate cancer is usually a disease of older men, it escaped selection acting against the development of malignant cells in the prostate gland.

Infectious Diseases, Allergy, and Autoimmune Diseases

Infectious diseases have certainly contributed much to selection of human traits. In fact, infectious diseases and diseases of the immune system are the prime example in medicine, which simply cannot be fully understood without an evolutionary approach. The problem is that pathogens evolve much faster than their hosts' immune systems, such that an arms race has emerged from which there is virtually no escape. In addition to germs that were already around in ancestral conditions of the EEAs, it is estimated that the domestication of animals has led to the transmission of some 700 new pathogens from animals to humans (Torrey & Yolken, 2005). Differences in sialic acid coding genes between our closest extant relative, the chimpanzee, and humans seem to have brought about greater susceptibility to malaria and cholera infection (Varki, 2001). One of the most well-known examples of a protective mutation against malaria was detected much earlier. The gene that codes for sickle-cell anemia evolved in malaria infested regions, because heterozygous carriers possess relative immunity against malaria, and hence, enjoy a reproductive advantage (Allison, 1954). The costly side is, however, that homozygous carriers of the sickle-cell allele die early in infancy. Cultural factors such as the introduction of farming and agriculture in West Africa have probably aggravated the situation, because this brought about new breeding grounds for *Anopheles gambiae*, which is the main vector of *Plasmodium falciparum* in West Africa (Livingstone, 1958). More recent examples for balancing selection (i.e., heterozygous advantage) include cystic fibrosis and Tay-Sachs disease, both of which are assumed to relatively protect against tuberculosis (Gluckman, Beedle, & Hanson, 2010).

In developed countries, the scourge by infectious diseases such as malaria and other epidemics has partially been replaced by diseases of the immune system that act against the body's own tissue. It is quite obvious that as the incidence of infectious disease has declined, the incidence of autoimmune disorders has increased (Bach, 2002). A plausible, fundamentally evolution-based, explanation for this apparent paradox is that the immune system attacks one's own body cells, because it has to deal less with infectious diseases. In other words, according to the "hygiene hypothesis," appropriate exposure to pathogens early in life is critical for adaptive activation of immunological pathways. In line with this proposition, it has been shown that children from rural areas suffer less often from asthma and atopic disorders compared to children from urbanized environments. Likewise, inflammatory bowel disease, including Crohn's disease, is less common in unhygienic environments than highly sanitized ones. In the case of asthma, the prevalence is particularly inversely correlated with helminth exposure, such that the normal immunoglobulin IgE to helminths may overreact to allergens such as dust mites when helminths were eliminated from environment (Barnes, Armelagos, & Morreale, 1999).

Gynecology and Obstetrics

Morning Sickness and Hyperemesis Gravidarum

At least in developed countries, morning sickness during early pregnancy occurs in 50–90% of women. Morning sickness is clearly not a disease in the strict sense, but subjectively highly unpleasant. Early morning sickness occurs in traditional cultures as well, such that an evolutionary explanation seems warranted. Early morning sickness peaks during the most sensitive period of embryogenesis, which has given rise to the hypothesis that it evolved to better protect the embryo from toxins. In fact, one characteristic of early morning sickness is that women avoid certain foods and prefer others, sometimes to their own surprise, because such foods do not necessarily comply with women's preferences outside pregnancy. In addition, women perhaps benefit from increased social support during the period of early morning sickness. In support of the hypothesis that early morning sickness could have been selected for, studies have shown that the condition is linked with better pregnancy outcome (Kohl, Kainer, & Schiefenhövel, 2009).

However, a more severe condition, known as Hyperemesis gravidarum, is certainly no longer adaptive. Hyperemesis is often associated with preeclampsia or edema-proteinuria-hypertension (EPH) gestosis. Evolutionary theorists have linked EPH with parent-offspring conflict (Trivers, 1974), which naturally occurs between fetus and mother, because both organisms may differ regarding their "interests" how to allocate resources. For example, it is in the fetus's interest that the maternal organism raises its blood sugar level to optimize resource extraction from the fetus's perspective. If driven to the extreme, these differences in metabolic optima may cause disease in the mother, and this situation may, in part, be triggered by genomic imprinting, a process that causes silencing of genes from one parent to the benefit of genes from the other parent (Haig, 1993; recently updated in Haig, 2010). Put differently, paternally inherited genes may have selected to extract a greater amount of resources than is the optimum for the mother. By contrast, maternally inherited genes may be selected to demand an amount of resources closer to the mother's optimum. Imprinted genes comprise only 1% of the genome, but they may exert major effects because they are often involved in growth regulation and are highly pleiotropic, that is, they influence multiple phenotypic expressions. Hyperemesis and EPH gestosis may illustrate that health and well-being are not necessarily targets of selection. Moreover, conflict over investment of parental resources persist after birth, and is expressed through infant's behavior such as tantrums during weaning and "regressive" behavior at later ages.

Postpartum Blues and Postpartum Depression

Postpartum blues is a common phenomenon in developed countries, affecting roughly 50% of women. This affective state is associated with dysphoric mood, emotional lability, and feelings of helplessness. In evolutionary perspective such a reaction to childbirth does not seem to make sense. The etiology of postpartum blues probably resides much less in endocrinological changes after birth than previously though, but more in the psychosocial environment. Postpartum blues is largely absent in developing countries. Childbirth is usually given in secluded, though familiar surroundings, in which the childbearing woman feels safe and secure (Schiefenhövel, 1993). In developed countries, this is often not the case. Moreover, separation of the newborn from the mother has been widely practiced in "modern" obstetric medicine, but obviously runs counter to evolved psychological mechanisms that foster close mother-child proximity (Hrdy, 2000). In support of this assumption, it could be shown that postpartum blues is less frequent in women who could practice "bedding-in," whereas "rooming-in" had no such effect (Schiefenhövel, 2007). So, it seems that postpartum blues belongs to the category of evolutionary mismatch, which should give rise to considerations of changing birth practices, including more restrictive use of cesarean section (because it suppresses the secretion of oxytocin under birth), introducing more "natural" environments for childbirth, and perhaps the restricted use of oxytocin in accelerating parturition. The latter consideration resides in the observation that primipara who received exogenous oxytocin had shortened duration of their first birth, however apparently at the expense of longer parturition in subsequent pregnancies, compared to women who did not receive parenteral oxytocin (Trevathan, 1987).

Postpartum depression is more frequent in women who experiences postpartum blues, but the relationship of the two is obscure. Postpartum depression is typical in terms of depressive symptomatology. However, it poses particular risks to both the mother and the child related to neonaticide and infanticide. Neonaticide needs to be distinguished from infanticide, as the former occurs within the first 24 hr after birth. The first hours and days after birth constitute a sensitive period for the formation of attachment and bonding. In evolutionary perspective, neonaticide has been a function of differential parental investment throughout human history. Unlike other mammals, humans are unable to abort undesired offspring, if environmental conditions are unfavorable (such as during times of food shortage), such that neonaticide is not necessarily linked with psychopathology. In contrast, filicide, the killing of older infants and children, deviates from this evolutionary explanation, as filicidal mothers are usually older, more frequently married, socially isolated or have been victims of domestic violence. Moreover, filicidal mothers are frequently depressed, psychotic or diagnosed with substance abuse. Suicidal thoughts may occur in up to 50% of filicidal women. In women with postpartum depression infanticidal ideation may occur in over 40%, and in one study actual infanticidal behavior happened in one third of patients, sometimes originally planned as homicide-suicide (Stone, Steinmeyer,

Dreher, & Krischer, 2005). These figures clearly indicate that the risk of infanticide should be closely monitored in women with postpartum depression, and alert clinicians to thoroughly diagnose depression postpartum.

Polycystic Ovary Disease

Polycystic ovary syndrome (PCOS) is the most common endocrine cause of infertility in women in developed countries, affecting 5–10% of women of reproductive age (Balen, 1999). Clinically, PCOS is characterized by menstrual irregularities, hyperandrogenism, and multiple cysts that develop in the ovary, preventing regular ovulation. Polycystic ovaries are even more common in the West, with prevalence rates of up to 20%, without meeting the full criteria for PCOS (Dunaif, 1997). Women who become pregnant have an increased risk of developing preeclampsia and gestational diabetes.

PCOS as a major cause of reduced fecundity is strongly linked with insulin resistance, hyperinsulinemia, and overweight (Pollard & Unwin, 2008). Hyperinsulinemia does not directly influence ovarian secretion of estrogen and progesterone, but rather, the production of testosterone and the sex-hormone binding protein. Low levels of the sex-hormone binding protein lead to increased levels of free testosterone, hence causing the symptoms associated with hyperandrogenism, which in turn increases insulin resistance. Women who recently migrated from developing countries to Western countries seem to be especially prone to developing hyperinsulinemia, which could relate to their "thrifty genotype." Alternatively, this metabolic change may be associated with a "thrifty phenotype" suggesting that slow intrauterine growth of the fetus may increase the risk for insulin resistance later in life (Pollard & Unwin, 2008).

In summary, PCOS is likely another example of evolutionary mismatch, through which reproductive disadvantage is caused by environmental conditions associated with a Westernized lifestyle.

Cancer of Reproductive Organs

A similar point can be made even with regard to cancers of the female reproductive organs. Women in developed countries have, on average, much higher estrogen and progesterone levels than women in developing countries, however, relative to estrogen, progesterone levels tend to be higher in women in developing countries. High estrogen levels are a common risk factor for breast, uterus, and ovarian cancers (Eaton et al., 1994). Early menarche, delayed first birth, reduced number of pregnancies, and refusal of breastfeeding are also linked with an increased risk of cancer of the female reproductive organs, especially breast cancer (Eaton et al., 1994). Breast cancer (and perhaps also other cancers of the reproductive organs) is much more common in developed countries compared to developing countries. A plausible explanation informed by evolutionary theory and human life history is that the exposure of the female reproductive organs to high levels of sex hormones differs from the ancestral pattern in many ways. Put differently, women are not adapted to nonpregnant states (Short, 1976). For example, the lifetime number of menstrual cycles of women who use hormonal contraception revolves around 350–400, whereas in ancestral conditions it was probably a third of that. In conditions that resemble those of the environment of evolutionary adaptedness, women were, for the most part of their reproductive lives, either pregnant or lactating, which exposed their reproductive organs to steroid hormones in different ways as compared to women in developed countries today (Sievert, 2008). So, again, considering evolutionary aspects of human reproduction, it is likely that some cancers of the female reproductive organs are caused by an evolutionary mismatch regarding exposure to steroid hormones, or cultural habits relating to child upbringing such as breastfeeding.

Psychiatry

Depression

According to WHO estimates, by 2020 depression will have dramatically increased in prevalence and rank #2 among the most debilitating illnesses worldwide (WHO, 2004). Phenomenologically, the behavioral correlates of depression resemble defeat and submission observed in animals after lost struggles over social rank. Depressed patients often avoid eye-to-eye contact, show little movements of eye and mouth region, reduce the amount of speech and affective tone of voice, and behave socially inactive. These nonverbal behaviors aim at reducing aggression of others that could be oriented towards the self, and avoiding harm by displaying de-escalating appeasement strategies in situations of (perceived) defeat or inferiority (Price et al., 2007). Submission and dominance are inherent to socially living species with complex hierarchies. Asymmetries in social status and competition for resources and mates, social rank, and relationships need to be negotiated. In ancestral environments, social exclusion from the community was probably one of the most important real threats to an individual, and potentially equivalent to a death sentence. Thus, submission in conflict-laden situations may in the first place be considered a life-saving strategy that evolved under ancestral condition despite its obvious, though perhaps transient, disadvantage in terms of reproductive success. In other words, a decision over fight or flight critically depends on the evaluation of one's own power and potential alliances, and in situations where success is unlikely, or escape impossible, submission and acceptance of subordination may be the best option, at least for the time being. Depression, in this line of reasoning, represents the extreme of submission or an appeasement strategy, however inappropriate in terms of context, duration and/or intensity compared to adaptive submissive behavior, and occurs foremost in situations associated with acute or chronic social stress (Gilbert, Allan, Brough, Melley, & Mikes, 2002). Abundant primate research has shown that defeat in social competition or fall in social rank produces a steep decline in serotonin levels in the brain. Subordinate individuals have on average much lower serotonin levels than dominant individuals, and the former are more aggressive and emotionally labile, but explore their environment less compared to the latter. In addition, research in nonhuman primates has shown that early abuse or neglect may stimulate proinflammatory immune responses, which in turn increase the activation of the serotonin transporter, thus leading to reduced serotonin availability (Suomi, 2006).

Increasing prevalence rates of depression have manifold causes. In line with an evolutionary mismatch scenario, it is conceivable that some of the reasons why depression is on the rise relates to increasing social pressures, such as competing with strangers in many different arenas (workplace, mating, etc.), and pressure to constantly present oneself as attractive and desirable. Moreover, at least in Western societies, individualism prevails over mutual cooperation, which reduces the chance of getting social support.

Schizophrenia

Schizophrenia has puzzled evolutionary theorists for a long time, because an apparent paradox resides in the way why schizophrenia is preserved in human populations, despite the marked reproductive disadvantage of affected individuals. Accordingly, it has been proposed that a selective advantage of traits may exist, of which only the extremes of variation are disadvantageous (Huxley, Mayr, Osmond, & Hoffer, 1964). The number and diversity of evolutionary hypotheses of schizophrenia, however, is unparalleled in other major psychiatric disorders. They span as divergently as the advantages of schizotypal traits in relation to group selection, schizophrenia as a trade-off of human language acquisition or creativity, reduced risk of cancer in relatives of schizophrenic patients, schizophrenia as extreme negative variation of sexually selected traits, and the effects of maternally imprinted genes (overview in Brüne, 2004). To date, none of these hypotheses has been proved by the evidence. However, it could be that genes that were positively selected during human evolution also have a role in schizophrenia, especially those that exert effects on brain metabolism during early ontogeny such as DISC1 – Disrupted in Schizophrenia I (Crespi, Summers, & Dorus, 2007).

For example, genes involved in neurodevelopment help to "buffer" against negative effects of multiple mutations, pathogens, and toxins. Variation at these loci may lead to increased "fluctuating asymmetry" (FA), that is, a near-normally distributed asymmetry of bilateral characters that are on average symmetrical in the population. In schizophrenia, FA is greater in twin pairs concordant for schizophrenia than in discordant pairs, which suggests that greater FA may indicate an imprecise expression of the developmental design due to genetically or environmentally caused developmental disruption (Yeo, Gangestad, Edgar, & Thoma, 1999). FA is under partial control of sexual selection, as small FA is usually perceived more attractive than large FA. It could therefore be that, in a general vein, the broad spectrum of schizophrenia represents the unattractive extreme of variation of sexually selected traits including increased FA (Shaner, Miller, & Mintz, 2004).

Consistent, though not identical with, the hypothesis of schizophrenia as maladaptive extreme of variation of sexually selected traits, some physical and behavioral characteristics indicate that genomic imprinting may play a role in the expression of schizophrenia-associated features. Generally speaking, several characteristics seem to support the assumption that maternal imprinting leads to a pattern of general undergrowth and "femaleness" of the brain in schizophrenia. This could include reduction of gray matter, reduced lateralization, and overactive mechanisms involved in social cognition – quasi, the opposite of what is found in autism (Crespi & Badcock, 2008). These general evolutionary hypotheses of schizophrenia are, in part, flawed by the fact that they hardly cover the majority of clinical aspects of schizophrenia. Thus, in addition to these broad approaches to understand the heterogeneous nature of the schizophrenia spectrum phenotype, it is useful to analyze individual symptoms based on evolutionary theory as pathological exaggerations of adaptive mechanisms, such as delusional belief formation or catatonia (Brüne, 2004).

Mismatch also seems to have a role in the manifestation of schizophrenia, because it has been observed that the incidence of schizophrenia dramatically increases in populations, which have made the transition from a more "traditional" to a Western lifestyle (Torrey, Torrey, & Burton-Bradley, 1974).

Dementia

In aging societies, dementia is causing a pressing problem. Dementia is ultimately linked to aging and senescence; processes that sexually reproducing organisms inevitably undergo. By definition, senescence, as opposed to aging, is characterized by increasing deterioration of body functions. One reason why senescence occurs is that natural selection has fostered the evolution of genes that exert balanced polymorphic effects: They convey fitness advantages early in life while having deleterious effects at advanced ages. For instance, a hypothetical gene that acts on calcium metabolism by facilitating bone calcification, thus making young individuals more resistant against fractures, may trigger atherosclerosis in older adults (Williams, 1957). Conversely, selection for longevity should be balanced against selection for genes that cause senescence. With respect to senescence and longevity in humans, the evolution of ApoE polymorphisms in primates reveals interesting insights. Recent research in nonhuman primates and other vertebrates suggests that an ApoE4-like allele is the ancestral form from which ApoE3, and subsequently ApoE2 are derived. The human isoforms E2 and E3 differ from ApoE4 by only two amino acids. Although the fossil record of early humans does not contain sufficient genetic material to exactly date back the evolutionary origin of the ApoE3 and ApoE2 variants, it is plausible to assume that these polymorphisms emerged at some point in human evolution that was accompanied by a rapid increase in brain size. Since brain size correlates with longevity, it is plausible to assume that longevity was also a target of selection. This scenario suggests that the increasing duration of dependence of infants on their mothers (and their mother's survival) created a selection pressure of expanding the human life span (Finch & Sapolsky, 1999). It is then reasonable to assume that it became advantageous for early humans to survive sufficiently long enough beyond ceasing reproduction to raise offspring born shortly before menopause. A life history of a female who gave birth at age 40 and died before her offspring was socially mature (some 20 years later) would certainly not have been favored by natural selection. In addition to experiencing longer life spans themselves, mothers (and their offspring) could have benefited from additional help from their own mothers – grandmothering evolved (Hrdy, 2000). Moreover, an increasing meat intake of human ancestors, which was probably advantageous in terms of protein supply for growing big brains, would predict, in reverse, a shorter life span – given the atherogenic effect and high load of infectious particles of (raw) meat. The differential binding potential of ApoE variants to cholesterol fractions may therefore be an adaptive response to both changing diet in early humans, and the need of postponing senescence (Finch & Stanford, 2004). However, these evolutionary changes have also created a burden in both economic and interpersonal terms. In light of the demographic development in Western countries, the expenses for care for the elderly will rise considerably in the next 50–100 years.

What Can Medicine Gain From an Understanding of Evolution? Conclusions and Future Directions

The above-mentioned examples may illustrate how evolutionary medicine may inform clinicians and researchers alike. It is important to note that the evolutionary approach is nothing new or something that is inconsistent with more "traditional" approaches to disease. Rather, evolutionary theory adds another dimension to the understanding of illness. This so-called "ultimate" level inquires into questions of adaptation and phylogenetic history of traits, whereas the traditional medical approach is confined to the "proximate" level of analysis, that is, mechanism and ontogeny (Tinbergen, 1963). Put differently, the ultimate and the proximate level are by no means mutually exclusive, but complimentary, and medicine ought to make use of both. This is much less radical as it seems at first sight, even though medicine has been regrettably slow in putting this into practice, and to include evolutionary topics in medical curricula (Nesse et al., 2010). In recent years several textbooks and seminal articles have highlighted the need for evolutionary explanations of human disease in great detail (e.g., Brüne, 2008; Gluckman et al., 2010; Nesse & Williams, 1994; Stearns & Koella, 2008; Trevathan et al., 2008) such that it can be hoped that the situation will change in the near future.

As shown in the previous paragraphs, the most powerful causal mechanism to explain illness and disease from an ultimate evolutionary point of view resides in environmental mismatch of evolved traits with current environmental conditions. Mismatch ranges from maladaptation to "modern" diet, exposure to new pathogens, lifestyle associated issues such as reduced physical exercise, elevated levels of social stress, "modern" habits of child upbringing, and perhaps even false medical interventions. With regard to the latter, the view that fever is primarily an adaptive defense mechanism to reduce reproduction rates of pathogens (Kluger, Kozak, Conn, Leon, & Soszynski, 1998), unwarranted prescription of antibiotics may contribute to antibiotic resistance. Similarly, anemia and iron deficiency can be seen as a defense against pathogens, because iron is needed by many germs to reproduce. Consequently, iron substitution may worsen infection, for example, in HIV (Weinberg, Friis, Boelaert, & Weinberg, 2001). Finally, although it is desirable to eradicate dangerous pathogens by immunization of at-risk populations, cessation of vaccination after successful elimination of certain strains can potentially produce even more virulent strains. It is therefore debated among evolutionary medical professionals, if immunization only against the most virulent strains, leaving out milder strains, might be a better strategy than immunization against all strains, because infection with a live mild strain may protect those who are not vaccinated or develop insufficient immunity to the vaccine from severe forms of the disease (Read et al., 1999).

Emphasizing the mismatch problem does not mean that individual variation in genetic make-up is irrelevant in causing disease. On the contrary, it seems quite obvious that at a population level some people are more vulnerable to develop disease such as type-II diabetes than others. Such between-population differences may, for example, reside in a differential expression of "thrifty" genotypes. However, from a therapeutic perspective, it seems currently more advisable to target environmental causes of disease, rather than genes. In comparison to dietary changes, physical exercise has been disregarded in importance to reduce the risk for diseases as diverse as cardiovascular disease, cancer, and mental illness. Research has shown that regular physical exercise such as jogging has the potential to simulate the energy expenditure found in extant hunter-gatherer populations (Cordain, Gotshall, & Eaton, 1997; Cordain, Gotshall, Eaton, & Eaton, 1998). In light of the almost absence of cardiovascular disease in traditional societies, physical exercise could therefore substantially contribute to the reduction of risk factors for a broad spectrum of diseases. Moreover, a recent study revealed immunological effects of regular exercise, which in turn had a modulating influence on food intake, and hence, body weight (Ropelle et al., 2010). Physical activity and exercise also have a well-established role in the secondary prevention of cardiovascular disease and several cancers (Kruk, 2007). In addition, physical exercise can have beneficial effects on depression, although findings are somewhat inconclusive to date (Mead et al., 2008). In any event, there is evidence to suggest that physical exercise is a suitable means to reduce the risk for quite a spectrum of diseases and disorders (O'Keefe, Vogel, Lavie, & Cordain, 2010).

In summary, these examples may show that evolutionary medicine has a lot to offer in thinking about how disease can be prevented, by reducing the effects of mismatch between adaptations that originated in the evolutionary past of our species and mainly cultural effects that fundamentally changed our environments, including the social environment. As a take-home message, evolutionary medicine has the potential to influence a broad array of issues pertaining to both human health and disease. Knowledge about the evolutionary forces that shaped the human body and mind can help prevent, diagnose, and cure disease (Nesse & Stearns, 2008). So, clearly, the Art and Science of Health Care ought to make use of this knowledge in the interest of our patients.

References

Allison, A. C. (1954). Protection afforded by sickle-cell trait against subtertian malarial infection. *British Medical Journal, 1*, 290–294.

Atkinson, L., Chester, I. C., Smyth, F. G., & ten Seldam, R. E. J. (1964). Oral cancer in New Guinea. A study in demography and etiology. *Cancer, 17*, 1289–1298.

Bach, J. F. (2002). The effect of infections on susceptibility to autoimmune and allergic diseases. *New England Journal of Medicine, 347*, 911–920.

Balen, A. (1999). Pathogenesis of polycystic ovary syndrome – the enigma unravels. *Lancet, 354*, 966–967.

Barnes, K. C., Armelagos, G. J., & Morreale, S. C. (1999). Darwinian medicine and the emergence of allergy. In W. R. Trevathan, E. O. Smith, & J. J. McKenna (Eds.), *Evolutionary medicine* (pp. 209–243). New York, NY: Oxford University Press.

Belsky, J., Jonassaint, C., Pluess, M., Stanton, M., Brummett, B., & Williams, R. (2009). Vulnerability genes or plasticity genes? *Molecular Psychiatry, 14*, 746–754.

Bowlby, (1969). Attachment and loss. In *Attachment* (Vol. 1). New York, NY: Basic Books.

Boyle, P., Macfarlane, G. J., Maisonneuve, P., Zheng, T., Scully, C., & Tedesco, B. (1990). Epidemiology of mouth cancer in 1989: A review. *Journal of the Royal Society of Medicine, 83*, 724–730.

Breinl, A. (1915). On the occurence and prevalence of diseases in British New Guinea. *Annals of Tropical Medicine and Parasitology, 9*, 285.

Brothers, L. (1990). The social brain: A project for integrating primate behavior and neurophysiology in a new domain. *Concepts in Neuroscience, 1*, 27–51.

Brüne, M. (2001). Evolutionary fallacies of Nazi psychiatry: Implications for current research. *Perspectives in Biology and Medicine, 44*, 426–433.

Brüne, M. (2004). Schizophrenia – an evolutionary enigma? *Neuroscience and Biobehavioral Reviews, 28*, 41–53.

Brüne, M. (2007). On human self-domestication, psychiatry, and eugenics. *Philosophy, Ethics, and Humanities in Medicine, 2*, 21.

Brüne, M. (2008). *Textbook of evolutionary psychiatry. The origins of psychopathology*. Oxford, UK: Oxford University Press.

Buss, D. M. (1999). *Evolutionary psychology. The new science of the mind*. Boston: Allyn & Bacon.

Cardno, A., & Mc Guffin, P. (2005). Quantitative genetics. In P. McGuffin, M. J. Owen, & I. I. Gottesman (Eds.), *Psychiatric genetics and genomics* (pp. 31–53). Oxford, UK: Oxford University Press.

Center for Disease Control and Prevention. Retrieved from http://www.cdc.gov/.

Cordain, L., Gotshall, R. W., & Eaton, S. B. (1997). Evolutionary aspects of exercise. *World Review of Nutrition and Dietetics, 81*, 49–60.

Cordain, L., Gotshall, R. W., Eaton, S. B., & Eaton, S. B. III (1998). Physical activity, energy expenditure and fitness: An evolutionary perspective. *International Journal of Sports Medicine, 19*, 328–335.

Crespi, B., & Badcock, C. (2008). Psychosis and autism as diametrical disorders of the social brain. *Behavioral and Brain Sciences, 31*, 241–320.

Crespi, B., Summers, K., & Dorus, S. (2007). Adaptive evolution of genes underlying schizophrenia. *Proceedings of the Royal Society of London Series B, 274*, 2801–2810.

Darwin, C. (1871). *The descent of man, and selection in relation to sex*. London, UK: Murray.

Day, M. H. (1992). Posture and childbirth. In S. Jones, R. Martin, & D. Pilbeam (Eds.), *The Cambridge Encyclopedia of human evolution* (p. 88). Cambridge University Press.

Dunaif, A. (1997). Insulin resistance and the polycystic ovary syndrome: Mechanism and implications for pathogenesis. *Endocrine Reviews, 18*, 774–800.

Dunbar, R. (2003). Evolution of the social brain. *Science, 302*, 1160–1161.

Eaton, S. B., Konner, M., & Shostak, M. (1988). Stone agers in the fast lane: Chronic degenerative diseases in evolutionary perspective. *American Journal of Medicine, 84*, 739–749.

Eaton, S. B., Pike, M. C., Short, R. V., Lee, N. C., Trussell, J., Hatcher, R. A., ... Bailey, R. (1994). Women's reproductive cancers in evolutionary context. *The Quarterly Review of Biology, 69*, 353–367.

Ehrlich, P. R. (2000). Human natures. *Genes, cultures and the human prospect*. Harmondsworth, UK: Penguin Books.

Finch, C. A., & Sapolsky, R. M. (1999). The evolution of Alzheimer disease, the reproductive schedule, and apoE insoforms. *Neurobiology of Aging, 20*, 407–428.

Finch, C. E., & Stanford, C. B. (2004). Meat-adaptive genes and the evolution of slower aging in humans. *The Quarterly Review of Biology, 79*, 3–50.

Fleagle, J. G. (1992). Primate locomotion and posture. In S. Jones, R. Martin, & D. Pilbeam (Eds.), *The Cambridge Encyclopedia of Human Evolution* (pp. 76–79). Cambridge, UK: Cambridge University Press.

Gilbert, P., Allan, S., Brough, S., Melley, S., & Mikes, J. N. V. (2002). Relationship of anhedonia and anxiety to social rank, defeat and entrapment. *Journal of Affective Disorders, 71*, 141–151.

Gluckman, P., Beedle, A., & Hanson, M. (2010). *Principles of evolutionary medicine*. New York, NY: Oxford University Press.

Greaves, M. F. (2000). *Cancer: The evolutionary legacy*. Oxford, UK: Oxford University Press.

Haig, D. (1993). Genetic conflicts in human pregnancy. *The Quarterly Review of Biology, 68*, 495–532.

Haig, D. (2010). Transfers and transitions: Parent-offspring conflict, genomic imprinting, and the evolution of human life history. *Proceedings of the National Academy of Sciences, 107*, Suppl. 1 1731–1735.

Hrdy, S. B. (2000). *Mother nature*. London, UK: Vintage.

Huxley, J., Mayr, E., Osmond, H., & Hoffer, A. (1964). Schizophrenia as a genetic morphism. *Nature, 204*, 220–221.

INTERHEALTH Steering Committee. (1991). Demonstration projects for the integrated prevention and control of noncommunicable diseases (INTERHEALTH programme): Epidemiological background and rationale. *World Health Statistics Quarterly, 44*, 48–54.

Joffe, B. I., Jackson, W. P., Thomas, M. E., Toyer, M. G., Keller, P., & Pimstone, B. L. (1971). Metabolic responses to oral glucose in the Kalahari Bushmen. *British Medical Journal, 4*, 206–208.

Keller, M. C., & Miller, G. (2006). Resolving the paradox of common, harmful, heritable mental disorders: Which evolutionary genetic models work best? *Behavioral and Brain Sciences, 29*, 385–404.

Kluger, M. J., Kozak, W., Conn, C. A., Leon, L. R., & Soszynski, D. (1998). Role of fever in disease. *Annals of the New York Academy of Sciences, 856*, 224–233.

Kohl, S., Kainer, F., & Schiefenhövel, W. (2009). Übelkeit und Erbrechen als evolutionäre Mechanismen der vielschichtigen Anpassungsreaktion an die Schwangerschaft [Nausea and vomiting as evolutionary mechanisms of the complex adaptation reaction to pregnancy]. *Zeitschrift für Geburtshilfe und Neonatologie, 213*, 186–193.

Kruk, J. (2007). Physical activity in the prevention of the most frequent chronic diseases: An analysis of the recent evidence. *Asian Pacific Journal of Cancer Prevention, 8*, 325–338.

Lende, D. H., & Smith, E. O. (2002). Evolution meets biopsychosociality: An analysis of addictive behaviour. *Addiction, 97*, 447–458.

Lindeberg, S. (2010). Food-related health in the Trobriand Islands. In M. Brüne, F. K. Salter, & W. C. McGrew (Eds.), *Building bridges between anthropology, medicine and human ethology. Tributes to Wulf Schiefenhövel* (pp. 189–210). Bochum, Germany: European University Press.

Lindeberg, S., & Lundh, B. (1993). Apparent absence of stroke and ischaemic heart disease in a traditional Melanesian island: A clinical study in Kitava. *Journal of Internal Medicine, 233*, 269–275.

Lindeberg, S., Nilsson-Ehle, P., Terént, A., Vessby, B., & Scherstén, B. (1994). Cardiovascular risk factors in a Melanesian population apparently free from stroke and ischaemic heart disease – the Kitava study. *Journal of Internal Medicine, 236*, 331–340.

Livingstone, F. B. (1958). The distribution of the sickle cell gene in Liberia. *American Journal of Human Genetics, 10*, 33–41.

MacLennan, R., Paissat, D., Ring, A., & Thomas, S. (1985). Possible aetiology of oral cancer in Papua New Guinea. *Papua New Guinea Medical Journal, 28*, 3–8.

Mead, G. E., Morley, W., Campbell, P., Greig, C. A., McMurdo, M., & Lawlor, D. A. (2008). Exercise for depression. *Cochrane Database Systematic Reviews, 4*, CD004366.

Morel, B. A. (1857). *Traité des dégénerescances physique, intellectuelles et morales de l'espèce humaine et des causes qui produisent ces variétés maladives* [Essays on physical, intellectual, and moral degenerations in the human domain and the cause which produce these various maladies]. Paris: Bailliere.

Neel, J. V. (1962). Diabetes mellitus: A "thrifty" genotype rendered detrimental by "progress"? *American Journal of Human Genetics, 14*, 353–362.

Nesse, R. M., Bergstrom, C. T., Ellison, P. T., Flier, J. S., Gluckman, P., Govindaraju, D. R., . . . Valle, D. (2010). Evolution in health and medicine Sackler colloquium: Making evolutionary biology a basic science for medicine. *Proceedings of the National Academy of Sciences of the United States of America, 107*, 1800–1807. Epub 2009 Nov 16.

Nesse, R. M., & Stearns, S. C. (2008). The great opportunity: Evolutionary applications to medicine and public health. *Evolutionary Applications, 1*, 28–48.

Nesse, R. M., & Williams, G. C. (1994). *Why we get sick. The new science of Darwinian medicine.* New York, NY: Times Books.

O'Keefe, J. H., Vogel, R., Lavie, C. J., & Cordain, L. (2010). Achieving hunter-gatherer fitness in the 21(st) century: Back to the future. *American Journal of Medicine* [Epub ahead of print].

Omenn, G. S. (2010). Evolution and public health. *Proceedings of the National Academy of Sciences, 107*, Suppl. 1 1702–1709.

Pollard, T. S., & Unwin, N. (2008). Impaired reproductive function in women in Western and "Westernizing" populations: An evolutionary approach. In W. R. Trevathan, E. O. Smith, & J. J. McKenna (Eds.), *Evolutionary medicine and health. New perspectives* (pp. 169–180). New York, NY: Oxford University Press.

Price, J. S., Gardner, R. Jr., Wilson, D. R., Sloman, L., Rohde, P., & Erickson, M. (2007). Territory, rank and mental health: The history of an idea. *Evolutionary Psychology, 5*, 531–554.

Radcliffe-Brown, A. R. (1948). *The Andaman Islanders: A study in social anthropology.* Cambridge, MA: Cambridge University Press.

Read, A. F., Aaby, P., Antia, R., Ebert, D., Ewald, P. W., Gupta, S., . . . Moxon, R. (1999). What can evolutionary biology contribute to understanding virulence? In S. C. Stearns (Ed.), *Evolution in health and disease* (pp. 205–215). Oxford, UK: Oxford University Press.

Roehlke, V. (1997). Biologizing social facts: An early 20th century debate on Kraepelin's concepts of culture, neurasthenia, and degeneration. *Culture, Medicine and Psychiatry, 21*, 383–403.

Ropelle, E. R., Flores, M. B., Cintra, D. E., Rocha, G. Z., Pauli, J. R., Morari, J., . . . Carvalheira, J. B. (2010). IL-6 and IL-10 anti-inflammatory activity links exercise to hypothalamic insulin and leptin sensitivity through IKKbeta and ER stress inhibition. *PLoS Biology, 8.* pii: e1000465.

Schiefenhövel, W. (1993). Ethnomedizinische und evolutionsbiologische Befunde zur Geburt [Ethnomedical and evolution biology findings at birth]. *Curare, 16*, 179–188.

Schiefenhövel, W. (1995). Aggression und Aggressionskontrolle am Beispiel der Eipo aus dem Hochland von West-Neuguinea [Aggression and aggression control using the example of the Eipo from the highlands of New West Guinea]. In H. von Stietencron & J. Rüpke (Eds.), *Töten im Krieg Freiburg* [Killing in the Freiburg War] (pp. 339–362). München: Verlag Karl Alber.

Schiefenhövel, W. (2000). Leid ohne Sinn? Krankheit, Schmerz und Tod. Entwurf einer evolutionären Medizin [Suffering without any sense? Disease, pain, and death. Blueprint of an evolutionary medicine]. *Gesundheitswesen (Sonderheft 1), 62*, S3–S8.

Schiefenhövel, W. (2007). Bedding-in als Prophylaxe gegen Baby-Blues? [Bedding-in as prophylaxis against baby blues?] In K.-H. Brisch & T. Hellbrügge (Eds.), *Die Anfänge der Eltern-Kind-Bindung* [The beginning of parent-child attachment] (pp. 100–114). Stuttgart, Germany: Klett-Cotta.

Shaner, A., Miller, G., & Mintz, J. (2004). Schizophrenia as one extreme of a sexually selected fitness indicator. *Schizophrenia Research, 70*, 101–09.

Short, R. V. (1976). The evolution of human reproduction. *Proceedings of the Royal Society of London. Series B, Biological Sciences, 195*, 3–24.

Sievert, L. L. (2008). Should women menstruate? An evolutionary perspective on menstrual-suppressing oral contraceptives. In W. R. Trevathan, E. O. Smith, & J. J. McKenna (Eds.), *Evolutionary medicine and health. New perspectives* (pp. 181–195). New York, NY: Oxford University Press.

Spielman, R. S., Fajans, S. S., Neel, J. V., Pek, S., Floyd, J. C., & Oliver, W. J. (1982). Glucose tolerance in two unacculturated Indian tribes of Brazil. *Diabetologia, 23*, 90–93.

Stearns, S. C., & Koella, J. C. (2008). *Evolution in health and disease* (2nd ed.). Oxford, UK: Oxford University Press.

Stone, M. H., Steinmeyer, E., Dreher, J., & Krischer, M. (2005). Infanticide in female forensic patients: The view from the evolutionary standpoint. *Journal of Psychiatric Practice, 11*, 35–45.

Suomi, S. J. (2006). Risk, resilience, and gene × environment interactions in rhesus monkeys. *Annals of the New York Academy of Sciences, 1094*, 52–62.

Tinbergen, N. (1963). On aims and methods of ethology. *Zeitschrift für Tierpsychologie, 20*, 410–433.

Torrey, E. F., Torrey, B. B., & Burton-Bradley, B. (1974). The epidemiology of schizophrenia in Papua New Guinea. *American Journal of Psychiatry, 131*, 567–573.

Torrey, E. F., & Yolken, R. H. (2005). *Beasts of Earth*. New Brunswick, NJ: Rutgers University Press.

Trevathan, W. (1987). *Human birth: An evolutionary perspective*. New York, NY: Aldine de Gruyter.

Trevathan, W. R., Smith E. O., & McKenna, J. J. (Eds.). (2008). *Evolutionary medicine and health. New perspectives*. New York, NY: Oxford University Press.

Trivers, R. L. (1974). Parent-offspring conflict. *American Zoologist, 14*, 249–264.

Trowell, H. C. & Burkitt D. P. (Eds.). (1981). *Western diseases: Their emergence and prevention*. Cambridge, MA: Harvard University Press.

Varki, A. (2001). Loss of N-glycolylneuraminic acid in humans: Mechanisms, consequences, and implications for hominid evolution. *American Journal of Physical Anthropology, 54*–69.

Wallington, M. (1986). Cancer in Papua New Guinea, 1985. *Papua New Guinea Medical Journal, 29*, 333–336.

Weinberg, G. A., Friis, H., Boelaert, J. R., & Weinberg, E. D. (2001). Iron status and the severity of HIV infection in pregnant women. *Clinical Infectious Disease, 33*, 2098–2100.

Williams, G. C. (1957). Pleiotropy, natural selection and the evolution of senescence. *Evolution, 11*, 391–411.

World Health Organization (WHO). (2004). *Prevention of Mental Disorders. Effective Interventions and Policy Options*. Geneva: World Health Organization.

Yeo, R. A., Gangestad, S. W., Edgar, C., & Thoma, R. (1999). The evolutionary genetic underpinnings of schizophrenia: The developmental instability model. *Schizophrenia Research, 39*, 197–206.

Zhang, Y., Galloway, J. M., Welty, T. K., Wiebers, D. O., Whisnant, J. P., Devereux, R. B., . . . Lee, E. T. (2008). Incidence and risk factors for stroke in American Indians: The Strong Heart Study. *Circulation, 118*, 1577–1584.

Circadian Misalignment and Its Impact on the Medical Profession

Timo Partonen[1,2]

[1]University of Helsinki, Finland
[2]National Institute for Health and Welfare, Finland

To everything there is a season. Our hectic life in urban cities does not however follow the time signals of nature anymore. Because of the way we nowadays use artificial lighting, trees are dropping their leaves later when the fall arrives and we are exposed to irregularity in the sleep-wake cycle and delays in sleep phase. In modern societies people tend to work and socialize around the clock and therefore it is not surprising that circadian rhythm disruptions are increasingly common (Rajaratnam & Arendt, 2001). Circadian rhythm disruptions easily lead to sleep deprivation and may lower mood, motivation, attention, and alertness. Lack of alertness and attention may predispose individuals to accidents. Lowered mood or motivation may trigger, for example, the emergence of depressive or manic episodes.

Thanks to their biological clocks, organisms are alert at specific times of the day and rest at others, so that overall, activity is at its highest level when there is a need for food not to be missed. The circadian rhythms regulate vital functions from unicellular organisms to humans. Circadian clocks guide the metabolic and cell-division cycles. They also generate the circadian rhythms, the sleep-wake cycle and the seasonal variations in mood and behavior. All these rhythmic fluctuations represent biological or physiological rhythms that range from ultradian (shorter than 24 hr in their period) to infradian (longer than 24 hr in their period). Circadian rhythms are approximate 24-hr oscillations, that is, the circadian (from the Latin words "circa dies") cycle, in behavioral or physiological processes that allow organisms to anticipate routine environmental changes and to prepare for the appropriate alignment in order to adapt. These biological rhythms are of key importance for medical personnel and health-care professionals, more particularly for clinical competency and for treatment of patients, since alertness and performance fluctuate by the time of day and because clinical status and course of illness are also affected by the circadian clocks.

Circadian rhythms are generated by the intrinsic clocks whose principal pacemaker is located in the suprachiasmatic nuclei of the anterior hypothalamus in the brain. This internal clock is synchronized to the external 24-hr clock by following time-giving cues, primarily the daily light-dark transitions, in the habitat. The principal circadian clock coordinates peripheral oscillators that maintain the timing for a range of physiological functions, such as hormone release, core body temperature, cardiovascular function, and physical activity. Exposures to light-dark transitions have its effect through the eyes on the phase position of circadian rhythms. The magnitude and direction of the phase shifts of circadian rhythms are dependent on the time of the day, the intensity of the contrast between light and darkness, and the duration of the exposures. The phase-response curve for light exposures has been characterized, and the correctly scheduled exposures to light have a high efficacy in synchronizing the circadian rhythms and avoiding the circadian misalignment.

Recently, there has been growing interest in the impact of disruption of the circadian clocks on health. Abnormalities in the circadian clocks or their functions may be a health hazard. So far, such abnormalities have been linked to metabolic, sleep, and mood disorders that have a substantial influence on public health and need attention in terms of prevention. Preventative measures which have their mechanisms of action directly on or through the functions of the circadian clocks may therefore be effective against these health hazards and beneficial to health promotion as operated by the medical profession, as well as among, but not restricted to, members of it.

Without light, metabolism synchronizes our circadian rhythm. Fluctuation of metabolic activities is a natural time signal for the organism and consequently regulates the sleep-wake cycle. The three-oscillator model of the human circadian system was derived from free-running experiments where subjects had lived isolated in caves or cellars and thus did not receive any timing signals from the external environment. According to this model, the circadian oscillator controls the duration of sleep by influencing the sleep oscillator which in turn determines the timing of wake onset (see Figure 1). The wake oscillator influences the timing of sleep onset and therefore mainly controls the duration of the waking state (Kawato, Fujita, Suzuki, & Winfree, 1982). Because the circadian oscillator regulates the sleep-wake cycle, disruptions in this cycle indicates a dysfunction in the oscillator. Thus, by studying the sleep-wake cycle, we can gather information about how and when the oscillator is disrupted. It also provides us with knowledge about the mechanisms which can synchronize the circadian oscillator after disruption and establishes the duration of the synchronization of the oscillator.

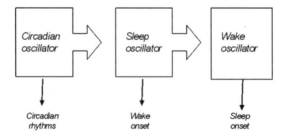

Figure 1. The three-oscillator model of the circadian rhythms and the sleep-wake cycle.

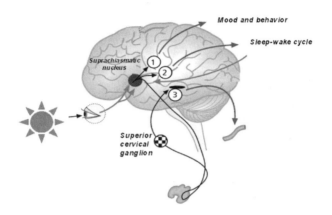

Figure 2. The principal circadian pacemaker in the suprachiasmatic nuclei of the anterior hypothalamus in the brain.

Light exposures or the constant lighting conditions in the evening delay the phase of the circadian rhythms, and in the early morning their effect is opposite, leading to advance of the circadian rhythms. Light through the eyes in the morning synchronizes the circadian pacemaker and this synchronization regulates wakefulness (see Figure 2). And wakefulness in turn regulates sleep patterns. Both wakefulness and sleep give feedback to the circadian pacemaker and thus participate in the regulation of the circadian clockwork. Hence, the external environment influences our endogenous rhythms. The circadian misalignment may emerge between the phase of the circadian rhythms and our behavior concerning the timing of sleep, or in other words, the time when we decide to, or can go to bed, and the time when we want or need to wake up.

Occupational perturbations of the homeostatic sleep process and of the oscillating circadian process systems can be profoundly detrimental to health-care professionals and their patients. These disruptions can emerge from prolonged working hours, or from a mismatch between the sleep duration and sleep requirements, or from mismatch between the internal and external clocks. Here, acute total sleep deprivation concerns primarily the medical profession on-call and thereafter, whereas prolonged work hours, chronic partial sleep deprivation, circadian misalignment, and seasonal misalignment apply to both practitioners and patients equally.

Prolonged Work Hours

Prolonged working hours have roots in the 24/7 nature of medical emergency and intensive care practices in hospital settings, and they are taken for granted during internship and residency training. In addition, overnight call is common in many residency programs.

Despite the economic, educational, and professional arguments that are used to justify these schedules, in fact the current evidence reveals that they are not only demanding, but also exhausting and have a significant negative impact on the physical and psychological well-being of both medical professionals and their patients.

Working shifts, fragmented sleep due to realized or threatened interruptions, additional tasks and extra jobs, and insufficient recovery sleep contribute most to acute as well as chronic sleep deprivation in physicians, particularly those in training (Akerstedt, Arnetz, & Anderzen, 1990; for review, see Olson, Drage, & Auger, 2009). This is consistent with findings that extended work and shift schedules in today's 24/7 global economy and modern society, combined with long commutes and other demands on the individual's time, restrict the time available and spent for sleep, and subsequently jeopardize safety. On the one hand, night work shifts force physicians to perform and resist the increasing sleep propensity, which can endanger the waking function. On the other hand, rotating work shifts disrupt the circadian alignment and sleep consolidation. Naps may be an effective countermeasure (Arora et al., 2006), but if taken in the context of sleep deprivation and against the circadian signal of increasing sleep propensity, sleep inertia may in fact unfavorably impair performance on awakening from a nap and thereafter.

When the substantial effect of sleep loss on trainee performance, their learning, errors, and well-being became evident (Owens, 2001; Veasey, Rosen, Baransky, Rosen, & Owens, 2002; Weinger & Ancoli-Israel, 2002), the US Accreditation Council for Graduate Medical Education reacted and decided to limit resident duty hours. For instance, 41% of internal medicine residents attributed tiredness to contributing to their most significant medical mistake, with a third resulting in a patient fatality (Wu, Folkman, McPhee, & Lo, 1991). Moreover, surgical residents "performed" twice as many errors during a simulated laparoscopy post-overnight call than after a night of sleep, displaying the loss of fine motor skills due to sleep deprivation (Eastridge et al., 2003; Grantcharov, Bardram, Funch-Jensen, & Rosenberg, 2001). Furthermore, anesthesia residents displayed sleepiness to a similar extent to patients with narcolepsy, in fact even without any on-call duty during the past two days (Howard, Gaba, Rosekind, & Zarcone, 2002; Howard et al., 2003).

Acute Total Sleep Restriction

Overnight call results in acute sleep deprivation that often approaches 24 hr or more without sleep. Sleep loss consistently reduces cognitive performance, impairs concentration, and lowers mood after 24 hr without sleep (Veasey et al., 2002; Weinger & Ancoli-Israel, 2002). Studies clearly demonstrate that alertness remains at a higher level and errors occur less frequently, if continuous wakefulness is limited to 16 hr (Gottlieb, Parenti, Peterson, & Lofgren, 1991; Landrigan et al., 2004; Lockley et al., 2004).

The harmful iatrogenic effect of acute total sleep restriction on clinical competency has been demonstrated in a series of elegant studies. Sleep deprived anesthesia residents demonstrated progressive psychomotor deficits in vigilance and working memory, were slower to process and give their responses to vigilance probes than their rested counterparts, and approximately a third fell asleep during 4-hr simulated cases (Howard et al., 2003).

A modified schedule (shifts no longer than 16 hr) seems to have benefits as compared with a traditional schedule with extended (24 hr or more) work shifts every other shift (an "every third night" call schedule) as far as intern errors in the intensive care unit setting are concerned (Landrigan et al., 2004). This modified schedule resulted in 19.5 hr less work and 5.8 hr more sleep per week, with interns on the traditional schedule making 21% more serious medication errors and 5.6 times more serious diagnostic errors compared with the modified schedule. It is not surprising that interns on the traditional schedule experienced twice the rate of attention failures, as documented with work logs and daily sleep logs that were validated with regular weekly episodes (72–96 hr) of continuous ambulatory polysomnography, while working during on-call nights (Lockley et al., 2004).

The odds of a motor vehicle crash or a near-miss incident during the home commute after an extended work shift is increased compared with those working nonextended shifts (Barger et al., 2005; Kirkcaldy, Martin, van den Eeden, & Trimpop, 1999; Trimpop, Austin, & Kirkcaldy, 2000). More in detail, each extended work shift in a month that was scheduled for interns increased the monthly risk of a motor vehicle crash by 9%, and the monthly risk of a crash during the commute from work increased by 16% (Barger et al., 2005). In months in which interns worked 5 or more extended shifts, the risk that they would fall asleep while driving or while stopped in traffic increased, with the odds ratios of 2.4 and 3.7, respectively. As compared with an identical time on the previous day, the risk of sustaining a cutting injury the day after working overnight was 1.6-fold greater (Ayas et al., 2006). On average, extended work injuries occurred after 29 consecutive work hours. Medical errors due to tiredness were reported during 4% of months with no extended shifts, 10% of months with 1–4 extended work shifts, and 16% of months with 5 or more extended work shifts, with the odds ratio for adverse events that were due to tiredness and preventable being 7.0 (Barger et al., 2006). In addition, falling asleep during educational activities and duties, for example, during surgery, occurred in proportion to the number of extended shifts to which one was exposed.

The impact of total sleep deprivation on physicians has been subjected to a meta-analysis whose conclusion was that acute sleep loss in the range of 24–30 hr reduces overall and clinical performances markedly (Philibert, 2005). A period of 30 hr is the period of continuous duty that is permitted under the US Accreditation Council for Graduate Medical Education's standards. This fact needs to be understood in the context that there are two basic traits of individual characteristic in sleep: The night-time sleep duration ranges from 6–9 hr and the best time for falling asleep has a range from 9–12 pm for 95% of the adult population. In terms of the period of the circadian rhythms, the duration of the internal day ranges from 23 hr 52 min to 24 hr 29 min, being on average 24 hr 11 min and not exactly 24 hr, for 95% of the adult population. In contrast, the structure of sleep in terms of sleep stages, whether short or long, is similar or nearly stereotypic between individuals, whether morning larks or evening owls, everywhere in the globe. These two endogenous traits greatly influence the degree of resilience the individual has against the effects of acute loss of sleep and of chronic sleep debt, and on the extent of their consequences in real life situations.

Chronic Partial Sleep Restriction

Chronic partial reductions in sleep duration in trainees reflects wider social trends, with chronic partial sleep debts presenting a greater hazard to health and well-being than acute total sleep deprivation. The average self-reported sleep duration among adults in the United States of America is 6 hr 42 min on weekdays, trending downward. Similarly, the average self-reported sleep duration is 7 hr 18 min and has shortened by 18 min among the adult population in Finland in 33 years (Kronholm et al., 2008).

Chronic partial sleep deprivation is defined as sleep duration of less than 5–6 hr for several consecutive nights. Chronic partial sleep loss is common in residency, with 20% of residents reporting sleep of 5 hr or less per night, and 66% indicating that they sleep 6 hr or less. Residents who report sleeping 5 hr or less are more likely to report having worked in an "impaired condition" and having made medical errors (Baldwin & Daugherty, 2004). A national survey of residents across specialties discovered average self-reported sleep durations of less than 6 hr per night (Baldwin, Daugherty, Tsai, & Scotti, 2003). It also assessed the degree to which chronic sleep debt influenced the personal and professional lives of residents. Those working extended hours were more susceptible to experiencing serious conflicts with attending physicians, other residents and nurses, in addition to an increase in alcohol use and instances of unethical behavior (Baldwin et al., 2003). Residents during an inpatient rotation performing call every 4th or 5th night had a markedly greater impairment in sustained attention and vigilance in a simulated driving task as compared with those involved in an outpatient rotation with a limited call (Arnedt, Owens, Crouch, Stahl, & Carskadon, 2005). During heavy call, the impairments were equal to the effects associated with, for example, blood alcohol concentrations of 0.04–0.05 g%. Compared with light call, heavy call performance was characterized by slower and more variable reaction times and by more commission errors. Heavy call residents were less able to maintain a consistent lane position and speed, and ran off the road more often on a simulated driving task. The effect of heavy call was equal to that of alcohol ingestion on reaction time, attention lapses, omission errors, and crashes. These results were independent of training year and of the self-ratings of greater effort in the heavy call. Moreover, the residents' ability to judge their level of impairment was limited, the finding that should be of alarm to all whom it may concern. The aforementioned results should also be disturbing since there is nowadays a sound basis of evidence that links both chronic insomnia and chronic hypersomnia to increased mortality rates (Cappuccio, D'Elia, Strazzullo, & Miller, 2010).

A substantial number of trainees from a range of specialties reported profoundly adverse effects of sleep restriction on personal life, well-being, work performance, learning ability, and motivation (Papp et al., 2004). Here, for example, 64% of residents agreed that sleep deprivation and fatigue had a major impact on their personal life, and 46% agreed that sleep loss and fatigue had a potentially deleterious effect on their work behavior. Furthermore, alarmingly, internal medicine interns were likely to be predisposed to the development of chronic sleep deprivation and subsequently to depressive disorder of moderate severity during the internship (Rosen, Gimotty, Shea, & Bellini, 2006).

Circadian Misalignment

Shift work is currently one of the most important disrupters of the circadian rhythms, since it has become more common during the past years and affects a substantial proportion of people of working age. The medical profession is no exception. For example, approximately 24% of Finns of working age engage in shift work and approximately 10% of working aged Finns are employed in night shifts at least once a month, according to the Finnish Institute of Occupational Health. Thus, approximately 624,480 Finnish people, according to Statistics Finland, may suffer from circadian disorders due to shift work. The most detrimental form of shift work is night work. From the physiological point of view the night is the most unnatural time to work. Yet night work is very common in health-care settings.

Recent data emphasize the relevance and importance of the circadian clocks with respect to health-care provider outcomes. For example, the self-reported cutting injuries are twice as common in interns during the night hours as compared with the daytime (Ayas et al., 2006), and among junior doctors night work and irregular work schedules both served as significant risk factors for medical errors due to tiredness, whereas the total work hours per week was not (Gander, Purnell, Garden, & Woodward, 2007). However, the impact of circadian related factors on patient safety is not known in detail yet.

Seasonal Misalignment

In the fall, the days start getting shorter. The shortening length of the day tends to affect mental well-being and to trigger the occurrence of season-bound symptoms at the population level. The natural daylight is considered to improve mental well-being, or the feeling of general well-being, with artificial light exposures also being beneficial. Modern citizens spend around 80% of their time indoors such as in houses, schools, offices, malls, and public transportations. This may lead to the circadian misalignment not only due to the seasonal changes in mood and behavior, but also due to poor illumination levels at home or in the work place, and it may therefore have a negative effect on the quality of life in general, the health-related quality of life in particular and more specifically, on mental well-being (Grimaldi, Partonen, Saarni, Aromaa, & Lönnqvist, 2008).

The sun is not only the dominant object in the sky during the day, but it is the source of virtually all of the light and the heat that fuels life on earth. In addition, nobody can resist a sunset nor help feeling the most intense emotions while observing the striking hues that paint the sky during a sunrise or sunset. It is an inexpensive resource that increases motivation as well as improves health. Concerning the health-related quality of life, to visualize the negative effect of poor illumination indoors, it has been estimated to be equal in degree to the positive effect that can be gained with regular physical exercise having the intensity of fitness training (Grimaldi et al., 2008). The intensity of seasonal changes in mood and behavior, especially those in energy level, mood, and social activity, has a negative effect on the health-related quality of life, and it is second to the intensity of depressive symptoms only and greater than, for example, that of age.

Clearly, indoor lighting is of importance to psychological well-being. They may therefore stimulate further research aimed at designing optimal working and living environments in terms of lighting conditions. Current indoor lighting standards are based on specifications concerning the visual requirements. If the nonvisual effects of light exposure to the eyes which contribute to the seasonal changes in mood and behavior were to be considered, novel codes and standards that influence the choice of lighting technologies and the design of indoor environments could be developed and implemented. Lighting levels indoors may be enhanced with architectural and design solutions, and the season-bound changes in mood and behavior could be alleviated or even prevented with the use of scheduled light exposures. These practices may even converge, as poor illumination indoors and the risk of negative seasonal changes in mood and behavior could be alleviated with innovations taking advantage of light exposure schedules that modulate the intensity of lighting as a function of time. Subsequent research activities on the design of indoor environments may bear relevance to the assessment and programming considerations for community-dwelling older adults and those living in long-term care settings.

Greater social activities, more activities outdoors and living together are positively associated with better mental well-being. On the other hand, greater seasonal changes and poor illumination indoors associate with worse mental well-being. The intensity of seasonal changes in mood and behavior has an adverse effect on mental well-being that is second to none (Grimaldi et al., 2008). In other words, its effect is greater than that of gender, age, education, outdoor, or social activities, for example, and the degree of these seasonal changes similar to that of winter blues yields the odds ratio of 2.97 for suffering from mental ill-being to a marked extent. Of the seasonal changes in mood and behavior, especially those in mood, appetite, social activity, and energy level, are of relevance to mental well-being. Here, the negative effect of poor illumination indoors is greater than the positive effect gained with regular physical exercise having the intensity of sports activities, and bears the odds ratio of 1.39 for suffering from mental ill-being to a marked extent.

Not more than 80 years ago doctors in Europe and North America were using sunlight to treat potentially fatal diseases on a routine basis, and a number of hospitals were built specifically for sunlight treatment. More recently in two Nordic countries, Finland and Sweden, light therapy was originally given for patients with winter depression in a room, not with portable devices, but designed for use in the treatment and equipped with lighting fixtures in the ceiling that produce light intense enough even at floor level.

Seasonal changes in mood and behavior are common in the general population, thereby being of relevance to public health (for review, see Partonen & Lönnqvist,

1998). This may give a rationale for administrating of light exposures with an intensity that is similar to light therapy to population at large. Such solutions concerning the use of indoor lighting applications will be of clear benefit to the approximately 1,226,531 persons, equaling 39% of the whole Finnish population aged 30 and over, who routinely suffer from the seasonal changes that emerge during winter and lead to winter blues (Grimaldi et al., 2008). This line of thinking is also supported by findings which demonstrate the efficacy of light exposures to be similar in patients with the winter type of seasonal affective disorder and individuals having its sub-clinical form. With a light intensity of less than 5,000 lx, optimal durations for treatment were 45–60 min daily. However, a shorter duration may well also be effective, for example, 15 min per day (Partonen, 1994). In fact, daily exposures to light in the morning may help relatively healthy as well as blind individuals to improve their vitality and to reduce their depressive symptoms (Partonen & Lönnqvist, 2000; Partonen, Vakkuri, & Lamberg-Allardt, 1995).

Light is not for vision only, but it also has "nonvisual" influences on us. These nonvisual effects in specific have gained growing attention in research during past years. They involve the function of the intrinsic body clocks, or the circadian clocks. The human core body temperature follows its approximate rhythm of 24 hr and thereby guides both melatonin production and sleep induction. Although the core body temperature follows the length of day across the year, it has a much smaller range of seasonal variation than sleep. The circadian rhythm of the core body temperature is phase-delayed by about 45 min and the onset of slow-wave sleep by about 40 min in winter compared with summer (Van Dongen, Kerkhof, & Kloppel, 1997). Under isolation from time cues, or to some extent under weak in-sync signals by the light-dark transitions as well, sleep tends to become longer in the fall and shorter in the spring (Wirz-Justice, Wever, & Aschoff, 1984). The onset of sleep phase is also delayed by about 90 min in the winter compared with summer (Kohsaka, Fukuda, Honma, Honma, & Morita, 1992). Under these conditions, healthy individuals go to bed earlier in the summer, at an intermediate time in the spring and fall, and later in the winter. There is a similar, but more robust, change in the wake-up time, which is earlier in the summer compared with winter (Honma, Honma, Kohsaka, & Fukuda, 1992).

Whereas the sleep phase, or the daily rest-activity cycle, is primarily reset by the work schedule, the circadian clockwork is substantially influenced by natural daylight. First, there is a seasonal pattern in the phases of circadian temperature and melatonin rhythms, peaking at an earlier time of day in the summer compared with winter. Second, there is also a seasonal pattern in the phase relation, or angle, between temperature rhythm and sleep: The relatively low core body temperature preceding sleep in the spring and summer (Honma et al., 1992). The mismatch therefore emerges most often during summer (Wirz-Justice et al., 1984). In six weeks, for example, most individuals may develop a free-running sleep-wake cycle longer than 24 hr and exhibit no harmony in rhythms under isolated conditions (Steel, Callaway, Suedfeld, & Palinkas, 1995). Interestingly, the temporal relationship between the circadian phase of core body temperature and the timing of slow-wave sleep is usually well preserved throughout the year (Van Dongen et al., 1997).

It seems that not only the external (the circadian pacemaker in relation to the local time) but also the internal (a circadian rhythm in relation to another) phase relations of the circadian rhythms are dependent on the season. These experimental results can be simulated with dual oscillators that are reset separately to dawn and dusk, or with a model of the circadian and sleep processes that has a lowered threshold for the onset of sleep in the dark period.

Since the endogenous seasonal variations are generated by the principal circadian pacemaker whose function produces the circadian rhythms as well (VanderLeest et al., 2007), the assessment of seasonal variations in mood and behavior gives us an estimate of the function, or malfunction, of the circadian clocks. The principal circadian clock located in the suprachiasmatic nuclei of the anterior hypothalamus receives stimuli and feedback from the light-dark transitions, the rest-activity cycles or physical exercise (Buxton, Lee, L'Hermite-Baleriaux, Turek, & Van Cauter, 2003), the fasting-eating cycles or nutrient intake as well as particular sleep stages (Deboer, Vansteensel, Détári, & Meijer, 2003). This master clock has plasticity in function (Scheer, Wright, Kronauer, & Czeisler, 2007) in order to coordinate this information and to pass it downstream and outwards, for instance to sense metabolic cues (for review, see Sakurai, 2007) and to control the rest-activity cycles (Abrahamson & Moore, 2006). In individuals having seasonal variations in mood and behavior, the circadian clockwork tends to produce elastic rest-activity cycles (Teicher et al., 1997), suggesting abnormalities in the reset or in the entrainment of oscillations.

Seasons challenge the circadian pacemaker functions. A change of seasons may challenge a switch between the metabolic and circadian based time-keeping mechanisms of action. Light-dark transitions are needed for the reset of the master circadian clock on a daily basis. When these signals are missed as occurs with the decreasing photoperiod in general and the shortage of light exposure in the morning hours during winter in particular, the circadian clock tends to delay and the circadian clockwork may start relying more on the metabolic cycles producing time-giving signals needed for adaptation (van Oort, Tyler, Gerkema, Folkow, & Stokkan, 2007). Fall and spring are the periods of the year which challenge the circadian clockwork and its integration. Studies in animals have demonstrated that in spring the morning-tagged or morning-active cells yield dominance to the evening-active cells (Stoleru et al., 2007), or from the wake-up to sleep onset process, within the master circadian clock. This may need the input from the intrinsic clock which reacts to a change of seasons and drives its targets (Lincoln, Clarke, Hut, & Hazlerigg, 2006).

In individuals with seasonal variations in their mood and behavior, physical activities are usually reduced, whereby the effect of exercise on, and the feedback from a peripheral circadian clock of the skeletal muscle to the master circadian clock are altered (Zambon et al., 2003). This may predispose these individuals to delays in the circadian clockwork. Indeed, scheduled bouts of physical exercise can advance the phase positions of circadian rhythms and synchronize them with each other, and regular fitness training does alleviate the seasonal symptoms. Furthermore, carbohydrate craving in the evening is a usual sign (Rosenthal et al., 1989), which may lead to delays in the circadian clockwork (Kräuchi, Cajochen, Werth, & Wirz-Justice, 2002). In patients with seasonal affective disorder, there are also increases in the resting metabolic rate (Gaist et al., 1990) during a depressive episode in winter, with this finding being similar to what is seen with the double knocked-out genes encoding CRY1 and CRY2 proteins.

Concerning a plausible network or a potential pathway that might link the light-exposure and food-intake responsive oscillators to a range of affective and behavioral outputs, the mechanisms of action remain to be elucidated at molecular level. At the molecular level, circadian rhythms are generated by a network of proteins. The clock protein (CLOCK) pairs up with aryl hydrocarbon receptor nuclear translocator-like (ARNTL or BMAL1) protein. Neuronal PAS domain protein 2 (NPAS2) can substitute for CLOCK and aryl hydrocarbon receptor nuclear translocator-like 2 (ARNTL2 or BMAL2) for ARNTL. Paired heterodimers thereafter activate the transcription of their target genes among others a number of canonical circadian clock genes of key importance including the period PER1, PER, PER3 genes and the cryptochrome CRY1 and CRY2 genes (for review, see Baggs & Hogenesch, 2010).

Since mood is influenced by a complex interaction of circadian phase and the duration of prior wakefulness, even moderate changes in the timing of the sleep-wake cycle may have profound effects on mood (Boivin et al., 1997). Transcriptional networks that include the circadian clock and have control of downstream pathways by circadian oscillators implicate the potential and importance of clock genes to the pathogenesis of seasonal affective disorder. For instance, cells in the limbic system are strategically positioned to modulate the clockwork downstream from the principal clock and exhibit rhythmic oscillations in PER2 levels (Lamont, Robinson, Stewart, & Amir, 2005). Disruption of circadian transcription concerning this loop may affect mood and cognitive performance, possibly in a similar way to what is seen in episodes of depressive disorder.

Whereas abnormalities of circadian clockwork may indicate a direct causative role of circadian clock genes in the pathogenesis, the PER2-mediated regulation of synaptic concentrations of glutamate which influence, for example, alcohol intake, suggests a mechanism of action for regulation of a secondary set of genes which affect directly the depressive phenotype. Two recent studies have addressed this issue. To establish a molecular link between the circadian-clock mechanism and dopamine metabolism, the promoters of genes encoding key enzymes important in dopamine metabolism have been analyzed in mice (Hampp et al., 2008). Transcription of the monoamine oxidase A (MAOA) promoter is regulated by the clock components ARNTL, NPAS2, and PER2. A mutation in the mPer2 gene leads to reduced expression and activity of MAOA in the mesolimbic dopaminergic system. Furthermore, there are increased levels of dopamine and altered neuronal activity in the striatum, leading to behavioral alterations observed in despair-based tests in Per2 mutant mice. These findings indicate that core components of the circadian clockwork influence dopamine metabolism and transmission, thereby highlighting a role of the circadian clock in regulation of mood and behavior (Albrecht, 2010).

The absence of light not only damages brain monoamine systems, but also induces depression-like behavioral symptoms as has been demonstrated in rats (Gonzalez & Aston-Jones, 2008). Long-term constant darkness appears to cause profound changes in neurons in the noradrenergic locus coeruleus, the serotonergic raphé and the dopaminergic ventral tegmental area that include increases in apoptotic markers and loss of cortical noradrenergic fibers or boutons. Next, the threshold for constant darkness concerning the development of these abnormalities needs to be measured, and whether subsequent light exposure can reverse these changes. Constant darkness may be less harmful for nocturnal wild rats adapted to long periods of darkness than for laboratory rats born and raised under constant light-dark transitions, and diurnal animals may be more sensitive to constant darkness than nocturnal animals, so that such harmful effects may occur in humans with less extreme light environments. However, these findings indicate the involvement of a light-dependent mechanism in the etiology of depression and suggest, if phenomena similar to these hold true in humans as well, that there is a light-dependent mechanism in the etiology of depressive disorder.

Although two basic phases, daytime and night-time, can be regenerated in addition to four phases near the subjective noon, dawn, dusk and late night, from the three basic circadian phases, one basic circadian phase, morning, escapes the transcriptional logic of mammalian clocks as analyzed using an in-cellulo mammalian cell-culture system (Ukai-Tadenuma, Kasukawa, & Ueda, 2008). Thus, morning transcriptional regulation is still a "missing link" in the mammalian circadian system. Because a strong repressor at evening phase seems indispensable to the reconstruction of the morning phase, a candidate transcription factor is CRY1 (Ukai-Tadenuma et al., 2008), or it could be CRY2 instead. Both CRY1 and CRY2 have been indicated to contribute to depressive disorders (Lavebratt et al., 2010; Soria et al., 2010).

In addition to these hypothesis-driven studies, microarrays whether they have or have not a prior focus on a system of interest will elucidate further the logic concerning the circadian clockwork. For fruitful data mining, recent published work has demonstrated the effect of light exposure, sleep induction, deprivation of sleep, and physical exercise on genome-wide expression patterns as a function of time (Partonen, 2009).

Forecast for Sleep Debt Induced Performance

It may be of real benefit to accurately predict individual differences in resilience against the adverse effects of sleep loss. A relatively small proportion of individuals may in fact account for most of the risk caused by tiredness in the working place (Mitler, Miller, Lipsitz, Walsh, & Wylie, 1997). Valid and reliable identification of workers who are most at risk of errors and accidents due to sleep loss could allow prevention, targeted countermeasures or removal of these individuals from harm's way. There is a broad search ongoing for predictors of the trait for vulnerability to sleep loss (Van Dongen, Baynard, Maislin, & Dinges, 2004; for review, see Van Dongen & Belenky, 2009).

So far, analysis of socio-demographics, sleep traits and habits, usual clinical outcomes of blood and urine test results, psychological traits such as personality, baseline cognitive functioning, global brain activation as measured with functional magnetic resonance imaging, or the circadian rhythm profiles has produced no viable candidate predictors of this vulnerability. The impact of age in the range encountered in the work environment remains relatively small as well. Mood or sleep disorders or some other clinical conditions can indeed increase the individual's risk of performance impairment during sleep deprivation, but the variance among individuals in the degree of impairment may remain substantial and therefore be of no help in risk assessment.

In the future, valid and reliable genetic predictors of responses to sleep deprivation, if any, may revolutionize the assessment protocols concerning the evaluation of sleep debt induced performance. Studies of genetic predictors have thus far involved a comparison of groups of individuals who were selected a priori to differ by the one single-nucleotide polymorphism under analysis. It does not tell us how much of the between-subjects variance in responses to sleep debt induced performance each genetic predictor can explain in the general population. However, the first of the eligible candidates for further validation exist already, including the circadian clock gene PER3 (Dijk & Archer, 2010) and the sleep need indicators salivary alpha-amylase 1 and homer homolog 1 (Maret et al., 2007; Seugnet, Boero, Gottschalk, Duntley, & Shaw, 2006). In addition to this kind of single gene and its protein isomer analysis, there is a future option enabling us to assess the internal time by using a number of simultaneous assays on the basis of blood-derived assessment of metabolites (Minami et al., 2009). In principle, such assessment can be obtained from one sample and only a drop of blood.

With no baseline predictors a way to the assessment of individual differences in response to sleep debt is to subject individuals to sleep deprivation, to measure their cognitive impairment under laboratory conditions or otherwise controlled circumstances, and to quantify their resilience to sleep deprivation. Since this resilience is a trait, not a state, the results should be predictive of the individual's subsequent responses to sleep deprivation. This strategy may be of use in such operational settings where there are structured training programs during which the trait can be measured with ambulatory tools.

Another way of utilizing information about individual differences in resilience to sleep debt is the use of mathematical modeling of performance with a forecasting technique to tailor the parameters for relevant characteristics such as the individual sleep need and circadian phase as well as the habitual sleep duration and circadian preference to the daily activities. This kind of technique depends on the closed-loop feedback of quantitative performance measures from embedded performance meters to improve the individualized prediction, and it is suitable for confined environments such as the cabin of a truck or the deck of a plane or a ship. However, the individual differences in performance impairment may not generalize from one performance task to another. Therefore, performance tests, even when performed during prolonged or shift work hours in the actual occupational setting, may not yield an accurate enough estimate of a person's resilience to distress in the job at hand. With regard to the example of anesthesia residents working with a simulated case, there were no group differences in clinical skills or error rates (Howard et al., 2003), suggesting that statistical extrapolation from psychomotor cognitive test performances into clinical performance may not be valid but needs a verification at bedside.

Evidently, in modern societies, there is an increasing need to have a medical screen for and identification of sleeping disorders, based on the assessment of sleep duration, quality of sleep, and responses to sleep debt, among individuals with physical and psychological health problems. Medical professionals and their personnel need to be aware of these health hazards personally and therefore constantly sensitive to potentially hazardous sleeping patterns in their life.

References

Abrahamson, E. E., & Moore, R. Y. (2006). Lesions of suprachiasmatic nucleus efferents selectively affect rest-activity rhythm. *Molecular and Cellular Endocrinology, 252*, 46–56.

Akerstedt, T., Arnetz, B. B., & Anderzen, I. (1990). Physicians during and following night call duty: 41 hour ambulatory recording of sleep. *Electroencephalography and Clinical Neurophysiology, 76*, 193–196.

Albrecht, U. (2010). Circadian clocks in mood-related behaviors. *Annals of Medicine, 42*, 241–251.

Arnedt, J. T., Owens, J., Crouch, M., Stahl, J., & Carskadon, M. A. (2005). Neurobehavioral performance of residents after heavy night call vs after alcohol ingestion. *JAMA: The Journal of the American Medical Association, 294*, 1025–1033.

Arora, V., Dunphy, C., Chang, V. Y., Ahmad, F., Humphrey, H. J., & Meltzer, D. (2006). The effects of on-duty napping on intern sleep time and fatigue. *Annals of Internal Medicine, 144*, 792–798.

Ayas, N. T., Barger, L. K., Cade, B. E., Hashimoto, D. M., Rosner, B., Cronin, J. W., . . . Czeisler, C. A. (2006). Extended work duration and the risk of self-reported percutaneous injuries in interns. *JAMA: The Journal of the American Medical Association, 296*, 1055–1062.

Baggs, J. E., & Hogenesch, J. B. (2010). Genomics and systems approaches in the mammalian circadian clock. *Current Opinion in Genetics & Development* [Epub ahead of print; doi:10.1016/j.gde.2010.08.009].

Baldwin, D. C. Jr., & Daugherty, S. R. (2004). Sleep deprivation and fatigue in residency training: Results of a national survey of first- and second-year residents. *Sleep, 27*, 217–223.

Baldwin, D. C. Jr., Daugherty, S. R., Tsai, R., & Scotti, M. J. Jr. (2003). A national survey of residents' self-reported work hours: Thinking beyond specialty. *Academic Medicine, 78*, 1154–1163.

Barger, L. K., Ayas, N. T., Cade, B. E., Cronin, J. W., Rosner, B., Speizer, F. E., & Czeisler, C. A. (2006). Impact of extended duration shifts on medical errors, adverse events, and attentional failures. *PLoS Medicine, 3*, 2440–2448.

Barger, L. K., Cade, B. E., Ayas, N. T., Cronin, J. W., Rosner, (2005). B., Speizer, F. E., & Czeisler, C. A. Harvard Work Hours, Health, and Safety Group. Extended work shifts and the risk of motor vehicle crashes among interns. *New England Journal of Medicine, 352*, 125–134.

Boivin, D. B., Czeisler, C. A., Dijk, D. J., Duffy, J. F., Folkard, S., Minors, D. S., . . . Waterhouse, J. M. (1997). Complex interaction of the sleep-wake cycle and circadian phase modulates mood in healthy subjects. *Archives of General Psychiatry, 54*, 145–152.

Buxton, O. M., Lee, C. W., L'Hermite-Baleriaux, M., Turek, F. W., & Van Cauter, E. (2003). Exercise elicits phase shifts and acute alterations of melatonin that vary with circadian phase. *American Journal of Physiology – Regulatory, Integrative, and Comparative Physiology, 284*, R714–R724.

Cappuccio, F. P., D'Elia, L., Strazzullo, P., & Miller, M. A. (2010). Sleep duration and all-cause mortality: A systematic review and meta-analysis of prospective studies. *Sleep, 33*, 585–592.

Deboer, T., Vansteensel, M. J., Détári, L., & Meijer, J. H. (2003). Sleep states alter activity of suprachiasmatic nucleus neurons. *Nature Neuroscience, 6*, 1086–1090.

Dijk, D. J., & Archer, S. N. (2010). PERIOD3, circadian phenotypes, and sleep homeostasis. *Sleep Medicine Reviews, 14*, 151–160.

Eastridge, B. J., Hamilton, E. C., O'Keefe, G. E., Rege, R. V., Valentine, R. J., Jones, D. J., ... Thal, E. R. (2003). Effect of sleep deprivation on the performance of simulated laparoscopic surgical skill. *American Journal of Surgery, 186*, 169–174.

Gaist, P. A., Obarzanek, E., Skwerer, R. G., Duncan, C. C., Shultz, P. M., & Rosenthal, N. E. (1990). Effects of bright light on resting metabolic rate in patients with seasonal affective disorder and control subjects. *Biological Psychiatry, 28*, 989–996.

Gander, P., Purnell, H., Garden, A., & Woodward, A. (2007). Work patterns and fatigue-related risk among junior doctors. *Occupational and Environmental Medicine, 64*, 733–738.

Gonzalez, M. M., & Aston-Jones, G. (2008). Light deprivation damages monoamine neurons and produces a depressive behavioral phenotype in rats. *Proceedings of the National Academy of Sciences of the United States of America, 105*, 4898–4903.

Gottlieb, D. J., Parenti, C. M., Peterson, C. A., & Lofgren, R. P. (1991). Effect of a change in house staff work schedule on resource utilization and patient care. *Archives of Internal Medicine, 151*, 2065–2070.

Grantcharov, T. P., Bardram, L., Funch-Jensen, P., & Rosenberg, J. (2001). Laparoscopic performance after one night on call in a surgical department: Prospective study. *British Medical Journal, 323*, 1222–1223.

Grimaldi, S., Partonen, T., Saarni, S. I., Aromaa, A., & Lönnqvist, J. (2008). Indoors illumination and seasonal changes in mood and behavior are associated with the health-related quality of life. *Health and Quality of Life Outcomes, 6*, 56.

Hampp, G., Ripperger, J. A., Houben, T., Schmutz, I., Blex, C., Perreau-Lenz, S., ... Albrecht, U. (2008). Regulation of monoamine oxidase A by circadian-clock components implies clock influence on mood. *Current Biology, 18*, 678–683.

Honma, K., Honma, S., Kohsaka, M., & Fukuda, N. (1992). Seasonal variation in the human circadian rhythm: Dissociation between sleep and temperature rhythm. *American Journal of Physiology, 262*, R885–R891.

Howard, S. K., Gaba, D. M., Rosekind, M. R., & Zarcone, V. P. (2002). The risks and implications of excessive daytime sleepiness in resident physicians. *Academic Medicine, 77*, 1019–1025.

Howard, S. K., Gaba, D. M., Smith, B. E., Weinger, M. B., Herndon, C., Keshavacharya, S., & Rosekind, M. R. (2003). Simulation study of rested versus sleep-deprived anesthesiologists. *Anesthesiology, 98*, 1345–1355.

Kawato, M., Fujita, K., Suzuki, R., & Winfree, A. T. (1982). A three-oscillator model of the human circadian system controlling the core temperature rhythm and the sleep-wake cycle. *Journal of Theoretical Biology, 98*, 369–392.

Kirkcaldy, B., Martin, T., van den Eeden, P., & Trimpop, R. (1999). Modelling psychological and work-situation processes that lead to traffic and on-site accidents. *Disaster Prevention and Management: An International Journal, 8*, 342–350.

Kohsaka, M., Fukuda, N., Honma, K., Honma, S., & Morita, N. (1992). Seasonality in human sleep. *Experientia, 48*, 231–233.

Kronholm, E., Partonen, T., Laatikainen, T., Peltonen, M., Härmä, M., Hublin, C., ... Sutela, H. (2008). Trends in self-reported sleep duration and insomnia-related symptoms in Finland from 1972 to 2005: A comparative review and re-analysis of Finnish population samples. *Journal of Sleep Research, 17*, 54–62.

Kräuchi, K., Cajochen, C., Werth, E., & Wirz-Justice, A. (2002). Alteration of internal circadian phase relationships after morning versus evening carbohydrate-rich meals in humans. *Journal of Biological Rhythms, 17*, 364–376.

Lamont, E. W., Robinson, B., Stewart, J., & Amir, S. (2005). The central and basolateral nuclei of the amygdala exhibit opposite diurnal rhythms of expression of the clock protein Period2. *Proceedings of the National Academy of Sciences of the United States of America, 102*, 4180–4184.

Landrigan, C. P., Rothschild, J. M., Cronin, J. W., Kaushal, R., Burdick, E., Katz, J. T., . . . Czeisler, C. A. (2004). Effect of reducing interns' work hours on serious medical errors in intensive care units. *New England Journal of Medicine, 351*, 1838–1848.

Lavebratt, C., Sjöholm, L. K., Soronen, P., Paunio, T., Vawter, M. P., Bunney, W. E., . . . Schalling, M. (2010). CRY2 is associated with depression. *PLoS ONE, 5*, e9407.

Lincoln, G. A., Clarke, I. J., Hut, R. A., & Hazlerigg, D. G. (2006). Characterizing a mammalian circannual pacemaker. *Science, 314*, 1941–1944.

Lockley, S. W., Cronin, J. W., Evans, E. E., Cade, B. E., Lee, C. J., & Landrigan, C. P., . . . Harvard Work Hours, Health and Safety Group. (2004). Effect of reducing interns' work hours on sleep and attentional failures. *New England Journal of Medicine, 351*, 1829–1837.

Maret, S., Dorsaz, S., Gurcel, L., Pradervand, S., Petit, B., Pfister, C., . . . Tafti, M. (2007). Homer1a is a core brain molecular correlate of sleep loss. *Proceedings of the National Academy of Sciences of the United States of America, 104*, 20090–20095.

Minami, Y., Kasukawa, T., Kakazu, Y., Iigo, M., Sugimoto, M., Ikeda, S., . . . & Ueda, H. R. (2009). Measurement of internal body time by blood metabolomics. *Proceedings of the National Academy of Sciences of the United States of America, 106*, 9890–9895.

Mitler, M. M., Miller, J. C., Lipsitz, J. J., Walsh, J. K., & Wylie, C. D. (1997). The sleep of long-haul truck drivers. *New England Journal of Medicine, 337*, 755–761.

Olson, E. J., Drage, L. A., & Auger, R. R. (2009). Sleep deprivation, physician performance, and patient safety. *Chest, 136*, 1389–1396.

Owens, J. A. (2001). Sleep loss and fatigue in medical training. *Current Opinion in Pulmonary Medicine, 7*, 411–418.

Papp, K. K., Stoller, E. P., Sage, P., Aikens, J. E., Owens, J., Avidan, A., . . . Strohl, K. P. (2004). The effects of sleep loss and fatigue on resident-physicians: A multi-institutional, mixed-method study. *Academic Medicine, 79*, 394–406.

Partonen, T. (1994). Effects of morning light treatment on subjective sleepiness and mood in winter depression. *Journal of Affective Disorders, 30*, 47–56.

Partonen, T. (2009). Circadian systems biology in seasonal affective disorder. In T. Partonen & S. R. Pandi-Perumal (Eds.), *Seasonal affective disorder: Practice and research* (2nd ed., pp. 113–128). Oxford, UK: Oxford University Press.

Partonen, T., & Lönnqvist, J. (1998). Seasonal affective disorder. *Lancet, 352*, 1369–1374.

Partonen, T., & Lönnqvist, J. (2000). Bright light improves vitality and alleviates distress in healthy people. *Journal of Affective Disorders, 57*, 55–61.

Partonen, T., Vakkuri, O., & Lamberg-Allardt, C. (1995). Effects of exposure to morning bright light in the blind and sighted controls. *Clinical Physiology, 15*, 637–646.

Philibert, I. (2005). Sleep loss and performance in residents and nonphysicians: A meta-analytic examination. *Sleep, 28*, 1392–1402.

Rajaratnam, S. M., & Arendt, J. (2001). Health in a 24-h society. *Lancet, 358*, 999–1005.

Rosen, I. M., Gimotty, P. A., Shea, J. A., & Bellini, L. M. (2006). Evolution of sleep quality, sleep deprivation, mood disturbances, empathy, and burnout among interns. *Academic Medicine, 81*, 82–85.

Rosenthal, N. E., Genhart, M. J., Caballero, B., Jacobsen, F. M., Skwerer, R. G., Coursey, R. D., . . . Spring, B. J. (1989). Psychobiological effects of carbohydrate- and protein-rich meals in patients with seasonal affective disorder and normal controls. *Biological Psychiatry, 25*, 1029–1040.

Sakurai, T. (2007). The neural circuit of orexin (hypocretin): Maintaining sleep and wakefulness. *Nature Reviews Neuroscience, 8*, 171–181.

Scheer, F. A., Wright, K. P. Jr., Kronauer, R. E., & Czeisler, C. A. (2007). Plasticity of the intrinsic period of the human circadian timing system. *PLoS ONE, 2*, e721.

Seugnet, L., Boero, J., Gottschalk, L., Duntley, S. P., & Shaw, P. J. (2006). Identification of a biomarker for sleep drive in flies and humans. *Proceedings of the National Academy of Sciences of the United States of America, 103*, 19913–19918.

Soria, V., Martínez-Amorós, E., Escaramís, G., Valero, J., Pérez-Egea, R., García, C., . . . Urretavizcaya, M. (2010). Differential association of circadian genes with mood disorders: CRY1 and NPAS2 are associated with unipolar major depression and CLOCK and VIP with bipolar disorder. *Neuropsychopharmacology, 35*, 1279–1289.

Steel, G. D., Callaway, M., Suedfeld, P., & Palinkas, L. (1995). Human sleep-wake cycles in the high Arctic: Effects of unusual photoperiodicity in a natural setting. *Biological Rhythm Research, 26*, 582–592.

Stoleru, D., Nawathean, P., Fernández, M. P., Menet, J. S., Ceriani, M. F., & Rosbash, M. (2007). The Drosophila circadian network is a seasonal timer. *Cell, 129*, 207–219.

Teicher, M. H., Glod, C. A., Magnus, E., Harper, D., Benson, G., Krueger, K., & McGreenery, C. E. (1997). Circadian rest-activity disturbances in seasonal affective disorder. *Archives of General Psychiatry, 54*, 124–130.

Trimpop, R., Austin, E. J., & Kirkcaldy, B. D. (2000). Occupational and traffic accidents among veterinary surgeons. *Stress Medicine, 16*, 243–257.

Ukai-Tadenuma, M., Kasukawa, T., & Ueda, H. R. (2008). Proof-by-synthesis of the transcriptional logic of mammalian circadian clocks. *Nature Cell Biology, 10*, 1154–1163.

Van Dongen, H. P. A., & Belenky, G. (2009). Individual differences in vulnerability to sleep loss in the work environment. *Industrial Health, 47*, 518–526.

Van Dongen, H. P. A., Kerkhof, G. A., & Kloppel, H. B. (1997). Seasonal covariation of the circadian phases of rectal temperature and slow wave sleep onset. *Journal of Sleep Research, 6*, 19–25.

Van Dongen, H. P. A., Baynard, M. D., Maislin, G., & Dinges, D. F. (2004). Systematic interindividual differences in neurobehavioral impairment from sleep loss: Evidence of trait-like differential vulnerability. *Sleep, 27*, 423–433.

van Oort, B. E., Tyler, N. J., Gerkema, M. P., Folkow, L., & Stokkan, K. A. (2007). Where clocks are redundant: Weak circadian mechanisms in reindeer living under polar photic conditions. *Naturwissenschaften, 94*, 183–194.

VanderLeest, H. T., Houben, T., Michel, S., Deboer, T., Albus, H., Vansteensel, M. J., . . . Meijer, J. H. (2007). Seasonal encoding by the circadian pacemaker of the SCN. *Current Biology, 17*, 468–473.

Veasey, S., Rosen, R., Baransky, B., Rosen, I., & Owens, J. (2002). Sleep loss and fatigue in residency training: A reappraisal. *JAMA: The Journal of the American Medical Association, 288*, 1116–1124.

Weinger, M. B., & Ancoli-Israel, S. (2002). Sleep deprivation and clinical performance. *JAMA: The Journal of the American Medical Association, 287*, 955–957.

Wirz-Justice, A., Wever, R. A., & Aschoff, J. (1984). Seasonality in free-running circadian rhythms in man. *Naturwissenschaften, 71*, 316–319.

Wu, A. W., Folkman, S., McPhee, S. J., & Lo, B. (1991). Do house officers learn from their mistakes? *JAMA: The Journal of the American Medical Association, 265*, 2089–2094.

Zambon, A. C., McDearmon, E. L., Salomonis, N., Vranizan, K. M., Johansen, K. L., Adey, D., . . . Conklin, B. R. (2003). Time- and exercise-dependent gene regulation in human skeletal muscle. *Genome Biology, 4*, R61.

Culture, Psychopharmacology, and Well-Being

Bruce D. Kirkcaldy,[1] Adrian F. Furnham,[2] and Rainer G. Siefen[3]

[1]International Centre for the Study of Occupational and Mental Health, Düsseldorf, Germany
[2]Department of Psychology, University College London, UK
[3]Department of Pediatrics, University of Bochum, Germany

> "On Prozac, Sisyphus might well push the boulder back up the mountain with
> more enthusiasm and more creativity.
> I do not want to deny the benefits of psychoactive medication.
> I just want to point out that Sisyphus is not a patient with a mental health problem.
> To see him as a patient with a mental health problem is to ignore certain larger aspects of
> his predicament connected to boulders, mountains, and eternity"
> Carl Elliott (2003)

The increase in the use of pharmaceuticals, particularly in the West, in the treatment of physical ill-health and psychological disorders has been significant during the last decades. Since the 1980s new psychotherapies, including psychotropic drugs for such disorders as schizophrenia, bipolar disorder, and depression, have been developed. In the 5 years leading up to 2001, there has been a tripling in the use of psychotropic drugs, with evidence that their sales outstrip any other therapeutic class of medication (Huskamp, 2005). Moran (2006) reported that medication costs continue to outpace inflation, with antipsychotics displaying the highest mean percent price change (6.6%) in the first months of 2006, more than 1.5 times the 3.5% general inflation rate. This was followed by the antidementia agents with a 6.0% increase, followed by anticonvulsants (5.9%). In Canada about 53% of total medicinal spending went on prescription drugs for the period 1980–1991 and 48.1% on over-the-counter medicaments (Madore, 1993). The expenditure of both types increased at an average annual rate of 10%. Substantial national differences were observed. For instance, Germany was spending approximately 22% of total healthcare purchasing medication, whilst the US and Sweden spent significantly less despite high spending in other areas.

The growth in pharmaceutical expenditures throughout the 1990s significantly exceeded the rate of growth in other types of health expenditures (Organisation for Economic Co-operation and Development – OECD, 2008a, 2008b). In addition to the soaring costs of expenditure in medicinal care are the personal costs. In an executive summary of the OECD (2008b), there were substantial variations across countries in the amount of pharmaceutical consumption. It was found that an average OECD country spent the equivalent of 401 US $ per currency per inhabitant on medication. Expenditure on this occasion was highest for the US (792 $) and lowest for Mexico (144 $). Among the countries with the lowest average retail price for pharmaceuticals were Poland, Turkey, the Slovak Republic, the Czech Republic, Korea, Greece, Hungary, and Spain. On the other hand, it has been claimed that the pharmaceutical sector accounts for an average of around 17% of the share of total government (or private) health expenditure in most OECD countries. Eighty percent of global pharmaceutical sales are made in nine OECD countries, with the US having the largest share (45% of global sales), followed by Japan (9%), then France (6%), Germany (5%), United Kingdom (4%), and Italy (4%).

Diverse theories exist trying to explain this growth in psychopharmacological use. Among such theories is the idea of economic and social change impacting on the belief in the "chemical miracle." Giedratis (2003) examined the enormous social anxiety, both culturally and financially, in Lithuania (and presumably other former Soviet-Bloc nations) as a result of the fragmentation of the Soviet Union, and the resulting difficulties associated with adaptation to a world economy. During the period from 1997 to 1998, for example, there was a substantial increase in the incidence of affective mood disorders (25.1–101.6 cases per 100,000), and in behavioral syndromes associated with physiological disturbances and physical factors (0.6–1.8 persons per 100,000), as well as neurotic and stress-related disorders (16.1–24.3 cases per 100,000). Lithuania also had previously shown to have one of the lowest rates of suicides in the world and became one of the highest. At the same time, there was a significant growth in the marketing of psychopharmaceuticals. It was argued that there was a strong association between the economic factors and the observed increments in such ailments as depression in Lithuania. More specifically, the changes in economy allow more western advertising associated with more disposable cash and plausibly greater consumption.

There is extensive literature in medical anthropology and cross-cultural psychology that indicates wide national and cultural differences in health beliefs and behaviors (Helman, 2001). Although recognizing the biopsychosocial origin of all medical conditions it is possible to differentiate very crudely between those with more psychological causes and symptoms, like depression, and those with more physical causes, like stomach complaints (Furnham & Kirkcaldy, 1996). Many factors play a part in the cultural preferences for using particular drugs to encourage health by preventing certain illnesses or curing particular diseases or other problems. These include the availability and cost of drugs, the extent to which they are advertised, prescription patterns of medical staff, as well as cultural beliefs about health and illness.

Lehtinen, Katschnig, Kovess-Masfety, and Goldberg (2007), in their review of the developments in the treatment of mental disorders, report that there has indeed been a dramatic increase in the use of antidepressants, and that this is, in part, attributable to the better recognition of depression by primary care physicians and the general public; the development of a new generation of antidepressants available with fewer adverse

B. D. Kirkcaldy et al.
Culture, Psychopharmacology, and Well-Being

53

side-effects; the better acceptance among the public and their accessibility to treatment, and the aggressive marketing style of the drug industry. Some of the disadvantages of the increased interest in psychotropic medication include the tendency by some doctors to offer prescriptions without clear clinical diagnoses, thus offering something akin to a "happiness pill," and the neglect or undervaluing of alternative treatments such as behavioral psychotherapy. To some extent the prescription rates will be dependent on the particular professional groups and their training and experience in providing the services, which vary from nation to nation. A European survey of psychotherapists found that of the psychotherapists 33% were psychiatrists, 47% psychologists, 4% social workers, 6% nurses, and 10% other trained personnel. On the other hand, health professionals, if they are not medical doctors, can at most recommend medication but not legally prescribe.

Rose (2006; 2007) noted several possible reasons for the increase in the diagnosis of mental disorders and the use of psychopharmacology. It may reflect a kind of "disease awareness campaign" resulting in "illness mongering" in which increased attention is directed towards the misery caused by apparent symptoms of undiagnosed or untreated conditions. Furthermore, there is frequently an inclination to interpret data in order to maximize the belief about the prevalence of a disorder. He also noted that the goal is to focus the attention of laypersons and medical professionals to the existence of a disease and the availability of appropriate treatment, and in the process shaping fears and anxieties into a clinical mold. Thus, the pharmaceutical industry may be eager to sell medicinal products, and/or psychiatrists could be agents ("moral entrepreneurs") focusing awareness and bringing attention to life's suffering, which they claim to best comprehend and to treat. Alternatively, it may be a problem of social and cultural malaise, that is, contemporary societies' inclination to perceive daily problems as disorders requiring treatment.

There are other reasons why variation may be found in medication, including differences in individuals, groups and nations' preferences. An individual's medical history, personality and history of self-medication no doubt are important factors in his/her patterns of seeking out drugs and medical drug taking. Furthermore, certain drugs are prescribed by medical practitioners (doctors and chemists) and recommended by relations, friends and others in their social network. Certain cultures develop folk diagnoses and remedies for particular drugs which over time make them distinctive. Additionally, the history of drug company advertising and merchandising in a country has a great impact on what, when, and why particular drugs are consumed. Some countries have a long history of pharmaceutical intervention dating back to nonproven potions thought to prevent or bring relief from certain symptoms. For instance, the history of alternative and complementary medicine shows that certain cultures favor certain therapies over others (Vincent & Furnham, 1997).

There is also some evidence that national socio-economic factors (i.e., gross domestic product – GDP) play a significant role in the use of psychotropic drugs. For example, Ketting (1989) examined the economic factors that may be related to the consumption of psychopharmaceuticals in Western Europe. He assumed that an increase in the use of psychotropic medicaments would be associated with the financial uncertainty coupled with economic recession and that sales of psychopharmaceuticals would increase specifically in times of recession. The analyses did show some evidence for tranquilizers, but no significant changes were observed in the use of hypnotics and sedatives, antidepressants and neuroleptics for the eight countries studied. Although variations in the intensity of economic decline could not explain differences in psychotropic drug use, differences in social security payments do appear to have an impact: Nations with a high level of social security displayed an increase in the consumption of neuroleptics during the recession. On the other hand, tranquilizer use remained stable for the low social security countries, but increased for those with a high level of social security.

Hirth, Piette, Greer, Albert, and Young (2006) reported a disproportionate amount of general health spending associated with pharmaceutical spending, with differences depending on the varying degrees of financial contributions from government health insurances, private insurances, and the patients (personal costs). The authors focused on a single illness (haemolytic patients) across 10 countries. Out-of-pocket costs ranged from 29% (France) to 99% (Argentina). Furthermore, 3.1% of Japanese and 28.6% of the Americans reported nonpurchase due to costs. The Swedes and Japanese were less likely to skip medication and Germans most likely to do so, suggesting that cultural and other health system related factors impact on cost-related compliance.

This chapter investigates, using archival data at a country/nation level, the relationship between pharmaceutical use and well-being. More specifically, the authors seek to examine national differences in the use of specific forms of medication, and to explore the relationship between specific pharmaceutical use (anxiolytics and antidepressives) and psychological well-being.

Several questions are addressed in this chapter. Firstly, are there differences in the daily consumption rate per inhabitant of specific categories of medication (anxiolytics, sedatives, antidepressants, and analgesics) across countries? Secondly, are there trends in their use observable over the last 5 years, and do these differ across European nations? Thirdly, is there a relationship between the use of psychopharmaceuticals and psychological health (e.g., suicide rate, subjective well-being, and life satisfaction) and/or physical health (e.g., longevity)? Finally, do socio-economic factors such as GDP/person, economic growth, and human development index, relate to consumption of psychopharmacology? In addition, the trends in "off-the-counter" expenditure for medication are examined for several countries.

Psychopharmaceutical Costs and Out-of-Pocket Expenditure

There is increasing concern about the escalating costs of medication especially psychotropic medicaments in nearly all developed Western countries. Penn and Zalesne (2007) reported over-the-counter medication sales between 1964 and 2005 for the US. There was a 10-fold increase reported, including analgesics, antihistamines, laxatives, antacids, etc. Patients spent substantial amounts on out-of-pocket fees for alternative medical treatment as well. A recent study of public and private expenditure of health per annum for each inhabitant of the population revealed that US spent the most (7,290 US $), followed by Norway (4,763 US $), Switzerland (4,417 US $), Luxemburg (4,162 US $), and Netherlands (3,837 US $), with the lowest spending displayed by Poland (1,035 US $), Hungary (1,388 US $), Czech Republic (1,626 US $), and Portugal (2,150 US $) (see www.healthpowerhouse.com for more detailed information about comparisons between health care systems). During this 15 year period, 1992–2007, costs seemed to increase linearly and progressively for the UK and USA, but this was not the case for Germany, the latter displaying a relatively stable value. The question is what could this imply about personal costs invested in medication?

The Figure 1 shows the per capita in US $ (purchasing power parity) expenditure for personal health costs (pharmaceutical and other medical nondurables, comprising pharmaceuticals such as medicinal preparations, branded and generic drugs, patent medicines, serums, vaccines, minerals, and oral contraceptives). Countries were selected from OECD (2008a, 2008b) for which complete data existed for the period 1995–2006. Expenditure was significantly higher in the US compared to Canada and other European countries (Germany, France, and Finland). France displayed substantially less expenditure than other nations until around 2002 when expenditure seemed to increase substantially to match other European countries. It is possible, however, that such marked increments in spending may be the result of changes in the rules and legislation introduced in a country associated

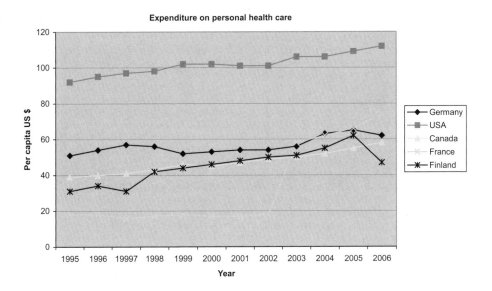

Figure 1. Trends in expenditure on personal healthcare (per capita US $) for several nations between the period 1995–2006 (Adapted from WHO, 2009 and OECD Health Data, 2008).

with health reforms. Certainly, some prudence must be exercised in the interpretation of cross-cultural data because of the accuracy and reliability of such data (Atkinson & Brandolini, 2001). Problems can arise due to national sources not being as easily accessible, and the absence of standardization (e.g., national sources may not always be harmonized; the absence or poor quality of anatomical therapeutic chemical [ATC] codes, that is, WHO standards, in some countries) (Folino-Gallo, 2003). On the other hand, in 2004, the OECD, WHO, and Eurostat joined forces to follow a common strategy to collate health data, increase international standards, and clarify definitions in healthcare.

Diener, Schneider, and Aicher (2008) explored per capita consumption based on sale figures of distributors by pharmaceutical companies in a sample of 1,000 pharmacies for nine different countries. Austria, Switzerland, and Germany displayed the lowest per-capita consumption of analgesics, with figures being three times higher for France and Sweden.

The figures for 2005 suggest that US appears to spend the most on private expenditure for personal health, almost double the cost of the next country, Switzerland, followed by the Netherlands and then Canada and Belgium. The least was spent by such nations as the Czech Republic, Poland, and the Slovak Republic (Figure 2).

Some of these effects may be influenced by the differences between health-care systems in the different countries (socialized vs. privatized healthcare). The majority of developed countries have universal healthcare with the exception of the US (at least still at present). On the other hand, there are those nations with some form of single payment policy

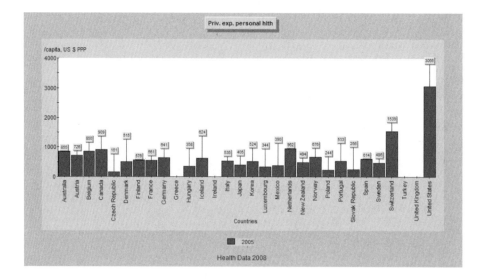

Figure 2. Private expenditure personal health (per capita, US $ PPP) for OECD nations for the year 2005 (Source: OECD Health Data, 2008).

(e.g., Norway, Japan, UK, Sweden, Finland, Spain, Portugal, Italy, and Iceland) and those in which governments mandate citizens to purchase insurance (whether private, public, or nonprofit), for example, Germany, Belgium, Austria, Greece, and Switzerland. Others adopt a type of dual structured medical insurance in which the government mandates a minimum insurance cover whilst permitting additional voluntary insurance, for example, New Zealand, Netherlands, France, Australia, and Ireland. Certainly, especially after the new legislation in the US, it is not easy to demarcate socialized and privatized health-care systems. Systems evolve out of time and each nation has its own "cocktail" of health funding.

Cross-Cultural Differences in the Use of Antidepressives

In an earlier review on mental health policy and practice, Rose (2004; 2007) explored differences in the prescription of psychopharmacologicals across countries. Over the decade 1990–2000, France displayed the highest use of antidepressives, followed by Belgium and the UK. The Mediterranean countries – Italy and Greece – showed relatively low prescription rates. Overall, across nations the rates of use per 1,000 inhabitants doubled in the decade from 1993 to 2002, with a 10-fold increase in the rates for selective serotonin reuptake inhibitors (SSRIs), which are widely prescribed for depression with agitation or comorbid anxiety. They have been shown to be effective with relatively low incidence of side-effects, although often patients report restlessness, anxiety, and insomnia during the initial week or two of taking them. But these side-effects usually are reduced within a couple of weeks (Preston & Johnson, 2009).

The Eurobarometer (2002) results revealed that among 16 countries the reported number of consultations with general practitioners (GPs) regarding mental health problems was highest for UK, France, Northern Ireland, and Portugal, and lowest for Italy, Greece, Finland, and Spain, to some extent supporting the findings reported by Rose. What possible explanations are there for these differences? This may in part be due to differences in consultation time and frequency of GPs. The high demand on doctors' time – German and Spanish GPs have more than 200 encounters with patients per week – could lead to a culture of abbreviated consultation times (Deveugele, Derese, van den Brik-Muinen, Bensing, & De Maeseneer, 2002). Those countries and health systems in which GPs spend more time thoroughly screening patients may be more likely to allow them to effectively screen out psychological disorders. An alternative explanation may be that in some countries there are better provisions – more psychotherapists, psychiatrists, and psychiatric social workers – for identifying and treating psychological disorders, and thus the GP is not necessarily the only professional consulted or indeed the sole "agent" of treatment for such disorders.

Using the latest data (OECD, 2008a, 2008b) and selecting the trends from 2000 to 2005 (when data were most complete), Siefen and Kirkcaldy (2009) found Iceland had the highest consumption of defined daily doses (ddd/1,000 inhabitants per day) of antidepressives, followed by Australia and Sweden then Denmark, while levels remained low

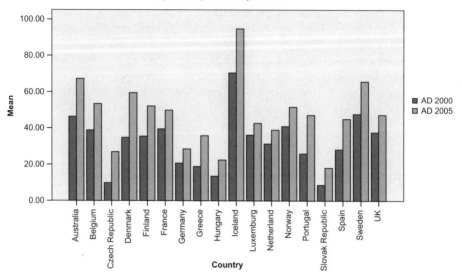

Figure 3. Use of antidepressives (ddd/1,000 inhabitants per day) across countries for the years 2000 and 2005 (statistics for Luxemburg 2001 and Netherlands 2003 replaced 2000 because of missing data and Greece 2004 instead of 2005). (Source: OECD Health Data, 2008).

for the Slovak Republic, Hungary, the Czech Republic, and Germany. In this same period, the use of antidepressants rates grew for all OECD listed nations, growth being most pronounced for the Czech Republic (175%), the Slovak Republic (111%), Portugal (81%), Denmark (71%), and Hungary (67%). The smallest increases were for the UK, Norway, and France. The intra-individual correlation coefficient for usage between 2002 and 2005 was $r = +.97$ across nations. These findings suggest that trends are not consistent across cultures and nations. They are no doubt caused by many factors including economic, political, and social. Thus pharmaceutical companies might decide to target particular countries as a function of their growing or declining economies (Figure 3).

In a recent cross-cultural study, Ploubidis and Grundy (2009) observed that among adult Europeans (over 50 years) the Scandinavian countries, Austria, and the Netherlands appear to display superior mental health scores (high well-being and low depression), followed by France, Austria, and Germany (medium or low depression coupled with either medium or high well-being). On the other hand, older persons in Italy, Greece, and Spain have the worst mental health (high depression and low well-being). Spain emerges as the nation with the highest mean depression scores, and Denmark as the highest on well-being. These national well-being scores may well be related to various medical variables including the taking of legal and illegal drugs.

B. D. Kirkcaldy et al.
Culture, Psychopharmacology, and Well-Being

59

Cross-Cultural Differences in Use of Anxiolytic Medication

The variation in prescription of anxiolytics across countries was relatively stable over a 10 year period (Rose, 2002); levels decreased somewhat in France, albeit usage there remained high. Portugal displayed the highest usage of all EU nations, with an increase of some 30% over that decade. A comparison of the data for 2000 and 2005 suggested a progressive increase in use in many countries, especially for Hungary (19%), Spain (17%), Norway (12%), and Iceland (5%). Overall, Portugal maintained its consistently high rates of prescription (70% vs. 73.1%) for the years 2000 and 2005. However, some European nations displayed a reduction in their prescription rates, for example, Germany (25%), Denmark (14%), and France (8%).

The question arises as to whether Portugal (and to a lesser extent Hungary, Spain, and France) are nations characterized by higher incidences of anxiety-related disorders compared to other nations. Equally interesting is the observation that the incidence of consumption of anxiolytics across countries does not match the levels of use of antidepressives, thus lending partial credence to the claim that anxiety-related disorders and depressive disorders are quite separate "phenomena" in spite of their substantial comorbidity.

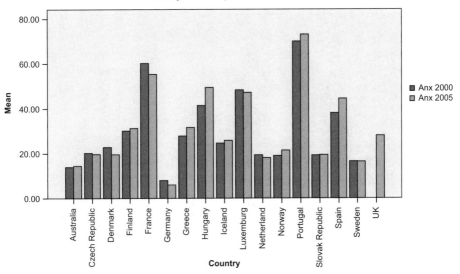

Figure 4. Consumption of anxiolytics for various countries for the years 2000 and 2005 (statistics for Luxemburg 2003 and Netherlands 2001 replaced 2000 because of missing data and Greece 2004 instead of 2005). (Source: OECD Data, 2008).

Examining the incidence rates reported by the WHO (Kessler, Haro, Huang, Ormel, Scott, Schoenbaum, & Alonso, 2009), and focusing on the US and European nations, anxiety disorders were reported to be highest in the US, then France, the Netherlands, Belgium, Germany, and Spain. Again there are some inconsistencies with the data presented in the figure for consumption of anxiolytics 2000–2005 (see Figure 4).

Cross-Cultural Differences in Use of Hypnotics/Sedatives Medication

An examination of Figure 5 reveals those countries which displayed the highest consumption of hypnotics and sedatives. They are Iceland, followed by Finland, Luxemburg, Sweden, Norway, and all Nordic countries, with the exception of Luxemburg. A comparison with the previous figures demonstrates marked differences in the use of such medication compared to anxiolytics. Later statistical analysis reveals there was no significant correlation between consumption of anxiolytics and that of hypnotics/sedatives. Why and under what conditions would medical practitioners prescribe anxiolytics compared to hypnotics/sedatives, and what might explain these subtle cultural differences is not clear and warrants further investigation.

The last group of psychopharmaceuticals are the hypnotics. For many nations data are lacking which renders it more difficult to understand and interpret the cross-cultural

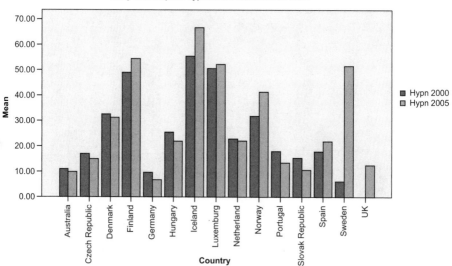

Figure 5. Daily consumption per inhabitant of hypnotics/sedatives across countries (2000 data for Luxemburg and Netherlands missing hence replaced by subsequent year). (Source: OECD Health Data, 2008).

differences. However, the Nordic nations would appear to use much more hypnotics (Iceland, Finland, Sweden, and Norway) than any other European countries with the exception of Luxemburg. Germany and Slovakia seem to show the lowest rates.

Prevalence of Psychological Disorders Across Countries

Some explanation as to the different prescriptions rates and different consumption of psychopharmaceuticals may be found in the differences across nations in the prevalence (or hospital discharge rate per 100,000 inhabitants) of the various categories of mental disorder.

In considering the prevalence rates of mental disorders per 100,000 of the population omitting Japan and Mexico (see Figure 6), we found nations with the highest rates were Finland (n = 1,614), Austria (n = 1,369), Hungary (n = 1,350), and Germany (n = 1,201). The lowest incidence was reported for Poland followed by Ireland and Portugal; interestingly countries with high proportions of Catholics in their communities. Making statements about causality is difficult here; that is, do these nations enjoy better mental health or is the willingness to cater for the needs of socially or emotionally deviant behavior less accepted and so these segments of the population are "neglected." Furthermore,

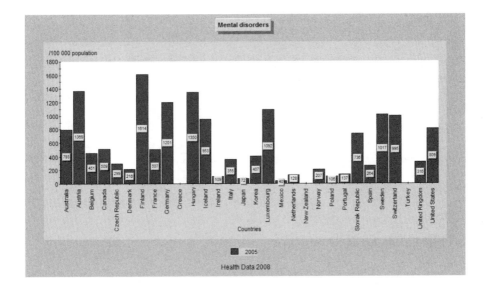

Figure 6. Incidence of mental disorders per 100,000 population across countries in the year 2005 (mental and behavioral disorders). Discharge rates by diagnostic categories/100,000 inhabitants. (Source: OECD Health Data, 2008).

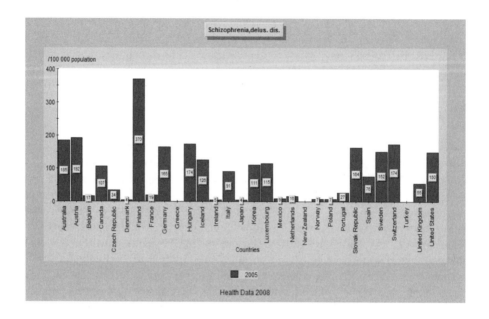

Figure 7. Incidence of schizophrenia and delusory disorders per 100,000 population across countries in the year 2005 (discharge rates by diagnostic categories/100,000 inhabitants). (Source: OECD Health Data, 2008).

other epidemiological data need to be explored to see whether the prevalence rates reflect cultural belief differences.

As mentioned, looking at the incidence rates of mental disorders across countries (OECD Health data, 2008a) the highest values are reported for Finland, Austria, Iceland, and Germany. The year 2005 was chosen as the reference because for this year most complete data were found for most countries. In an examination of the data in Figure 7, the incidence rate of discharge for schizophrenia (delusory disorders) per 100,000 appeared highest for Finland, then Austria, Australia, Hungary, and Switzerland. Data were missing apparently for Greece and Turkey for the year selected (2005).

Suicide Rates Across Countries

If the suicide rates (WHO, 2005) are examined, which may be associated with severe mental disorders, the rates were highest for Eastern European countries: Lithuania was followed closely by Russia, Hungary, and Latvia, then followed by Finland, Poland, France, and Iceland (see Figure 8). The lowest suicidal rates were reported for Greece, then Spain, Israel, UK, Luxemburg, and Denmark.

B. D. Kirkcaldy et al.
Culture, Psychopharmacology, and Well-Being

63

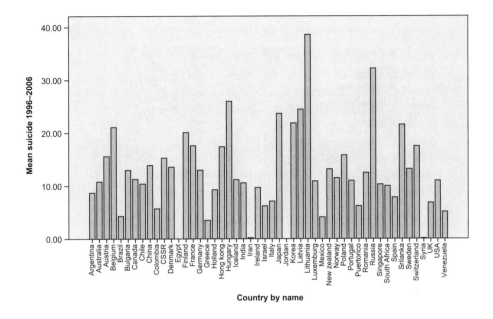

Figure 8. Mean suicide rates for the period 1996–2006 for various countries (Adapted from WHO, 2009).

Alcohol and Substance Abuse

Considering mental disorders of the category "alcohol abuse," figures were highest for Finland ($n = 347$), Germany ($n = 320$), and Luxemburg ($n = 293$). Rates were lowest for the Netherlands, Portugal, and then Spain. It is important to examine not only *how much* people drink but *how* they drink, that is, binge versus excessive regular drinking. It may be argued that if alcohol is used as a method for coping with stress, some nations may show a predilection for using this style of coping. Examining the statistics for the year 2008 presented by the Economist (2009), the following countries displayed the highest level of consumption of alcoholic drinks per head of the population: Germany (100.4), Czech Republic (98.0), Finland (97.1), Denmark (89.3), and Russia (88.5). Almost a decade earlier (WHO, 1999), the statistics for the percentage of 15–16 year olds who had been drunk by the age of 13 years was highest for Denmark (42%), followed by Finland (33%), UK (38%), and Russia (33%).

Examining substance abuse per 100,000 inhabitants, the rates were highest for Iceland, followed by Luxemburg, Sweden, and Germany and lowest for the predominantly Catholic communities such as Poland, Portugal, and Ireland. The question arises whether these are accurate cross-national differences of incidence or to what extent they also mirror

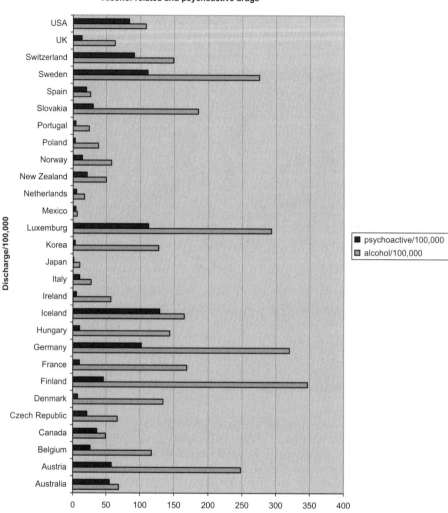

Figure 9. Incidence of mental disorders-discharge rates from hospital due to mental and behavioral disorder resulting from alcohol, and from psychoactive drugs, per 100,000 inhabitants across countries in the year 2005. (Source: OECD Health Data, 2008).

a cultural bias in diagnoses. Other large scale epidemiological surveys, for example, Kessler et al. (2009), have shown that the 12 month prevalence rates for substance disorders were highest for the Ukraine, followed by South Africa, US, New Zealand, Columbia, Mexico, and the Netherlands. Certainly, not only the European nations rate

B. D. Kirkcaldy et al.
Culture, Psychopharmacology, and Well-Being

65

among the highest in the world for alcohol consumption (c.f. hospital discharge rates across countries with regard to alcohol-related and psychoactive drugs. Figure 9).

Differences in the Structure of Healthcare and Medical Health Belief Models

Among health outcome variables of interest are national differences in acute bed care, number of staff per day/bed, number of inpatients (cases/bed turnover and duration of stay – all causes), all available in the OECD Data (June, 2008a). Moving to the "all causes" days ill in hospital (duration), again Korea is an exception (scoring high), otherwise, Finland (12.5), Switzerland (11.6), and then Germany (8.8) have the most days. It could be argued that just as the inpatients admissions differ dependent on which country and presumably on accessibility to healthcare, so does the tendency to keep people in hospital over longer periods of time compared to those countries where patients are hospitalized for shorter times. This too may be a function in part of the cases/bed turnover. In countries in which the rate is low it may be likely that the duration of hospitalization is longer, which in turn will be dependent on the number of beds available in a country. Medical practice has changed considerably over time, partly for financial reasons, with patients being discharged as soon as it is viable. Overall, these differences suggest significant cultural variations in the traditions of treatment care. In instances where many beds are available, there is an increased likelihood on the part of doctors and patients to conduct medical screening and treatment in a hospitalized setting. The in-patient stay will generally be perceived as more intense and superior qualitatively. The temporary transition from out-patient to in-patient care is also financially interesting for a health-care system – as in Germany – when the diagnostic and treatment costs are derived from different economic sources. The culture-specific preferences in methods of healthcare will probably be more determined through the interdependence of what appears are objective symptoms of the patient and the socio-economic resources than the "professional health actors" are aware. This area of conflict between medical bioethics and financial interests of doctors and hospitals has tended to be neglected. Instead the focus tends to be on the threatening reduction of aspects of healthcare for the patient due to escalating health expenditure costs.

Finally, the mood affective disorders per 100,000 inhabitants were analyzed. The countries with the highest incidence rates of affective disorders were Hungary, Austria, Luxemburg, and Finland (and rates were also very high for the US). The question remains as to why the incidence rates of affective disorders are much higher in these European countries? Are they an accurate reflection of the occurrence of such mental disorders in the general population, or are there more likely cultural biases in the diagnostic categories or "allocations" used by medical practitioners? One way of demonstrating this would be to compare migrant doctors, for example, from Hungary, Austria, and Luxemburg, in a novel culture with native practitioners and see whether their implementations of certain diagnoses are different. It may be that these doctors "transmit" some of their cultural biases in the new host nation. In fact, some of the guest practitioners may have a much more accurate diagnoses battery than their colleagues in the host country. A good starting point may be the US or other nations with a high migrant community. We would hypothesize that immigrant physicians use categories of illnesses differently based on both their cultural experiences and training.

Among the methodological reasons for possible variation in mental health diagnoses across countries (Kessler et al., 2009) are symptom threshold differences across nations; (un)willingness to report mental disorders; sensitivity to the health screening procedures and translations in operationalizing the DSM or ICD criteria in a country, and adequacy of the DSM or ICD system to characterize some forms of psycho-pathology in a given country or culture.

Preferences in certain medical health belief models may also influence the prescription of medication such as psychopharmacological agents. The figure showing the daily drug dosage per person per day indicates that medical doctors in countries like Portugal, France, and Hungary prescribe significantly more than their counterparts in nations at the lower end, such as Germany, Sweden, and the Netherlands. These data refer to the statistics for 2005 and it may be that trends can be observed over the next years that might lead to somewhat different results. Germany is the European country with the apparently lowest dosage per person on anxiolytical drugs of any of the European countries, albeit that some data is not available for some nations. These variables such as daily dosage per head of the population are much better figures for comparison because they take account of the population size of a nation. In absolute terms, Germany may exhibit a very high use of anxiolytics but distributed on the average individual it may be less than originally thought.

Analyses of Cross-Cultural Differences in the Prevalence Rates and Treatment Performances

The above findings suggest that exploring the associations between different health outcome variables and analyzing cross-cultural differences in prevalence rates of illnesses and medication may be a useful area of exploratory study for understanding the impact that national differences may have on health belief systems. This may in turn affect the patient's likelihood to seek such traditional solution to medical healthcare or the doctor's preference for treatment.

We move on to examine the relationship between psychopharmacology and mental health data including neuroticism, happiness, well-being, suicide, alcohol consumption, alcohol-related deaths, drug-related deaths, mental disorders, and psychiatric diagnoses. The data came in large part from the OECD Health Database (2008a), personality variables (Barrett & Eysenck, 1984), the WHO database (2001/2008), socio-economic and related data (The Economist, 2010), happiness and well-being data (Diener, 1984; Veenhoven, 2010), and quality of life data (European Foundation for the Improvement of Living and Working Conditions, 2009). These were chosen because they appear to offer some of the health outcome variables which we would assume are most associated with psychological/psychiatric disorders. The issue of the reliability and comparability of these figures must always be considered due to the possibility of error being introduced and this will be considered at the end of the chapter.

Overall, these analyses showed that consumption rates of analgesics, sedatives, anxiolytics, or antidepressives were not significantly correlated with suicide rates across countries nor with deaths caused through driving accidents. Moreover, there was no significant correlation between the trait neuroticism (anxiety, depression, and hypochondriasis) and any of the four categories of medication, with the exception of anxiolytics which almost reached statistical significance ($r = .51$, $p < .10$, $n = 12$ countries). Happiness significantly correlated with several of the classifications of medication consumed daily. For example, (high) anxiolytic consumption was negatively correlated with Veenhoven's index of happiness ($r = -.62$, $n = 15$, $p < .05$) and with antidepressives – albeit this time the correlation coefficient was positive ($r = +.68$, $p < .01$). Moreover, well-being was positively and significantly correlated with the consumption of antidepressives ($r = +.62$, $p < .05$), analgesics ($r = +.65$, $p < .05$), but again negatively with anxiolytics ($r = -.70$, $p < .05$).

The correlation coefficients between the category use of medication ranged from $r = -.19$ (anxiolytics and analgesics) through zero to $+.53$ (antidepressives and hypnotics/sedatives; $p < .05$, $n = 15$). The correlation between psychological well-being (happiness) and suicide rates (year 2005) was statistically significant ($r = -.51$, $n = 22$, $p < .02$) indicating that happy nations were those with lower levels of suicide rates. Moreover, living in colder countries (lower temperatures) was associated with higher happiness scores ($r = -.65$, $n = 31$, $p < .001$).

Clearly, countries have been shown to differ in their prevalence rates of psychological disorders. For example, Ayuso-Mateos et al. (2001) examined several countries and found the prevalence of depression was 8.56%, with figures of 10.05% for women and 6.61% for men. The prevalence rates were high for urban Ireland and the UK, and low for urban Spain.

As mentioned, there was a significant positive correlation between average daily consumption of antidepressives (for nations) and well-being as measured by Veenhoven's life satisfaction scales. The linear regression was statistically significant, $F(1, 14) = 11.93$, $p < .01$, $R^2 = 0.46$. Countries with high use of antidepressives were those that displayed the highest happiness scores (Iceland, Australia, Sweden, and Denmark; Figure 10). Of the two nations with lowest use of antidepressives, Hungary and the Czech Republic, life satisfaction scores were low. Countries with relatively low rates of consumption of antidepressives, such as Germany, Holland, and Luxemburg, all displayed fairly high scores in happiness. The direction of causality is unclear here, and raises the questions: Do those nations with a higher consumption of antidepressives display better health, or is it the case that happier nations have more people disposed to taking antidepressives – perhaps because being depressive in a country characterized by higher psychological well-being may produce significantly more need for medication to counter the adverse effects of negative affect? More importantly it could be that there are

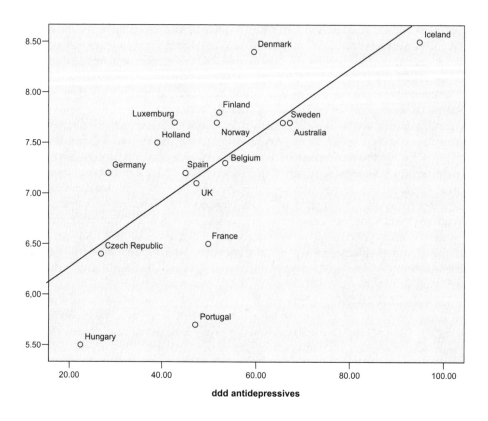

Figure 10. Psychological well-being (life satisfaction scores from Veenhoven) as a function of consumption of antidepressives (ddd in year 2005). (Source: OECD Health Data, 2008).

significant moderator or mediator variables that influence both drug consumption *and* well-being across nations.

Paradoxically, the curve for anxiolytica use and life satisfaction was reversed, that is, those countries with a higher use of antianxiolytic drugs were also likely to display lower happiness scores, these include nations such as Portugal, France, Hungary, and Spain (Figure 11).

The question remains as to why the relationship seems reversed. It clearly shows that those countries who report a high usage of antidepressives are not the same nations that exhibit a high use of anxiolytic medications, $R = .58$, adj. $R^2 = .27$, $F(1, 14) = 6.53$, $p < .03$.

The previous analyses suggest that there may be a relationship between consumption of specific types of psychotropic medicines and subjective reports of well-being. On the other hand, there was no significant correlation between incidence of suicides and consumption of psychopharmaceuticals such as antidepressives. Physical health, as measured

B. D. Kirkcaldy et al.
Culture, Psychopharmacology, and Well-Being

69

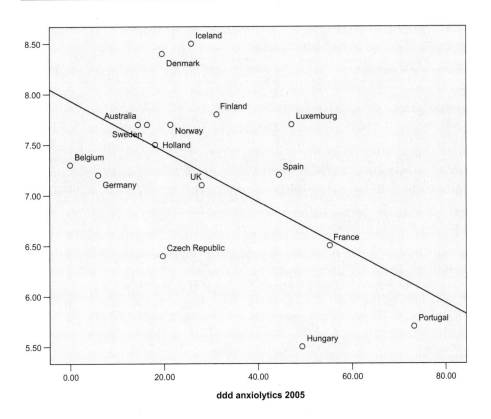

Figure 11. Psychological well-being (life satisfaction scores from Veenhoven) as a function of consumption of anxiolytics (ddd in year 2005) (Source: OECD Health data, 2008a).

Table 1. Correlations between four classes of psychopharmaceuticals and measures of physical and psychological well-being (longevity, suicide rates, subjective well-being, and trait neuroticism; let (*) $p < .10$, *$p < .05$, **$p < .01$)

	Analgesics	Hypnotics/sedatives	Anxiolytics	Antidepressives
Suicide	−.19	−.04	+.01	−.27
SWB (happiness)	+.52(*)	**+.54***	**−.56***	**+.68****
Neuroticism	−.18	−.28	+.51(*)	+.06
Longevity (men)	+.22	+.13	−.35	**+.70****
Longevity (women)	+.02	+.13	−.05	**+.62*(*)**

Note. SWB = Subjective Well-Being.

Table 2. Consumption of specific categories of psychopharmaceuticals as a function of economic factors (let (*) $p < .10$, *$p < .05$, and **$p < .01$)

Socio-economic variables	Analgesics	Hypnotics/sedatives	Anxiolytics	Antidepressives
GDP	0.28	**0.60***	−0.14	0.38
Economic growth	−0.11	0.40	0.03	−0.23
HDI	0.35	0.42	−0.41	**0.65***
% unemployed	−0.14	−0.29	0.16	0.30
Health spending % GDP 2009	0.09	−0.17	0.07	0.26
Total expenditure pharm. % GDP	**−0.53(*)**	**−0.53(*)**	0.40	−0.46
Doctors/1,000 inhabitants	−0.25	0.03	−0.20	−0.15

Note. HDI = Human Development Index.

by longevity (years), was significantly correlated with the consumption of antidepressives for both men and women. Aging appears to be associated with a higher risk of depressive mood changes, and this is more pronounced among men than women. Of course, it is also likely that inhabitants of richer countries tend to live longer and take more drugs, and that whatever relationship between longevity and medical use is spurious (Table 1).

Socio-Economic Factors Associated With Consumption of Psychopharmaceuticals

Table 2 shows clearly that economic factors may contribute a role in the use of medication. For most psychopharmaceuticals, GDP, and economic growth were unrelated to their consumption, with the exception of hypnotics/sedatives, which tended to be more frequently used among the richer nations.

There was no evidence suggesting that low economic growth in a nation was associated with elevated use of psychotropic drugs. Nor were unemployment rates associated with the use of psychopharmaceuticals.

Discussion

The first research question concerned whether there were clear differences in the consumption of specific categories of psychopharmaceutical medication across countries. This was partly supported by the results. What possible explanations may exist for the use of certain categories of medication? Helman (2001) claimed that the use of psychotropic drugs is "embedded in a matrix of social values and expectations," (p. 202) taken as a means of meeting social expectations. In many Western industrialized societies, "chemical coping" (Pellegrino, 1976; 1983) and chemical comforters – including tobacco, alcohol, vitamins, marijuana, and psychotropics – are consumed to enhance one's emotional state and social relationships and, as such, form a method for dealing with the vicissitudes of daily living.

Countries differ in which specific comforters are most commonly used. In some countries there is a tendency to consume more tobacco and alcohol, in others nonlegal drugs, and in yet others psychoactive medication. There are even cultural differences in the preference for certain types of psychotropic drugs. For example, Elliott (2003) has claimed that despite a growth in the market of SSRI prescriptions in Japan, where there is no shortage of psychiatrists or a cultural resistance to medication, Japanese psychiatrists seem more enthusiastic to offer antianxiety drugs such as benzodiazepines over SSRIs. He argued that it may be that the Japanese culture does not object to sedatives as much as to stimulants. The increase in self-confidence, lessening inhibition, and greater energizing impact of SSRIs may be perceived as beneficial for the American, but not so for the Japanese who are "expected to wear a mask of shy deference and modesty ... a lack of social inhibitions may be an advantage in a culture that values animated conviviality and the sparkling personality, but it may be a handicap in a culture that requires an exquisite sensitivity to matters of etiquette and social hierarchy" (pp. 75–76).

The countries that displayed the highest use of antidepressives in the 1990s were not necessarily the same ones that peaked in the early years of the new Millennium, 2000. Of course, our findings are restricted to the data for those countries assessed by the OECD (2008a, 2008b). Iceland, Australia, Sweden, and Denmark were the nations that displayed the highest level of daily consumption. Interestingly, these are not the countries with the highest level of suicide rates, which one may predict are related to depressive disorders which in turn may be associated with the consumption of antidepressives. It could be argued that the early recognition of symptoms and the early prescribing of antidepressives may contribute to the low prevalence rate of suicide in a country. There are clear cultural differences as to which provider is consulted for the initial treatment of a psychological disorder, and nations vary too on the providers of psychotherapy.

Secondly, there are significant trends across time in the use of psychopharmaceuticals across nations. These appear to vary between epochs, that is, the trends in 1990–2000 do not match those observed between 2000–2005/2006. Antidepressant use grew in the latter five-year period for all OECD countries, and was particularly pronounced for the Eastern European nations, Czech Republic, Slovak Republic, and Hungary, as well as Portugal and Denmark (see Kirkcaldy, Shephard, & Siefen, 2010).

Several plausible reasons can be offered for such trends in use. Firstly, it may be the influence of psychopharmaceutical marketing in a country, or an increased awareness of the problem of depression. This may be a reasonable argument for the former Eastern European nations. In the case of countries such as Denmark and Portugal, additional information would be necessary for a plausible interpretation. Secondly, it is possible that a change in consumption rates is related to the medical professionals' preference in implementing a certain medical health model and utilizing medicines as a way of alleviating or curing defined psychological ailments. For example, quite recently in Germany, medical agencies have initiated an "Alliance Against Depression" ("Buendnis gegen Depression"), aiming to raise the level of awareness of depressive ailments, which in turn may increase the screening of suicidal attempts and the prescription rates of antidepressives. Alternatively, it could be that the prevalence of mental disorders, especially anxiety and depression are commonplace in industrialized societies and demands on speedy and effective resolution are underlined.

Thirdly, is there a relationship between average daily consumption of a medication such as anxiolytics and/or antidepressants per 1,000 inhabitants, and other health outcome variables such as suicide rate, well-being, etc.?

There was some indication that of those countries examined, predominantly economically developed, industrialized nations, the level of consumption of antidepressives would appear associated with better psychological health as defined by subjective reports of life satisfaction/happiness, but this did not hold true for the use of anxiolytics. In fact here the relationship was reversed, people living in countries characterized by a high consumption of anxiolytics were likely to be less satisfied with their lives.

Why should people in countries with greater subjective well-being be consumers of more antidepressants? There are many reasons why national rates of self-medication differ. One is that the richer, democratic countries are more likely to have a well-established health service which dispenses drugs freely. Secondly, they are also likely to have a well-established pharmaceutical industry. Third, they also keep better records of, for example, health and prescription rates.

Another possibility, though less likely, is that this shows evidence of the efficacy of the drugs. If people who need them take antidepressants (and they work) then overall the happiness of the region should go up. This cross-cultural study showed no significant correlation between consumption of antidepressives and suicidal rates across countries.

Both anxiety and depression are symptoms of the trait neuroticism. It has been established that northern, light-deprived countries seem to have higher incidences of depression but not anxiety. Equally, temperamental Latin, Mediterranean countries show a high incidence of anxiety. If, for instance, we examine trait neuroticism scores, countries with high scores include Greece, (Russia), Italy, Spain, and Portugal. On the other hand, the results suggest that climate (average temperature) was significantly and negatively correlated with happiness, that is, colder countries were generally likely to be happier (higher SWB): High SWB countries (using Veenhoven's measure) include Denmark, Iceland, Switzerland, Canada, Finland, and Norway. Levels of suicide (associated with depression) are likely to be highest in Lithuania, Russia, Hungary, Latvia, and Japan, and lowest in countries such as Greece, (Jordan, Syria, and Mexico), Italy, and Spain, as well as the UK. Ploubidis and Grundy (2009) found that, at least for elderly persons (defined as a population over 50 years of age), countries such as Greece, Italy, and Spain also show higher scores of depression, and this may not relate to higher suicidal rates.

Theoretically, positive and negative affect are separate and not simply two sides of the same coin (Costa & McCrae, 1980). That is happiness and unhappiness are unrelated to each other. One early researcher suggesting this was Bradburn, who found that different factors influenced positive and negative effect. The construct of (subjective) well-being

B. D. Kirkcaldy et al.
Culture, Psychopharmacology, and Well-Being

73

was defined by Bradburn (1969) as the overall differences in the sum of positive minus negative effect. Watson (2000) has reviewed much of the research on mood and temperament and confirmed that negative affect (linked to basic affect of fear, guilt, sadness, and hostility) was strongly associated with neuroticism and only weakly with extraversion, in contrast to positive affect which was strongly related to extraversion (basic positive affect are joviality, self-assuredness, and to a lesser extent attentiveness) but not neuroticism. Neuroticism is related to the pervasive feelings of distress and dissatisfaction (nervousness, fear, guilt, shame, dissatisfaction, self-loathing, sadness, loneliness, anger, etc.). Certainly the measures of life satisfaction/happiness may not necessarily be related to depression (mistakenly assumed to be its opposite).

Added to this are findings suggesting that depression is associated with debilitating cognitions/worries about past events, in contrast to anxiety, which are related to concerns about the future (catastrophizing). Eysenck, Payne, and Santos (2006) examined the timing (past, present, and future) of negative events, levels of anxiety and depression in nonclinical populations. Depression was associated more with past events than future events, but the case was reversed for anxiety. Moreover, persons were required to monitor their emotional reactions to scenarios referring to negative events lying in the past or in the future (future events being either uncertain or probable). They found that past events were connected with more depression and less anxiety than future events, whether uncertain or probable. Conversely, probable future events were related with greater anxiety and depression than uncertain ones.

One aspect is that health may not be the obverse of illness. More obviously, a person may have marked physical ailments and yet still express positive well-being. An individual may be free of any apparent physical disorder and yet still feel (psychologically) burdened, as is the case in many forms of depression (displaying comorbid features such as pronounced or chronic physical disorders). Moreover, even subjective estimates of well-being and life satisfaction may not be monitoring the same aspects as those relevant for diagnosing a clinical depression. This may partly explain why nations may display a high overall level of happiness/well-being and yet also show strong negative effect in the form of depression or anxiety. It was interesting that countries with a high rate of completed suicides were indeed likely to have displayed lower overall well-being scores.

An alternative explanation for these national differences could be afforded by social comparison theory. Northern countries have the least differences between rich and poor, and more social mobility, which subsequently reduces alienation. Another possible artifact may arise from different criteria for health and medical data. Government statistics are possibly "massaged" to help ensure re-election.

The finding that physical health, or more specifically longevity, was correlated with antidepressives could most easily be seen as being a result of a relationship between aging and depression (see Blazer, Hughes, & George, 1987). Medical doctors in those nations with a higher proportion of elderly citizens may therefore also be most likely to be the ones prescribing most antidepressives. Presumably, these are also the richer nations which have more money to invest in healthcare and their citizens will enjoy "superior" lifestyles, including nutrition and comfortable housing, which in turn lead to longer life spans. It has been shown that depression is quite commonplace among the elderly and the over 65 year olds, especially men, accounting for some 30% of suicides in Germany (Statistisches Bundesamt, 2006. Statistics 23211 "Causes of death statistics"). More recent data would seem to offer further, albeit, indirect support for this, with an increased alcohol consumption being observed among older persons (70 years and older) (German Ministry of Health, News report 8.4.2010).

Fourth, this study investigated relationships between socio-economic variables, including GDP, economic growth and human development index and use of psychopharmacology. The OECD Executive Summary (2008b) reported that although income per capita was positively correlated across countries with the amount and expenditure per capita, differences in income were not sufficient in themselves to explain these differences in pharmacological consumption. It claims that these findings suggest "that pharmaceutical demand varies across countries and is relatively income-inelastic – meaning that expenditure changes with income, but not as fast as income does" (p. 10). Our findings, hardly surprising, underline this, although only for the four categories of psychotropic medicines this study focused on. For only one class of psychopharmaceuticals, the hypnotics/sedatives, did GDP correlate significantly with the defined daily dosage rates. Moreover, there was no indication that countries with greater economic growth were more or less likely to consume such medicines. There was also no evidence that the percentage of GDP in health spending was related to any of the consumption rates of the four classes of psychopharmaceuticals. As discussed, and perhaps somewhat paradoxically, those nations with a higher percent of GDP investment in pharmaceuticals were somewhat more likely to be consuming less of the analgesics and hypnotics/sedatives. One explanation is that such medication could be purchased over the counter without subsidy from the pertinent health insurance companies. Certainly, expenditure in medication per se, does not necessarily need to be related to the amount of consumption of psychopharmaceuticals.

The final question concerned whether countries differ in their out-of-pocket expenditure on medication and whether these differences are likely to change across time? Ploubidis and Grundy (2009) in addressing their study on depression among the elderly across nations reported "A common feature of previous studies is that they suffer from a major methodological limitation because none has formally addressed the issue of between-country measurement invariance. To engage in a meaningful country-level comparison of a mental health construct, the measurement invariance of the construct under study needs to be considered due to the possible influence of language, culture, different levels of expectations for the future, and other country-specific influences on mental health assessment." (p. 666). They add that most studies focus attention on either well-being or depression but not both, and suggest "Although it is clear that depressed individuals are not mentally healthy, it does not follow that nondepressed individuals have good mental health, and considering only one dimension may bias cross-country comparisons. If only depression is studied, relevant variation in positive aspects of mental health is not taken into account; similarly, if only information from well-being indices is used, low scorers on well-being are grouped with those who are depressed" (p. 666).

Overall, this study demonstrates the potential value of transcultural and transnational comparative analyses, particularly in exploring the idiosyncrasies of medical healthcare in individual nations and/or in a specific constellation of countries. Inevitably there are multiple factors that determine a countries' overall consumption of legal (and illegal) drugs aimed to improve medical and psychological health. Economic, legal, social, medical, as well as cultural factors together conspire to influence the decision how, when and why people in some countries personally choose to take and get prescribed drugs. Furthermore, the consequences of drug taking at a national level are also difficult to assess as outcomes like well-being are themselves equally affected by many factors. Despite the complexity of these issues the causes and consequences of national differences in psychopharmacological use are well worth pursuing.

It is of course important to point out that there may be considerable error variance in this data depending on how it was collected. National data gathering is unreliable and idiosyncratic. For instance, how a person is defined and categorized as unemployed may differ widely from one country to another. Equally the way in which medical statistics are gathered and logged can radically differ from one country to another. Nevertheless hypotheses maybe entertained and tested on the basis of these data.

In an era of international diagnostic and therapeutic legislations and evidence-based medicine, it is probable that the incidence rates of depression and the implementation of antidepressives (per head of the population) for its treatment will increase. When these predictions are not borne out, which has been partly demonstrated in this study, the first interpretation may be to focus on the methodological deficiencies of such comparative studies or to be skeptical towards the validity/significance and comparability of such data. Such criticism would appear justified because it stimulates increased efforts to generate more complete and reliable data, which is the goal of the OECD initiative.

The critical discussion concerning the validity of epidemiological comparisons between nations should not, however, blind us from the potential benefits of exploratory analyses, which reveal clear differences, both culturally and regionally, in the different patterns of healthcare. Such differences promote a critical reflection and understanding of existing preferences in a country's medical healthcare. On the other hand, medical and allied health professionals, including doctors and psychotherapists, in their roles on the "stage of health care" make decisions based on subjective beliefs "felt" derived from rigid scientific premises. This chapter suggests that treatment cultures and medical belief systems do vary across countries, and this insight to some extent challenges the subjective model of uniformity of healthcare – and this can generate novel and fruitful discussion. Moreover, specific diagnostic and treatment expectations of migrants can be better understood, and as a consequence improve healthcare. Possible areas of influence could include that exerted by the pharmaceutical industry. It is also feasible that more traditional values of certain kinds of diagnoses and treatments which may have been unfairly neglected in modern medicine could be revitalized. Future research may benefit by focusing on the varying treatment cultures and their different degree of effectiveness.

References

Aktinson, A. A., & Brandolini, A. (2001). Promises and pitfalls in the use of "secondary" data-sets: Income inequality in OECD countries a case study. *Journal of Economic Literature, XXXIX*, 771–799.

Ayuso-Mateos, J., Vazquez-Barquero, J. L., Dowrick, C., Lehtinen, V., Dalgard, O. S., Casey, P., ... Wilkinson, G. (2001). Depressive disorders in Europe: Prevalence figures from the ODIN study. *The British Journal of Psychiatry, 179*, 308–316.

Barrett, P., & Eysenck, S. B. G. (1984). The assessment of personality factors across 25 countries. *Personality and Individual Differences, 5*, 615–632.

Blazer, D., Hughes, D. C., & George, L. K. (1987). The epidemiology of depression in an elderly community population. *The Gerontologist, 27*, 281–287.

Bradburn, N. M. (1969). *The structure of subjective well-being*. Chicago: Aldine.

Costa, D., & McCrae, P. (1980). Influence of extraversion and neuroticism on subjective well-being. *Journal of Personality and Social Psychology, 38*, 668–678.

Deveugele, M., Derese, A., van den Brik-Muinen, A., Bensing, J., & De Maeseneer, J. (2002). Consultation length in general practice: Cross sectional study in six European countries. *British Medical Journal, 325*, 472.

Diener, E. (1984). Subjective well-being. *Psychological Bulletin, 95*, 545–575.

Diener, H.-C., Schneider, R., & Aicher, B. (2008). Per-capita consumption of analgesics: A nine country survey over 20 years. *Journal of Headache and Pain, 9*, 225–231.

Elliott, C. (2003). *Better than Well. American Medicine meets the American Dream*. New York and London: Norton.

EU. (2009). *Second European Quality of Life Survey*. Dublin: European Foundation for the Improvement of Living and Working Conditions.

Eysenck, M. (2006). Anxiety and depression: Past, present and future events. *Cognition and Emotions, 20*(2), 274–294.

Folino-Gallo, P. (2003). Euro-Med-Stat – a web based European data base of medicine. 11th EUPHA Conference, 21st NovemberRome.

Furnham, A., & Kirkcaldy, B. D. (1996). The health beliefs and behaviours of orthodox and complementary medicine clients. *British Journal of Clinical Psychology, 25*, 49–61.

Giedratis, V. (2003). Selling madness: Pharmaceutical companies in Lithuania 1990–2000. *Lithuania Journal of Arts and Sciences, 49*, 1.

Helman, C. G. (2001). *Culture, health and illness* (4th ed.). London, UK: Arnold.

Hirth, R., Piette, J., Greer, S., Albert, J., & Young, E. (2005). "International Comparison of Out-of-Pocket Costs and Medication Compliance". Paper presented at the annual meeting of the Economics of Population Health: Inaugural Conference of the American Society of Health Economists, June 04, 2006. TBA, Madison, WI, USA. Retrieved May 5, 2009, from http://www.allacademic.com/meta/p91512_index.html.

Huskamp, H. A. (2005). Pharmaceutical cost management and access to psychotropic drugs. The US context. *International Journal of Law Psychiatry, 28*, 484–495.

Kessler, R., Haro, J. M., Huang, Y., Ormel, J. H., Scott, K., Schoenbaum, M., & Alonso, J. (2009). THE WHO. *World Mental Health Survey Initiative IFPE Congress*. Vienna Austria: .

Ketting, E. (1989). Use of psychotropic drugs and economic recession in the EC-countries 1978–1987. Chapter 8. In Ruut Veenhoven & Aldi Hagenaars (Eds.), *Did the Crisis really hurt? Effects of the 1980 – 1982 economic recession on satisfaction, mental health and mortality*. The Netherlands: Universitaire Pers Rotterdam133152 ISBN nr. 90 237 2279 5.

B. D. Kirkcaldy et al.
Culture, Psychopharmacology, and Well-Being

77

Kirkcaldy, B. D., Shephard, R. J., & Siefen, R. G. (2010). *The making of a good doctor.* New York, NY: Nova Publishers.

Lehtinen, V., Katschnig, H., Kovess-Masfety, V., & Goldberg, D. (2007). Developments in the treatment of mental disorders. In M. Knapp, D. McDaid, & E. Mossialos (Eds.), *Mental health policy and practice across Europe.* McGraw-Hill, Berkshire, UK: European Observatory on Health Systems and Policy series.

Madore, O. (1993). *Medication costs in Canada.* Economics Division, Government of Canada.

Moran, M. (2006). Medication costs continue to outpace inflation. *Health Care Economics, 41,* 12.

OECD. (2008a). *OECD Health Data 2008.* June 08 version.

OECD. (2008b). *Pharmaceutical pricing policies in a global market.* Summary Executive.

Pellegrino, E. D. (1976). Prescribing and drug ingestion: Symbols and substances. *Drug Intelligence and Clinical Pharmacy, 10,* 624–630.

Pellegrino, E. D. (1983). The healing relationship: Architectonics of clinical medicine. In E. E. Shelp (Ed.), *The clinical encounter: The moral fabric of the physician-patient relationship.* Boston: Reidel.

Penn, M., & Zalesne, E. K. (2007). *Microtrends. Surprising tales of the way we live today.* London and New York: Penguin.

Ploubidis, G. B., & Grundy, E. (2009). Later-life mental health in Europe: A country-level comparison. *Journal of Gerontology: Social Sciences, 64B,* 666–676.

Preston, J., & Johnson, J. (2009). *Clinical psychopharmacology: Made ridiculously simple* (ed. 6). Miami: MedMaster.

Rose, N. (2004). Becoming neurochemical selves. In N. Stehr (Ed.), *Biotechnology, commerce and civil society.* Somerset, UK: Transaction Publishers. (pp. 89–128).

Rose, N. (2006). Disorders without borders? The expanding scope of psychiatric practise. *Biosocieties, 1,* 465–484.

Rose, N. (2007). Pharmaceuticals in Europe. Chapter 7. In M. Knapp, D. McDaid, & E. Mossialos (Eds.), *Mental health policy and practice across Europe.*

Siefen, R. G., & Kirkcaldy, B. D. (2009). *Transnationale und transkulturelle Aspekte der Psychopharmakotherapie* [Cross national and cross-cultural differences in psychopharmacological treatment] Migration und Gesundheit (Migration and Health). Gene, Umwelt und Gesundheit. 12. Kongress der Deutschen Gesellschaft für Verhaltensmedizin und Verhaltensmodifikation. Leipzig, 1–3 October.

Statistisches Bundesamt. (2006). *Statistiken 23211. "Todesursachenstatistik".* Wiesbaden.

The Economist. (2009). *Pocket world in figures* (2010 Edition). London, UK: Profile Books.

Veenhoven, R. (2010). *State of nations: World database for happiness.* Faculty of Social Sciences, Erasmus University of Rotterdam.

Vincent, C., & Furnham, A. (1997). *Complementary medicine: A research perspective.* Chichester, UK: Wiley.

Watson, D. (2000). *Mood and temperament.* New York, NY: Guilford Press.

World Health Organization. (2001). *The world health report.* Geneva: WHO.

World Health Organization. (2008). *Suicide statistics.* Geneva: WHO.

Personality and Health Outcome Determinants: Medical Professionals

Becoming, Being, and Excelling as a Physician

Physician Motivation, Satisfaction, Wellness, and Effectiveness

Richard J. Bogue,[1] Brian Fisak,[2] and Roy Lukman[3]

[1]Richard Bogue & Affliates, Orlando, FL, USA
[2]University of North Florida, Jacksonville, FL, USA
[3]Florida Hospital College of Health Sciences, Orlando, FL, USA

Physicians have been examined in many different contexts: as revenue producers, as cogs in the machinery of health services delivery, as business managers, as consumers of liability insurance, and of course as clinicians. This book has the ambitious aim of acknowledging all this and yet to also push beyond this, by shifting the focus toward the people whom we call physicians and examining the more human aspects of medical care and doctoring.

This chapter strives to push this focus on physicians as people based on existing and emerging research. We attempt to examine the physician experience from the perspective of those who are living their lives as physicians. To see physicians as people, working as physicians, we review previous and emerging research and pursue three interrelated themes: motivation, sustainability, and excellence *or* becoming, being, and excelling as a physician. In particular, the aim of this chapter is to address the following: Why people choose to become physicians? What factors are associated with choice of speciality? What matters most in physician satisfaction? How do people act if they seek to be excellent physicians?

Motivation: Choosing the Life of a Physician

This section provides an overview of the literature on physician motivation and motivating factors, with a particular focus on categorizing and quantifying motivation, choosing medicine as a career, the choice of particular specialties, and motivation throughout the career. Before providing an overview of the literature on physician motivation, it is relevant to make a general distinction between career satisfaction (discussed in the following section) and motivation. Motivation has been described as the factors that provide purpose and drive individuals towards specific decisions and goals, such as electing a career as a physician; in contrast, career satisfaction is a generalized response or appraisal of the one's work experience (Ratanawongsa et al., 2006).

Motivating Factors and Choosing Life as a Physician

Researchers have made efforts to categorize and quantify physician motivating factors. These studies tend to focus on factors related to interest in medicine as a career and generally focus on medical school applicants and students currently in medical school. For example, Vaglum, Wiers-Jennsen, and Ekeberg (1999) examined motivators in a sample of first year medical students. The authors conceptualized motivators into three basic categories: people-oriented, status/security oriented, and natural science oriented. In comparing the degree to which physicians endorse each of these motivating factors, it is not surprising that the highest scores were for the person-oriented index, suggesting that helping others is a primary motivating factor in the decision to become a physician. Further, females scored higher than males on the person-oriented index.

Two similar studies utilized factor analysis in attempt to categorize and quantify motivational factors. McManus, Livingston, and Katona (2006) surveyed medical school applicants regarding their motivation to become a physician. Participants completed the Medical Situations Questionnaire, which measures "generic" or general motivating factors. Based on a factor analysis, the authors found that motivation fell into four factors: helping people, respect, science, and indispensability. Interestingly, endorsement of particular motivating factors was related to personality traits (e.g., agreeableness and neuroticism) and gender. Helping people, as a motivating factor, was related to higher levels of agreeableness. In contrast, less agreeableness was found for those who were focused on science, respect, and indispensability. Further, respect and science as motivators were associated with higher levels of neuroticism, while indispensability was associated with lower levels of neuroticism. Regarding gender differences, females tended to place a greater emphasis on helping, and males rated science and indispensability as more important motivating factors.

In a second factor analytic study, Wright and Beasley (2004) examined associations between three motivating factors – self-expression (expressing one's own personality, as in conversation, behavior, music, or painting), helping others, and extrinsic rewards – and personal differences. Differences emerged based on gender and specialty. Affirming a central finding of both of the previously mentioned articles, females were more motivated by helping others. Further, clinician-researchers were more motivated by self-expression when compared to nonresearchers.

Overall, the above research indicates that a number of general themes appear in the literature in relation to motivating factors to become a physician. These themes include helping people/altruism, status/respect, intellectual challenge/interest in science, and security/indispensability. However, more research is on the empirical classification of motivating factors based on personal characteristics is needed.

In a comprehensive review by Ratanawongsa et al. (2006), motivating factors were conceptualized as two basic categories: intrinsic and extrinsic. Intrinsic motivation included internal factors that have the potential to make a career in medicine fulfilling and rewarding, such as altruism, intellectual challenge, professional growth, and a sense of competence. Regarding extrinsic motivating factors, an additional distinction was made between positive and negative extrinsic factors. Positive extrinsic factors included the incentives/rewards associated with a career as a physician, such as salary potential, job security, and promotion. Negative extrinsic factors were defined as general deterrents/ disincentives and included factors such as delayed compensation and prolonged training, personal time/lifestyle (the habits, attitudes, tastes, moral standards, economic level, etc., that together constitute the preferred mode of living of an individual or group), and medical school debt. In general, Ratanawongsa et al. (2006) concluded that intrinsic factors appear to be the primary motivators for those who enter medical school, and the strongest of these intrinsic factors appears to be helping others and intellectual challenge. The authors also suggested that limitations to one's preferred lifestyle can be a common deterrent to becoming a physician (a negative extrinsic factor). Overall, physicians appear to be initially motivated by intrinsic factors. Ratanawongsa et al. speculated that is possible that the degree to which these motivators are fulfilled may be related to long-term job satisfaction and motivation.

Motivation and Choice of Specialty

In addition to the initial motivation to enter medical school, researchers have also focused on the motivating factors related to the next major career decision for physicians – the choice of specialty. Motivation related to specialty choice is relevant to the field because the match or fit between motivation and specialty may be related to satisfaction with specialty choice and performance. Further, concerns about adequate recruitment for particular specialties (e.g., primary care) has led to interest in strategies to enhance motivation.

As with the decision to enter medical school, Ratanawongsa et al. (2006) suggest that both intrinsic and extrinsic motivating factors appear to be related to specialty choice. The authors reviewed commonly cited intrinsic motivating factors relevant to specialty choice, including the opportunity to make a difference, interest in helping people, the type of cases/intellectual stimulation, and the nature of the relationship with patients (e.g., long-term physician-patient relationships). Extrinsic factors are also important to career choice. Economic factors, including income potential and educational debt accrued, appear to be among the most commonly discussed and influential extrinsic factors. Another particularly relevant extrinsic factor is lifestyle (e.g., work hours, predictable schedule, and being on call). In general, the degree to which physicians prioritize economic and lifestyle factors seems to be important to specialty choice. Finally, experiences during medical school, including initial experiences and exposure to particular specialties and role models, both positive and negative, appear to be relevant to choice of specialty (Ratanawongsa et al., 2006). This finding emphasizes the importance of providing positive experiences in medical school in order to facilitate recruitment in particular specialties.

Perhaps because both groups are large and the apparent differences in the nature of their practice are substantial, the motivating factors for two particular specialties have received considerable attention in the research literature: primary care and surgery. An overview of the motivating factors for these respective areas of practice follows.

Motivations to Choose Primary Care/General Practice

Motivations for choosing primary care as a specialty have been of particular interest due to recent concerns regarding diminishing interest of this specialty and the burgeoning need for generalists. In a recent study, Thistlethwaite, Ajjawi, and Aslani (2008) examined the factors related to choice of general practice. Both role models and the student's experiences during medical school, including the quality of the primary care training experience in medical school, were considered relevant motivating factors in the decision to enter primary care as a specialty. Other relevant factors included the nature of patient-physician interactions (i.e., forming long-term relationships with patients), lifestyle, autonomy, variety of skills utilized, and the ability to practice holistic care. Deterring factors included negative role models, decreasing prestige, perceived lack of support, and inadequate time with patients.

Other studies have suggested that, relative to other specialties, helping others, being person-oriented, and the establishment of long-term physician-patient relationships appear to be of particular importance to those motivated to choose a primary care specialty (Kassler, Wartman, & Silliman, 1991; Vaglum et al., 1999). Further, lifestyle and extraprofessional concerns have been found to be of particular importance to those motivated to become primary care physicians. For example, when compared to other specialties, primary care physicians appear to be more focused on work-family/work-life balance, tend to be more part-time oriented, and to place less emphasis on career success (Buddeberg-Fischer, Klaghofer, Abel, & Buddeberg, 2006; Buddeberg-Fischer, Klaghofer, Stamm, Siegrist, & Buddeberg, 2008).

Motivations to Choose a Surgery Specialty

Barshes et al. (2004) provide a comprehensive review of the factors related to the decision to enter surgery as a specialty. The authors indicated that economic factors appeared to be a particularly relevant factor. Specifically, applicants to surgery programs expected to make more money, and anticipated educational debt was associated with an increased likelihood that one would apply to surgery over primary care programs. Prestige was also discussed as a relevant factor, as surgery is considered among the more prestigious specialties; students motivated by prestige were more likely to choose surgery over primary care. Although educational debt and prestige appeared to be relevant motivators, Barshes et al. (2004) indicated that lifestyle factors may be a deterrent and, sometimes, may be a more important consideration for medical students in deciding whether to enter surgery. As with primary care, role models and experiences in medical school were also found to be important. Regarding gender, research has indicated that many female medical students view surgery as unfavorable to their gender, which may be a deterrent for entering surgery as a specialty. Further, other reasons cited by females for avoiding a career in surgery have included perceived competition, lifestyle, and the negative attitudes of surgeons they have met (Richardson & Redfern, 2000).

Motivation Throughout the Physician's Life

Although several studies have focused on the motivation factors related to the decision to enter medical school and specialty choice, it appears that fewer studies have focused on the factors related to maintaining motivation throughout the physician's career, the stability of motivation over time, and the degree to which initial motivating factors relate to long-term satisfaction and success. However, research does indicate that burnout and decreased job satisfaction are common concerns. Moreover, an emerging area of research includes interventions to enhance motivation and decrease burnout (Ratanawongsa et al., 2006). Potential interventions include the use of motivational coaching, the use of written narrative reflection by which physicians renew their initial motivation, and related processes to enhance career insight (Ratanawongsa et al., 2006).

Overall, it is not surprising that physicians are initially motivated by intrinsic factors including helping others and intellectual stimulation. However, there appears to be substantial heterogeneity in motivating factors. Gender, personality, and lifestyle choices appear to be particularly relevant. Further, heterogeneity in motivating factors appears to become particularly salient when it comes to the selection of specialty. While intrinsic factors remain important, extrinsic factors may take on a more prominent role among the motivations for choosing a specialty. Interestingly, although burnout and decreased satisfaction appear to be common concerns for physicians throughout their career, little is known about the stability of motivation throughout the career and the degree to which a physician's initial motivation is related to long-term success and satisfaction. Because continued satisfaction and burnout are of concern throughout the career of the physician, interventions have been developed to enhance motivation. However, more research is needed that explains why the people who become physicians choose to do so, and how those motivations at the beginning of their lives as physicians shape their satisfaction throughout their career.

Living the Life of the Physician

Above, we reviewed recent literature on physician motivation. In this section, we review how physicians experience being physicians by examining research about physician satisfaction and physician well-being. We also summarize the results of two recent studies at the forefront of examining the experience of being a physician from the physician's viewpoint.

Satisfaction in the Life of the Physician

One productive area of research focused on the physician experience may generically be referred to as physician satisfaction research. It is noteworthy that the phrase "physician satisfaction" is widely and consistently used to refer to physicians' generalized appraisal of their experience as physicians (Ratanawongsa et al., 2006), yet in practice it does not refer to one theoretical stance on how to understand the physician's appraisal of his or her experience. In point of fact, "physician satisfaction" research has followed three general lines with distinct ways of understanding the scope of a physician's experience.

Organization-Centric and Work-Limited Satisfaction Physician Satisfaction

The most common type of physician satisfaction research includes requests for feedback from physicians about an organization, typically a hospital or hospital system. This type of physician satisfaction research where the physician is a source of information for appraising an organization might be defined as "organization-centric and work-limited." The purpose of this research centers on information for and about the organization and is limited in scope to the organizationally defined work context. This line of research, as important as it may be to hospital administrators, is not about what is satisfying to physicians as doctors, let alone as people. It is about soliciting information from physicians about an organizational work context to help the organization evaluate and become more satisfied with its own performance. In this type of physician satisfaction research, there typically is little or no emphasis on appraising those aspects of a physician's experience that the physician might use to make choices leading to greater satisfaction for the physician her- or himself.

This organization-centric and work-limited type of physician research is not prominent in peer-reviewed publications. It may be sufficient to illustrate the purpose and scope of this type of physician satisfaction research using descriptions of such surveys, as shown in Table 1.

Physician-Centric and Work-Limited Physician Satisfaction

Physician-centric and work-limited satisfaction research makes up the bulk of peer-reviewed physician satisfaction, physician job satisfaction, or physician career satisfaction research. This type of research focuses on how features of work and organization affect physician job satisfaction, and often includes personal demographic information.

R. J. Bogue et al.
Becoming, Being, and Excelling as a Physician

87

Table 1. Organization-centric and work-limited physician satisfaction research

Statement of purpose and scope	Source
A physician satisfaction survey offers hospital administrators the means to ensure outsourced physicians are providing a level of patient care that is consistent with hospital standards.	Direct Opinions (2010)
Gallup has studied the psychology of physician behavior for more than 50 years. Using this extensive understanding of the profession and its impact on the physical health of patients and the fiscal health of healthcare organizations, Gallup developed an improvement methodology that measures Physician Engagement and drives positive financial outcomes.	Gallup (2010)
Essential to any healthcare organization's bottom line is the physician. Knowing how physicians think and feel about your organization is critical to your success.	HealthStream Research (2010)

This type of physician satisfaction research has sometimes indicated that many physicians experience low levels of satisfaction with their profession (Demmy, Kivlahan, Stone, Teague, & Sapienza, 2002), or with specific aspects of their work context, such as the complexity of their patients' health issues (Wetterneck et al., 2002), bureaucratic controls that limit autonomy (Stoddard, Hargraves, Reed, &Vratil, 2001), or fee-for-service practice (Schulz, Scheckler, Moberg, & Johnson, 1997). One theme has been that dissatisfaction may be on the rise (Burns, Anderson, & Shortell, 1993; Landon et al., 2002; Shearer & Toedt, 2001). A recent, large scale meta-analytic study suggests a moderation in this trend, except perhaps among primary care providers, and concludes by emphasizing that physician satisfaction is "a dynamic entity mediated by both physician-related and job-related factors, the majority of which are modifiable." (Scheurer, McKean, Miller, & Wetterneck, 2009, p. 565).

Indeed, studies in this area have focused on a wide variety of potential sources of satisfaction and dissatisfaction among physicians. A modest sampling of studies is sufficient to highlight the dynamic and situational nature of physician satisfaction. For example, Leigh, Kravitz, Schembri, Samuels, and Mobley (2002) found that early and late career physicians were more satisfied than mid-career physicians, apparently a phase-of-life dynamic. Hadley, Mitchell, Sulmasy, and Bloche (1999) surveyed 1,549 physicians under age 52 and found incentives to limit service utilization to be the best predictor of dissatisfaction, which may be a generational dynamic. Cashman, Parks, Ash, Hemenway, and Bicknell (1990) found physicians formerly employed by a chain of clinics to be most dissatisfied with reimbursement, while those still employed identified constraints on autonomy as their top source of dissatisfaction; these results demonstrate that the same situation may be dynamically linked to satisfaction depending on whether physicians are still in the situation when asked about it. Hueston (1998) found overall satisfaction to be relatively high for family physicians, except when practicing in smaller groups, a situational factor.

Scheurer et al. (2009) concluded in their meta-analysis that four extrinsic factor areas (job characteristics exogenous to the physician) have shown the strongest associations with physician satisfaction: work demands, work control, colleague support, and income/incentives. Scheurer also reported weaker but largely consistent associations between physician satisfaction and four extrinsic factor areas, that is, practice characteristics, capitation, managed care training and long-term patient relations, and two intrinsic factors, age/years in practice and specialty.

Physician-centric and work-limited research has also produced information about the outcomes of physician work satisfaction on patients. The impact of low job satisfaction among physicians has been found to include lower quality of patient care, lower patient satisfaction with their treatment, and poorer patient compliance with treatment (Deckard, Meterko, & Field, 1994; Demmy et al., 2002; DiMatteo et al., 1993; Landon, Reschovsky, & Blumenthal, 2003; Zuger, 2004). Higher physician satisfaction has also been associated with lower patient care costs, apparently mediated by improved patient compliance with treatment (Beck et al., 1997; DiMatteo et al., 1993).

What differentiates this second line of research from the first type of physician satisfaction research identified above is that it is about physicians rather than about the organizations with which they interact. Its purpose, that is, is to garner information about physicians themselves. Yet, as in organization-centric and work-limited physician satisfaction research, the scope of understanding about physician satisfaction remains restricted to their work context.

Physician-Centric and Life-Oriented Satisfaction

Finally, a third and smaller body of physician satisfaction research has demonstrated that a broader view of the potential sources of physician satisfaction may produce a better understanding of workplace satisfaction, as well as about physicians' personal experiences, such as with stress (Kirkcaldy, Athanasou, & Trimpop, 2000; Murray et al., 2001; Shearer & Toedt, 2001; Wetterneck et al., 2002). This type of physician satisfaction research that is about physicians, and in which work issues are seen within the broader scope of the physician's overall life experience as a physician, may be defined as "physician-centric and life-oriented."

McMurray et al. (1997) identified eight facets of physician satisfaction through a Delphi-like, series of physician focus groups. Konrad et al. (1999) subsequently drew from a comprehensive examination of prior research to identify 10 facets of physician satisfaction. Based on these studies, Konrad and colleagues posited a broader scope of issues that are relevant to physician satisfaction. Combining the expert panel approach and the focus group results, the issues identified as related to satisfaction for physicians were, from most to less often mentioned, (1) day-to-day practice, (2) relationships, (3) administrative issues, (4) autonomy, (5) income, (6) personal and family issues, (7) quality of care, and (8) government concerns. Relationships and personal and family issues, it turns out, have a place among clinical practice issues, clinical autonomy or income if the aim is to understand not only the physician's work experience, but the larger life circumstances that may affect one's experience as a physician.

Drawing on this previous work examining the broader set of contributors to physician satisfaction, Bogue, Guarneri, Reed, Bradley, and Hughes (2006) developed a 17-item, four-factor measure to assess physician satisfaction, the Life of the Physician Satisfaction Scale (LPSS). Although a majority of the final items related to dimensions of physician satisfaction with their professional lives (e.g., satisfaction with organizational climate, office & hospital resources, medical decision-making, and relationships with colleagues), three of the items assessed physician satisfaction with their personal lives (i.e., satisfaction with personal time, family issues, and personal growth).

Kirkcaldy et al., Chapter 5 in this volume, provide a sweeping review of physicians' psychosocial issues, including stress. Here, we review a single study on the association between physician satisfaction and stress using the LPSS so as to continue explicating the emerging field of physician-centric and life-oriented physician satisfaction research. Utilizing the LPSS, Fisak, Bogue, and Paolini (2007) assessed relationships between physician-centric and life-oriented physician satisfaction and self-reported stress in a survey of 696 physicians. Hierarchical regression analysis was used to predict stress with (a) practice characteristics (e.g., type of practice (i.e., single specialty, multi-specialty, solo, and hospital-based), payer mix, and hours worked per week; (b) personal demographics (e.g., number of children living at home, marital status, and age), (c) the four factors of the LPSS (work-environment, work-tasks, work-relationships, and personal-life). The resulting model was significant, $F(4, 546) = 22.10$, $p < .001$, accounting for 24% of the variance in stress. Personal-life satisfaction scores were inversely and strongly associated with physician stress. In contrast, the work-related satisfaction factors of the LPSS did not add significantly to the multivariate model predicting physician stress. Indeed, as shown in Table 2, Personal-Life Satisfaction also predicted stress substantially better than any of the more traditional intrinsic (demographic) and extrinsic (practice characteristics), explaining nearly twice as much variance in physician stress as hours worked per week.

Table 2. Predictors of physician stress

	β
Female	$-.08^*$
Age	$-.15\ddagger$
Hours worked per week	$.16\ddagger$
Personal-life satisfaction	$-.30\ddagger$

$^*p < .05.$ $\ddagger p < .001.$

Well-Being in the Life of the Physician

Once one has acknowledged that, not only phenomenologically but also empirically, *a physician's work life operates within the context of a physician's overall life* – it becomes possible to see that understanding physician behavior in the work context may benefit substantially from a physician-centric and life-oriented perspective. Indeed, outside the realm of satisfaction research, the personal health and well-being of physicians has been documented to have many important implications. Numerous studies have examined areas of poor health and outcomes for physicians themselves (Goodman, 1975; Harms, Heise, Gould, & Starline, 2005; Ullman et al., 1991; Williams et al., 2002). Specific areas of concern for physicians' physical and emotional health include: occupational hazards (Dorevitch & Forst, 2000), lifestyle (Frank, 2004), substance abuse (Adams, Dart, Knisely, & Schnoll, 2004; Domino et al., 2005), cancer (Maitre, 2003), cardiovascular disease (Murphy et al., 2000), fatigue (Arora, 2006), motor vehicle accidents (Barger, 2005; Kirkcaldy et al., 1997), work-environment (Chan & Huak, 2004), and stress (Graske, 2003). Further, researchers have consistently documented a high suicide rate among physicians (Center et al., 2003; Frank & Dingle, 1999; Torre et al., 2005). Finally, when physicians are patients, they are known for a lack of good attention to their own health, along with self-diagnosis and self-doctoring (Brown & Schneidman, 2004; Fromme et al., 2004; Kay et al., 2004).

It is not only physicians and their families who suffer the consequences of poor health among physicians. The health of overall health systems is dependent, among other things, on well-functioning physicians, and under a physician-centric and life-oriented viewpoint, it is clear that "well-functioning" refers to much more than being competent at the technical aspects of work. This has led to two lines of research: (1) the identification and treatment of impaired physicians and (2) the impact of physician health, adjustment, and well-being on patient health. Identifying and treating impaired physicians may be the oldest and most mature thread in research on physician health (Baldisseri, 2007; Berliner, 1999). Averting or addressing disruptive behavior by physicians is widely accepted to require continuing vigilance (Piper, 2005). Despite a history of attention to physicians' physical and emotional health, when doctors leave their career the most common reasons are distress and burnout, depression, anxiety, and alcoholism (Shanafelt et al., 2003; Stanton & Caanwent, 2003). To give an idea about the prevalence of burnout, Shearer & Toedt (2004) found that about one-third of family practice doctors report they are burning out.

Beyond this, however, physicians' health and well-being can also have major consequences for patients' physical and psychological health. Physicians' own health behaviors can affect patient care quality and patient compliance with medical advice (Kay et al., 2004; Stuyt, 1998). Unprofessional behavior by physicians is another mature thread of study and intervention related to potentially devastating consequences for patients (Arnold, 2006; Dehlendorf & Wolfe, 1998). Physicians who attend better to psychosocial issues end up with more collaborative patient relationships, resulting in improved patient satisfaction and outcomes (Levinson & Roter, 1995). Physicians' own emotional engagement in the care process can help or harm them and has important consequences for the

R. J. Bogue et al.
Becoming, Being, and Excelling as a Physician

91

quality of patient care (Charon, 2001; Christakis & Iwashyna, 1998; Jackson et al., 2005; Meier, Back, & Morrison, 2001).

In short, evidence has begun to emerge on the relationships between a physician's broader well-being and consequences for physicians and their patients. As the scope has broadened to acknowledge additional human experiences, beyond the physical, that may affect physicians and their patients, increasing attention has been given to diagnosis and treatment that takes into account the philosophical and/or religious aspect of human experience. Attending to patients' religious and spiritual views in systematic and appropriate ways has been shown to improve patient satisfaction and may help doctors provide better care (Curlin, Chin, Sellergren, Roach, & Lantos, 2006; Curlin, Roach, Gorawara-Bhat, Lantos, & Chin, 2005; Deloney, Graham, & Erwin, 2000; Ehman et al., 1999; Koenig, 2001; Lo et al., 2002; McCord et al., 2004; Musick, Cheever, Quinlivan, & Nora, 2003; Post, Pulchaski, & Larson, 2000; Pulchaski & Larson, 1998). The field of medicine is beginning to recognize that a patient's philosophical orientation or religious views strongly influence how she or he processes the medical encounter, medicines, caregivers, and conceptions of health, life, and death. In turn, recently, increasing attention has been given to incorporating religio-spiritual understanding into medical school curricula (Fortin & Barnett, 2004; King, Blue, Mallin, & Thiedke, 2004) and other training for physicians (Koenig, 2004; Meier et al., 2001; Reilly & Ring, 2005).

A subset of the studies referenced above and others have attempted to integrate multiple domains of physician well-being. A broader literature heavily dependent on anecdote and opinion pieces or advocacy has promoted a more comprehensive approach to understanding and improving health and health care. These more comprehensive frameworks have become commonplace, using terms such as psychosocial, biopsychosocial, mindbody-spirit and whole person health. Sulmasy (2007, p. 123) notes that "a few physicians recently have written about the need for a model that goes even further – a biopsychosocial-spiritual model of health care." Yet, prior to completion of the development of Physician Wellness Self-Assessment Tool (PWSAT), described below, a practical and reliable method for measuring physician health and well-being across all four of these domains was not to be found in the published literature.

Development of the PWSAT was initiated in 2007 when Ted Hamilton, Vice President of Medical Mission for Adventist Health System, convened an expert panel to define a theory and approach to the measurement of physician health and well-being. To develop a measurement instrument, a team of researchers extracted 261 candidate items from a review of 115 peer-reviewed articles and research-based books from 1990 through 2007 reporting empirical evidence on factors affecting physician health in one or more of four domains: bio-physical, psycho-emotional, socio-relational, and religio-spiritual.[1] These were supplemented by 96 candidate items from the Behavioral Risk Factor Surveillance System (Centers for Disease Control and Prevention).

---

[1] A reference list related to PWSAT is under continual enhancement and may be requested by writing the lead author of this chapter.

After several steps of evaluation and ratings by an 11-member panel of physicians and researchers, 87 items about evenly distributed across the four domains of well-being were selected for use in a pilot study with a convenience sample of 120 physicians planning to attend a conference on physician well-being. Factor structure, item-factor correlations and scale reliability were used to identify the 10 items for each of four single-factor subscales that produce the highest reliability attainable with these data. The resulting 40-item scale was also subsequently used in a very small pilot survey of 29 medical residents. Across both pilots, Cronbach's Alpha measure of internal reliability ranged from .77 to .88 for the four subscales, with the overall scale producing Alpha of .93 (pilot1, $N = 120$) and .88 (pilot2, $N = 29$). In these small samples, PWSAT demonstrated excellent internal consistency for the overall scale, and good internal consistency for the four subscales. An initial assessment of the convergent validity of PWSAT was conducted by correlating subscale scales with global, single-item rating scales for each of the four domains; these four correlations were statistically significant above the 99th confidence level. The PWSAT instrument requires further testing with larger samples drawn randomly from more diverse populations of physicians, as well as more robust tests of validity.

Even when it is more fully tested for reliability and validity, PWSAT is not intended to be diagnostic. Feedback reports were sent to the respondents for personal reflection and discussion of aggregate results in group settings (see example feedback report in Figure 1). The first aim in this emergent research on a broad, four dimensional assessment of physician well-being is to allow physicians opportunities to transcend the technical and organizational limits they constantly face. Perhaps in this way, they might see themselves, and their patients, in a more completely human light. And gaining more balance between technical professional competencies and humanistic perspective and competencies, it can be theorized, might contribute to higher physician satisfaction as well as better outcomes for physicians and patients.

Excelling as a Physician

Above we have reviewed what motivates a person to become a physician and how seeing the physician as a person may add depth and clarity to understanding what it is like to be a physician, including physician satisfaction and well-being. We have given examples of evidence that a more physician-centric and broader conception of satisfaction might improve both the understanding of how physicians navigate the careers within their lives and the quality of the care their patients receive. We then introduced truly emergent work toward a more completely human conception of health and well-being for physicians and perhaps to strengthen their competencies with patients.

Here, we extend this line of thinking to the quality of excellence. For the current purpose, we take excellence as a physician to refer to the characteristics and behaviors of an effective physician, one who produces the best possible outcomes.

Defining physician effectiveness is a challenging task as we are faced with a broad spectrum of methodological strategies and operational definitions of effectiveness evident

R. J. Bogue et al.
Becoming, Being, and Excelling as a Physician

93

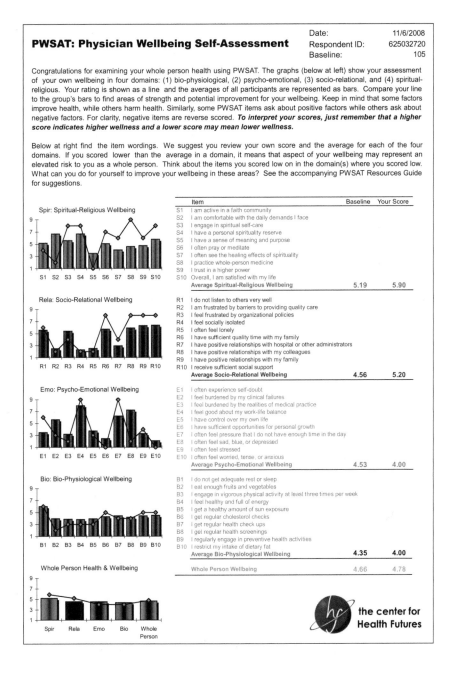

PWSAT: Physician Wellbeing Self-Assessment

Date: 11/6/2008
Respondent ID: 625032720
Baseline: 105

Congratulations for examining your whole person health using PWSAT. The graphs (below at left) show your assessment of your own wellbeing in four domains: (1) bio-physiological, (2) psycho-emotional, (3) socio-relational, and (4) spiritual-religious. Your rating is shown as a line and the averages of all participants are represented as bars. Compare your line to the group's bars to find areas of strength and potential improvement for your wellbeing. Keep in mind that some factors improve health, while others harm health. Similarly, some PWSAT items ask about positive factors while others ask about negative factors. For clarity, negative items are reverse scored. *To interpret your scores, just remember that a higher score indicates higher wellness and a lower score may mean lower wellness.*

Below at right find the item wordings. We suggest you review your own score and the average for each of the four domains. If you scored lower than the average in a domain, it means that aspect of your wellbeing may represent an elevated risk to you as a whole person. Think about the items you scored low on in the domain(s) where you scored low. What can you do for yourself to improve your wellbeing in these areas? See the accompanying PWSAT Resources Guide for suggestions.

Item		Baseline	Your Score
S1	I am active in a faith community		
S2	I am comfortable with the daily demands I face		
S3	I engage in spiritual self-care		
S4	I have a personal spirituality reserve		
S5	I have a sense of meaning and purpose		
S6	I often pray or meditate		
S7	I often see the healing effects of spirituality		
S8	I practice whole-person medicine		
S9	I trust in a higher power		
S10	Overall, I am satisfied with my life		
	Average Spiritual-Religious Wellbeing	5.19	5.90
R1	I do not listen to others very well		
R2	I am frustrated by barriers to providing quality care		
R3	I feel frustrated by organizational policies		
R4	I feel socially isolated		
R5	I often feel lonely		
R6	I have sufficient quality time with my family		
R7	I have positive relationships with hospital or other administrators		
R8	I have positive relationships with my colleagues		
R9	I have positive relationships with my family		
R10	I receive sufficient social support		
	Average Socio-Relational Wellbeing	4.56	5.20
E1	I often experience self-doubt		
E2	I feel burdened by my clinical failures		
E3	I feel burdened by the realities of medical practice		
E4	I feel good about my work-life balance		
E5	I have control over my own life		
E6	I have sufficient opportunities for personal growth		
E7	I often feel pressure that I do not have enough time in the day		
E8	I often feel sad, blue, or depressed		
E9	I often feel stressed		
E10	I often feel worried, tense, or anxious		
	Average Psycho-Emotional Wellbeing	4.53	4.00
B1	I do not get adequate rest or sleep		
B2	I eat enough fruits and vegetables		
B3	I engage in vigorous physical activity at least three times per week		
B4	I feel healthy and full of energy		
B5	I get a healthy amount of sun exposure		
B6	I get regular cholesterol checks		
B7	I get regular health check ups		
B8	I get regular health screenings		
B9	I regularly engage in preventive health activities		
B10	I restrict my intake of dietary fat		
	Average Bio-Physiological Wellbeing	4.35	4.00
	Whole Person Wellbeing	4.66	4.78

the center for Health Futures

Figure 1. Physician well-being self-assessment (PWSAT). © 2011, Adventist Health System/Sunbelt, Inc. d/b/a Florida Hospital. Reproduced with permission.

in the literature (see Chapter 6 by Furnham in this volume for a more complete examination of physician effectiveness). But we have attempted to demonstrate that some portion of the additional excellence available to physicians – whether this results in satisfaction or better well-being – may result from a most obvious, yet perhaps under-appreciated fact: beyond organizational policies, technical competencies, and the tools of medicine, there is a humanistic dimension to being a physician and to producing well-being. And this humanistic dimension may have important contributions to make to excellence.

A model of physician effectiveness may perhaps best be based on two general domains: professionalism and humanism (Cohen, 2007; Conti, 2005; Osler, 2008). According to Cohen, professionalism comprises a set of observable behaviors by which the physician fulfills the medical profession's social contract with society. In order for a physician to fulfill the professionalism obligation to provide cure, effectiveness stems from the rigors that are organized by accreditation competencies, passing qualifying examinations, and being and remaining fully licensed to practice. Humanism comprises a set of internalized personal convictions that motivate the physician to meet the highest standards of professionalism and, beyond this, to provide care beyond cure. Similarly, Osler argues that humanism is at least of equal importance to physician effectiveness as professionalism.

Internationally, medical societies, accrediting agencies and foundations have embraced the critical role of humanism in excellent medical practice. The core principles of three notable exemplars are presented in Table 3. In 2002, the American Board of Internal Medicine, the American College of Physicians Foundation and the European Federation of Internal Medicine jointly developed and endorsed a Physician Charter for Advancing Medical Professionalism to Improve Health Care (ABIM, ACPF, & EFIM, 2002). At present the Physician Charter is endorsed by 102 medical societies, academies, boards and royal colleges from Europe and the Americas. As shown in the first column of Table 3, the Charter includes several components that clearly emphasize humanism to advance medical professionalism and improve health care.

The Arnold P. Gold Foundation promotes humanism in medicine by supporting and recognizing educational and research efforts. The Foundation's principles for Humanism in Medicine are also presented in Table 3. As of 2007, the Accreditation Council for Graduate Medical Education requires all accredited graduate medical education programs to incorporate five common elements into their curricula. ACGME's Common Program Elements, listed in Table 3, also emphasize that to become excellent physicians, medical residents must learn and practice behaviors that express humanistic values.

Just as evidence is emerging that a broader conception of physician satisfaction and well-being might improve the experience of physicians and patients, the evidence is mounting in support of a broader conception of the competencies of medical excellence. To give only several examples, studies on patient preferences support the importance of humanism in medicine. Patients have been found to prefer physicians who show humaneness and support; moreover, patients' first priority is for the physician to respect their autonomy (Shattner, Rudin, & Jellin, 2004). Fung et al. (2005) demonstrated that if patients were forced to choose between technical quality and interpersonal quality in identifying a preferred physician in primary care, most selected the technically proficient

R. J. Bogue et al.
Becoming, Being, and Excelling as a Physician

95

Table 3. Principles supporting excellence in medicine

Advancing medical professionalism to improve health care (the Physician Charter)	Humanism in medicine (I.E., C.A.R.E.S.)	Accreditation Council of Graduate Medical Education (Common Program Requirements)
Professional competence	Integrity: The congruence between expressed values and behavior	Patient care
Honesty with patients	Excellence: Clinical expertise	Practice-based learning and improvement
Patient confidentiality	Compassion: The awareness and acknowledgement of the suffering of another and the desire to relieve it	Interpersonal and communication skills
Maintaining appropriate relations with patients	Altruism: The capacity to put the needs and interests of another before your own	Professionalism
Improving quality of care	Respect: The regard for the autonomy and values of another person	Systems-based practice
Improving access to care	Empathy: The ability to put oneself in another's situation,	
Just distribution of finite resources	Service: The sharing of one's talent, time and resources with those in need; giving beyond what is required	
Scientific knowledge		
Maintaining trust by managing conflicts of interest		
Professional responsibility		

physician; yet, about one-third were willing to sacrifice technical competence and instead would select a physician with interpersonal competencies. Bendapudi, Berry, Fery, Parish, and Rayburn (2006) interviewed patients to determine the behavioral characteristics they most desired in a physician; seven ideal behavioral themes were identified: confident, empathetic, humane, personal, forthright, respectful, and thorough.

In addition to patients' preferences, the evidence that the competencies of humanism are fundamental to medical excellence has become difficult to ignore. Communication competence is one relevant and burgeoning area of research and education in health care.

Within the 21st century, new research and education societies have formed in this area, including the European Association for Communication in Healthcare and the American Academy on Communication in Healthcare. There are good reasons for urgency in this communication component of humanism in medicine. For example, physician communication independently predicted the quality of 2,500 VA patients' diabetes self-management (Heisler, 2002). It is now widely acknowledged that human communication is at the root of medical errors. Woolf, Kuzel, Dovey, and Phillips (2004) found that 63% of medical errors had their root cause in human communication. In the United States, the Joint Commission has identified ineffective communication as the most frequent root cause of sentinel events causing serious harm or death. And as if to pour salt in the wound, Huycke and Huycke (1994) found that over one-half of potential plaintiffs in malpractice lawsuits complained, often in angry terms, of a poor relationship with the provider before the event that occasioned a legal consultation.

Policy positions and training requirements promulgated internationally, patients preferences about physicians, and mounting evidence support qualities of the effective physician that rest upon the twin pillars of professionalism and humanism. The effective physician intentionally operates in a network of technology and relationships. She or he employs those relationships as important tools for diagnosis and treatment as well the embodiment of the personal touch that leads to better information exchange and is sometimes as therapeutic as medical intervention. To be effective, a physician must meet the needs of patients on two basic dimensions, the cure and care of medicine. To build toward excellence on the first dimension, a physician strives to be a flawless technician. To build toward excellence on the latter dimension, a physician strives to be a complete person.

References

ABIM, ACPF, & EFIM: Medical Professionalism Project. (2002). Medical professionalism in the new millenium: A physician's charter. *Annals of Internal Medicine, 136*, 243–246.

Adams, E. H., Dart, R. C., Knisely, J. S., & Schnoll, S. H. (2004). Tramadol abuse and dependence among physicians. *The Journal of the American Medical Association, 292*, 1818–1819.

Arnold, L. (2006). Responding to the professionalism of learners and faculty in orthopaedic surgery. *Clinical Orthopaedics and Related Research, 449*, 205–213.

Arora, V., Dunphy, C., Change, V. Y., Ahmed, F., Humphrey, H. J., & Meltzer, D. (2006). The effects of on-duty napping on intern sleep time and fatigue. *Annals of Internal Medicine, 144*, 792–798.

Baldisseri, M. R. (2007). Impaired healthcare professional. *Critical Care Medicine, 35*, 106–116.

Barger, L. K., Cade, B. E., Ayas, J. T., Cronin, J. W., Rosner, B., Speizer, F. E., & Czeisler, C. A. (2005). Extended work shifts and the risk of motor vehicle crashes among interns. *New England Journal of Medicine, 352*, 125–134.

Barshes, N. R., Vavra, A. K., Miller, A., Brunicardi, F. C., Goss, J. A., & Sweeney, J. F. (2004). General surgery as a career: A contemporary review of factors central to medical student specialty choice. *Journal of the American College of Surgeons, 199*, 792–799.

R. J. Bogue et al.
Becoming, Being, and Excelling as a Physician

97

Beck, A., Scott, J., Williams, P., Robertson, B., Jackson, D., Gade, G., & Cowan, P. (1997). A randomized trial of group outpatient visits for chronically ill older HMO members: The Cooperative Health Care Clinic. *Journal of the American Geriatrics Society, 45*, 643–644.

Bendapudi, N., Berry, L., Fery, K., Parish, J., & Rayburn, W. (2006). Patients' perspectives on ideal physician behaviors. *Mayo Clinic Proceedings, 81*, 338–344.

Berliner, H. (1999). Underperforming doctors. Recovery services. *Health Service Journal, 109*, 28–29.

Bogue, R. J., Guarneri, J. G., Reed, M., Bradley, K., & Hughes, J. (2006). Secrets of physician satisfaction. *Physician Executive*, 30–39.

Brown, R. L., & Schneidman, B. S. (2004). Physicians' health programs – What's happening in the USA? *Medical Journal of Australia, 181*, 390–391.

Buddeberg-Fischer, B., Klaghofer, R., Abel, T., & Buddeberg, C. (2006). Swiss residents' specialty choices: Impact of gender, personality traits, career motivation and life goals. *BMC Health Services Research, 6*, Retrieved from http://www.biomedcentral.com/1472-6963/6/137.

Buddeberg-Fischer, B., Klaghofer, R., Stamm, M., Siegrist, J., & Buddeberg, C. (2008). Work stress and reduced health in young physicians: Prospective evidence from Swiss residents. *International Archives of Occupational and Environmental Health, 82*, 31–38.

Burns, L. R., Andersen, R. M., & Shortell, S. M. (1993). Trends in hospital/physician relations. *Health Affairs, 12*, 213–223.

Cashman, S. B., Parks, C. L., Ash, A., Hemenway, D., & Bicknell, W. J. (1990). Physician satisfaction in a major chain of investor-owned walk-in centers. *Health Care Management Review, 15*, 47–57.

Center, C., Davis, M., Detre, T., Ford, D. E., Hansbrough, W., Hendin, H., . . . Silverman, M. M. (2003). Confronting depression and suicide in physicians: A consensus statement. *The Journal of the American Medical Association, 289*, 3161–3166.

Charon, R. (2001). Narrative medicine: A model for empathy, reflection, profession, and trust. *JAMA: The Journal of the American Medical Association, 286*, 1897–1902.

Chan, A. O. M., & Huak, C. Y. (2004). Influence of work environment on emotional health in a health care setting. *Occupational Medicine, 54*, 207–212.

Christakis, N. A., & Iwashyna, T. J. (1998). Attitude and self-reported practice regarding prognostication in a national sample of internists. *Archives of Internal Medicine, 158*, 2389–2395.

Cohen, J. (2007). Linking professionalism to humanism: What it means, why it matters. *Academic Medicine, 82*, 1029–1032.

Conti, R. (2005). What makes a good doctor? *Clinical Cardiology, 28*, 496–498.

Curlin, F. A., Chin, M. H., Sellergren, S. A., Roach, C. J., & Lantos, J. D. (2006). The association of physicians' religious characteristics with their attitudes and self-reported behaviors regarding religion and spirituality in the clinical encounter. *Medical Care, 44*, 446–453.

Curlin, F. A., Roach, C. J., Gorawara-Bhat, R., Lantos, J. D., & Chin, M. H. (2005). How are religion and spirituality related to health? A study of physicians' perspectives. *Southern Medical Journal, 98*, 761–766.

Deckardi, G., Meterko, M., & Field, D. (1994). Physician burnout: An examination of personal, professional, and organizational relationships. *Medical Care, 32*, 745–754.

Dehlendorf, C. D., & Wolfe, S. M. (1998). Physicians disciplined for sex-related offenses. *The Journal of the American Medical Association, 279*, 1883–1888.

Deloney, L. A., Graham, C. J., & Erwin, D. O. (2000). Presenting cultural diversity and spirituality to first-year medical students. *Academic Medicine, 75*, 513–514.

Demmy, T. L., Kivlahan, C., Stone, T. T., Teague, L., & Sapienza, P. (2002). Physicians' perceptions of institutional and leadership factors influencing their job satisfaction at one academic medical center. *Academic Medicine, 77*, 1235–1240.

DiMatteo, M. R., Sherbourne, C. D., Hays, R. D., Ordway, L., Kravitz, R., McGlynn, E. A., . . . Rogers, W. H. (1993). Physicians' characteristics influence patients' adherence to medical treatment: Results from the medical outcomes study. *Health Psychology, 12*, 93–102.

Direct Opinions. (2010). Physician Satisfaction Survey: Telephone and Online Research [online]: Retrieved November 14, 2010, from http://www.directopinions.com/physician-satisfaction-survey.html.

Domino, K. B., Hornbein, T. F., Polissar, N. L., Genner, G., Johnson, J., Alberti, S., & Hankes, L. (2005). Risk factors for relapse in health care professional with substance use disorders. *JAMA: The Journal of the American Medical Association, 293*, 1453–1460.

Dorevitch, S., & Forst, L. (2000). The occupational hazards of emergency physicians. *American Journal of Emergency Medicine, 18*, 300–311.

Ehman, J. W., Ott, B. B., Short, T. H., Ciampa, R. C., & Hansen-Flaschen, J. (1999). Do patients want their physicians to inquire about their spiritual or religious beliefs if they become gravely ill? *Archives of Internal Medicine, 159*, 1803–1806.

Fisak, B., Bogue, R. J., & Paolini, H. (2007). Explaining physician stress: Is it work or is it life that harms the doctor? Center for Health Futures Working Paper. Available from the first author by writing to <b.fisak@unf.edu>.

Fortin, A., & Barnett, K. G. (2004). Medical school curricula in spirituality and medicine. (Reprinted from American Medical Association). *JAMA: The Journal of the American Medical Association, 291*, 2883.

Frank, E. (2004). Physician health and patient care. *JAMA: The Journal of the American Medical Association, 29*, 637.

Frank, E., & Dingle, A. D. (1999). Self-reported depression and suicide attempts among US women physicians. American *Journal of Psychiatry, 156*, 1887–1894.

Fromme, E. K., Hebert, R. S., & Carrese, J. A. (2004). Self-doctoring: A qualitative study of physicians with cancer. *Journal of Family Practice, 53*, 299–306.

Fung, C., Elliott, M., Hays, R., Kahn, K., Kanouse, D., McGlynn, E., . . . Shekelle, P. (2005). Patients' preference for technical versus interpersonal quality when selected a primary care physician. *Health Services Research, 40*, 957–977.

Gallup. (2010). Physician Engagement [online] (Updated November 13, 2010) Retrieved November 14, 2010, from http://www.gallup.com/consulting/healthcare/15385/Physician-Engagement.aspx.

Goodman, L. J. (1975). The longevity and mortality of American physicians, 1969–1973. *Milbank Memorial Fund Quarterly – Health & Society, 53*, 353–375.

Graske, J. (2003). Improving the mental health of doctors. *British Medical Journal, 327*, s188.

Hadley, J., Mitchell, J. M., Sulmasy, D. P., & Bloche, M. G. (1999). Perceived financial incentives, HMO market penetration & physicians' practice styles and satisfaction. *Health Services Research, 34*, 307–321.

Harms, B. A., Heise, C. P., Gould, J. C., & Starline, J. R. (2005). 25-year single institution analysis of health, practice, and fate of general surgeons. *Annals of Surgery, 242*, 520–529.

HealthStream Research. (2010). Physician Insights: Satisfaction Research [online]. Retrieved November 14, 2010, from http://www.healthstreamresearch.com/Products/research/Pages/physician.aspx.

Heisler, M., Bouknight, R. R., Hayward, R. A., Smith, D. M., & Kerr, E. A. (2002). The relative importance of physician communication, participatory decision making, and patient understanding in diabetes self-management. *Journal of General Internal Medicine, 17*, 243–252.

Hollis, R. (1994). Caring: A privilege and our responsibility. *Obstetrics & Gynecology, 83*, 1–4.

Hueston, W. J. (1998). Family physicians' satisfaction with practice. *Archives of Family Medicine, 7*, 242–247.

Huycke, L. I., & Huycke, M. M. (1994). Characteristics of potential plaintiffs in malpractice litigation. *Annals of Internal Medicine, 120*, 792–798.

R. J. Bogue et al.
Becoming, Being, and Excelling as a Physician

99

Jackson, V. A., Sullivan, A. M., Gadmer, N. M., Seltzer, D., Mitchell, A. M., Lakoma, M. D., . . . Block, S. D. (2005). "It was haunting . . .": Physicians' descriptions of emotionally powerful patient deaths. *Academic Medicine, 80*(7), 648–656.

Kassler, W. J., Wartman, S. A., & Silliman, R. A. (1991). Why medical students choose primary care careers. *Academic Medicine, 66,* 41–43.

Kay, M. P., Mitchell, G. K., & Del Mar, C. B. (2004). Doctors do not adequately look after their own physical health. *Medical Journal of Australia, 181,* 368–370.

King, D. E., Blue, A., Mallin, R., & Thiedke, C. (2004). Implementation and assessment of a spiritual history taking curriculum in the first year of medical school. *Teach Learn Medicine, 16,* 64–68.

Kirkcaldy, B. D., Athanasou, J., & Trimpop, R. (2000). The idiosyncratic construction of stress: Examples from medical work settings. *Stress Medicine, 16,* 315–326.

Kirkcaldy, B. D., Trimpop, R., & Cooper, C. L. (1997). Working hours, job stress, work satisfaction and accident rates among medical practitioners, consultants and allied personnel. *International Journal of Stress Management, 4,* 79–87.

Koenig, H. G. (2001). Spiritual assessment in medical practice. *American Family Physician, 63,* 30.

Koenig, H. G. (2004). Taking a spiritual history. *The Journal of the American Medical Association, 291,* 2881.

Konrad, T. R., Williams, E. S., Linzer, M., McMurray, J., Pathman, D. E., Gerrity, M., . . . Douglas, J. (1999). Measuring physician job satisfaction in a changing workplace and a challenging environment. *Medical Care, 37,* 1174–1182.

Landon, B. E., Aseltine, R., Shaul, J. A., Miller, Y., Auerbach, B. A., & Cleary, P. D. (2002). Evolving dissatisfaction among primary care physicians. *American Journal of Managed Care, 8,* 890–901.

Landon, B. E., Reschovsky, J., & Blumenthal, D. (2003). Changes in career satisfaction among primary care & specialists physicians, 1997–2001. *The Journal of the American Medical Association, 289,* 442–449.

Leigh, J. P., Kravitz, R. L., Schembri, M., Samuels, S. J., & Mobley, S. (2002). Physician career satisfaction across specialties. *Archives of Internal Medicine, 162,* 1577–1584.

Levinson, W., & Roter, D. (1995). Physicians' psychosocial beliefs correlate with their patient communication skills. *Journal of General Internal Medicine, 10,* 375–379.

Lo, B., Ruson, D., Kates, L. W., Arnold, R. M., Cohen, C. B., Faber-Langendoen, K., . . . Tulsky, J. A. (2002). Discussing religious and spiritual issues at the end of life: A practical guide for physicians. *JAMA: The Journal of the American Medical Association, 287,* 749–754.

Maitre, A., Colonna, M., Gressin, C., Menegoz, F., & de Guademaris, R. (2003). Increased incidence of haematological cancer among physicians in a university hospital. *International Archives of Occupational & Environmental Health, 76,* 24–28.

McCord, C., Gilchrist, V. J., Grossman, S. D., King, B. D., McCormick, K. F., Oprandi, A. M., . . . Srivastava, M. (2004). Discussing spirituality with patients: A rational and ethical approach. *Annals of Family Medicine, 2,* 356–361.

McManus, I. C., Livingston, G., & Katona, C. (2006). The attractions of medicine: The generic motivations of medical school applicants in relation to demography, personality and achievement. *BMC Medical Education, 6,* 1–15.

McMurray, J. E., Williams, E., Schwartz, M. D., Douglas, J., Van Kirk, J., Konrad, R., . . . Linzer, M. (1997). Physician job satisfaction: Developing a model using qualitative data. *Journal of General Internal Medicine, 12,* 711–714.

Meier, D. E., Back, A. L., & Morrison, R. S. (2001). The inner life of physicians and care of the seriously ill. *JAMA: The Journal of the American Medical Association, 286,* 3007–3014.

Murphy, K. A., Yeazel, M., & Center, B. A. (2000). Validity of residents' self-reported cardiovascular disease prevention activities: The Preventative Medicine Attitudes and Activities Questionnaire. *Preventative Medicine, 31,* 241–248.

Murray, A., Montgomery, J. E., Chang, H., Rogers, W. H., Inui, T., & Safran, D. G. (2001). Doctor discontent: A comparison of physician satisfaction in different delivery system settings, 1986 and 1997. *Journal of General Internal Medicine, 16*, 451–459.

Musick, D. W., Cheever, T. R., Quinlivan, S., & Nora, L. M. (2003). Spirituality in medicine: A comparison of medical students' attitudes and clinical performance. *Academic Psychiatry, 27*, 67–73.

Osler, W. (1909). *The principles and practice of medicine.* New York: D Appleton & Co.

Piper, L. E. (2005). Adressing the phenomenon of disruptive physician behaviour. *The Health Care Manager, 22(4),* 335–339..

Post, S. G., Pulchaski, C. M., & Larson, D. B. (2000). Physicians and patient spirituality: Professional boundaries, competency, and ethics. *Annals of Internal Medicine, 132*, 578–583.

Puchalski, C. M., & Larson, D. B. (1998). Developing curricula in spirituality and medicine. *Academic Medicine, 73*, 970–974.

Ratanawongsa, N., Bolen, S., Howell, E. E., Kern, D. E., Sisson, S. D., & Larriviere, D. (2006). Residents' perceptions of professionalism in training and practice: Barriers, promoters, and duty hour requirements. *Journal of General Internal Medicine, 21*, 758–763.

Reilly, J. M., & Ring, J. M. (2005). Healing and hopefulness: A tool for doctor well-being. *Medical Education, 39*, 1158–1159.

Richardson, H. C., & Redfern, N. (2000). Why do women reject surgical careers? *Annals of the Royal College of Surgeons of England, 89*, 290–293.

Scheurer, D., McKean S., Miller J., & Wetterneck, T. (2009). U.S. physician satisfaction: A systematic review. *Journal of Hospital Medicine 4*, 560–568.

Schulz, R., Scheckler, W. E., Moberg, D. P., & Johnson, P. R. (1997). Changing nature of physician satisfaction with HMO and fee-for-service practices. *Journal of Family Practice, 45*, 321–330.

Shanafelt, T. D., Sloan, J. A., & Habermann, T. M. (2003). The well-being of physicians. *American Journal of Medicine, 114*, 513–519.

Shattner, A., Rudin, D., & Jellin, N. (2004). Good physicians from the perspective of their patients. *BMC Health Services Research, 4*, 26.

Shearer, S., & Toedt, M. (2001). Family physicians' observations of their practice, well being, and health care in the United States. *Journal of Family Practice, 50*, 751–756.

Stanton, J., & Caanwent, W. (2003). How many doctors are sick? *British Medical Journal Career Focus, 326*, S97a–103.

Stoddard, J. J., Hargraves, J. L., Reed, M., & Vratil, A. (2001). Managed care, professional autonomy, and income: Effects on physician career satisfaction. *Journal of General Internal Medicine, 16*, 675–684.

Stuyt, E. B. (1998). Doctors who smoke: Can physician tobacco use constitute impairment? *Texas Medicine, 94*, 14.

Sulmasy, D. P. (2007). *Rebirth of the clinic: An introduction to spirituality in health care.* Washington, DC: Georgetown University Press.

Thistlethwaite, J. E., Ajjawi, R., & Aslani, P. (2008). The decision to prescribe: Influences and choice. *Oxford Journals Medicine InnovAiT, 3*, 237–243.

Torre, D. M., Wang, N. Y., Meoni, L. A., Young, J. H., Klag, M. J., & Ford, D. E. (2005). Suicide compared to other causes of mortality in physicians. *Suicide & Life-Threatening Behavior, 35*, 146–153.

Ullmann, D., Phyllips, R. L., Beeson, W. L., Dewey, H. G., Brin, B. N., Kusma, J. W., . . . Hirst, A. E. (1991). Cause-specific mortality among physicians with differing life-styles. *The Journal of the American Medical Association, 265*, 2352–2359.

Vaglum, P., Wiers-Jensen, J., & Ekeberg, Ø. (1999). Motivation for medical school: The relationship to gender and specialty preferences in a nation-wide sample. *Medical Education, 33*, 236–242.

Wetterneck, T. B., Linzer, M., McMurray, J. E., Douglas, J., Schwartz, M. D., Bigby, J., . . . Rhodes, E. (2002). Worklife and satisfaction of general internists. *Archives of Internal Medicine, 162,* 649–656.

Williams, E. S., Konrad, T. R., Linzer, M., McMurray, J., Pathman, D. E., Gerrity, M., . . . Douglas, J. (2002). Physician, practice, and patient characteristics related to primary care physician physical and mental health: Results from the physician worklife study. *Health Services Research, 37,* 121–143.

Woolf, S. H., Kuzel, A. J., Dovey, S. M., & Phillips, R. L. (2004). A string of mistakes: The importance of cascade analysis in describing, counting, and preventing medical errors. *Annals of Family Medicine, 2,* 317–326.

Wright, S. M., & Beasley, B. W. (2004). Motivating factors for academic physicians within departments of medicine. *Mayo Clinic Proceedings, 79,* 1145–1150.

Zuger, A. (2004). Dissatisfaction with medical practice. *New England Journal of Medicine, 350,* 69–75.

Stress and Its Impact on Psychosocial Well-Being Among Medical Professionals

Bruce D. Kirkcaldy,[1] Rüdiger Trimpop,[2] and Terry Martin[1]

[1]International Centre for the Study of Occupational and Mental Health, Düsseldorf, Germany and Den Haag, The Netherlands
[2]Department of Work and Organisational Psychology, Friedich Schiller Universität, Jena, Germany

The Changing Face of Medicine

There can be little argument that the scope of developments and changes surrounding traditional and nontraditional medical professions have been momentous. Waves of statutory, legislative, and technological innovations have produced wide-ranging reforms and resulted in new ways that medicine is practiced and delivered, with implications for the design and composition of the workforce. In recent times, particularly in many European countries such as Germany, these changes have sometimes been accompanied by a decline in the number of candidates entering medicine, and in some cases, an increase in the number of medical students who fail to complete their training. Once considered the ultimate ticket to success, commonly associated with a high status, professional kudos, and considerable social prestige, traditional high profile medical careers have been competing with computer science, information technology, and electrical engineering, where university graduates can earn substantial financial rewards from the onset. Today, medical organizations, like legal and accounting firms, must recruit fiercely and offer better compensation to retain talent. Certainly the issue of money, including the costs involved in getting trained as doctor, for example, may exert an influence in some cases. Indeed, the educational debt of the physician-in-training is steadily increasing, and seemingly does not affect specialty choice. As the cost of medical education continues to rise, the applicant pool has begun to shrink, thereby possibly affecting both the quantity and quality of future physicians.

The increase in the number of "drop outs" from medical schools has been of sufficient concern to warrant considerable investigation of other reasons for dropping out of medical school. For example, some discover that it is much more demanding than their undergraduate pre-med programs. Others find that family or other relationships conflict strongly with the academic workload of medical school. Some students opt to enter the workforce earlier, to pursue a different career in health care. In some cases students simply conclude that practicing medicine is not their "passion" and elect to pursue a career in another environment (Bogue et al.'s chapter in this book for more details of motivational aspects of medical careers). One German study by Kaiser, Kohler, Popovic, and Stilwe (2005) compared students who completed their medical studies with those who did not. The authors established that the principal reasons cited by the students who had failed to complete their training were adverse working conditions, together with a dissatisfaction with their working hours.

In another German study, this time looking at the attitudes of experienced physicians, Gefken (2008) found that although 73% claimed it was a desirable career – with the medical profession offering a high degree of autonomy and latitude for decision making – yet nearly three quarters of the respondents still stated that they would reconsider entering the profession. To add to these somewhat contradictory findings, the physicians also reported elevated levels of stress and admitted having limited time for their patients.

In its 2006 report, the World Health Organization (WHO) estimated that whilst there are nearly 59.2 million full-time paid health workers worldwide, there was a critical shortage of healthcare providers equivalent to a global deficit approaching 4.3 million health workers.

In spite of concerns surrounding the worldwide shortages, the number of women entering medical school and practicing medicine has grown steadily over recent decades. This is commonly borne out in statistics, which prove that what was once a male-dominated sphere has been transformed. Irrefutable evidence shows that women are increasingly gravitating towards medicine as a career. Indeed, women were not even admitted to London Medical Schools (except the "Royal Free Hospital") until 1947. The proportion of female medical students in the UK increased steadily from 20% to 25% in 1968 to above 50% by 1991. By 2002, 60.8% of students accepted to British medical or dental schools were women (Royal College of Physicians, 2006). In Germany, the proportion of female medical students rose from 46% to 59% between 1994 and 2004, and by 2006 56% of newly registered physicians were women (Forum Gesundheitspolitik, 2009). By 2003–2004, the number of applicants to US medical schools was higher for women (50.8%) than for men (American Medical Association [AMA], 2004). Female physicians were once a rarity early in the 20th century, yet by 1980, their proportionate representation was 17% for the USA, 19% for Germany, 20% France, and 32% (medical doctors and dentists) in Israel (Compton Interactive Encyclopaedia, 1995). One issue which was recently highlighted in a German study by Köhler, Napp, and Kaiser (2003) has been that in terms of specialist medicine women have tended to show a preference towards specialties of child and adolescent psychiatry, pediatrics, psychosomatics, skin, and sexual disorders, psychiatric and gynecology, whereas they are underrepresented in surgery and urology.

Stress – Magnitude of the Problem

Individuals and groups employed within and across the healthcare sectors have long been considered to be prone to stress in addition to occupational health risks (Agius, Blenkin,

B. D. Kirkcaldy et al.
Stress and Its Impact on Psychosocial Well-Being Among Medical Professionals

105

Deary, Zeally, & Wood, 1996). Not surprisingly there exists a voluminous literature surrounding the causes, effects, and consequences of stress within these professions. This has included a considerable and diverse investigation of stress research in professions and subprofessions within and across the broad healthcare sphere (BMJ, 2008). Some of the most prominent research has primarily focused on doctors, either in General Practice (GP) or based in hospital settings. Previous studies have frequently, if not invariably, uncovered a higher level of stress among doctors when compared to the general population. Firth-Cozens (2003) observed that the proportion of doctors demonstrating higher levels of stress was roughly 28% compared to around 18% in the general working population. The consequences of stress among doctors have also been associated with an increased rate of psychological morbidity, for example, depression, anxiety, and substance abuse (Wong, 2008).

Consequences

Emotional and Psychological Distress

In a correspondence in the British Medical Journal, Symons and Persuade (1995) agreed that doctors are frequently exposed to "sheer misery." They argue, however, that there had also been a tendency for researchers to focus on external factors (e.g., working hours, work conditions, etc.) and neglect the less comfortable questions relating to "stress among colleagues" or "gravitation of specific personality types" towards the health profession which may make them more vulnerable to stress. To compound the risk factors, many doctors like to perceive themselves as *invincible*. Thus, A'Brook (1990) noted the reluctance of doctors to disclose personal problems such as psychotic or depressive illnesses and the development of chemical dependencies. Nevertheless, in response to direct questioning, Fuchs (2008) noted that 39% of female doctors admitted to experiencing depression, compared with 30% of other females who had earned doctoral degrees. Psychiatric conditions common among physicians include major depression, ethanol and drug abuse, bipolar disorder, anxiety disorder, and various other personality disorders (Fung, 2007).

Irrespective of the causal or predictive determinants, the potentially damaging effects of chronic stress on health is substantially and widely verified by health statistics. For example, in their middle years, (female) nurses had a shorter life expectancy than other female-dominated occupations such as social workers, secretaries, and teachers (Elliott & Eisdorfer, 1982). Likewise, British physicians had an increased risk of dying from suicide, hepatic cirrhosis, accidental poisoning, and accidents in general (Registrar General, 1978). Various other authors have noted high levels of psychiatric illness among (male) doctors (Murray, 1977), borderline depression or depressive bouts (Caplan, 1994), sustained emotional distress among junior doctors (Cartwright, 1987), elevated job-related anxiety and depression (Belfer, 1989; Rucinski & Cybulska, 1985), up to seven times greater alcohol dependence for doctors than for control groups of similar social class

(Bissel, 1976; Brooke, Edwards, & Taylor, 1991), and a high proportion of physicians who smoked and drank to excess (Allibone, Oakes, & Shannon, 1981).

Job Burnout

Frequently, individuals and groups employed within the popularly defined helping/caring professions are supposedly prone to the negative effects of occupational stress, including an increased susceptibility to "burnout" (Felton, 1998). McCranie and Brandsma (1988) perceived burnout to be a "state of physical, emotional and mental exhaustion that occurs as a result of intense involvement over long periods of time in situations that are emotionally demanding. It is commonly characterized in its extreme form by physical depletion and chronic fatigue, feelings of helplessness and hopelessness, and the development of negative attitudes toward self, work, life and other people" (p. 30). Its frequent occurrence among health professions is anecdotally yet widely believed to result from a confrontation with the emotional aspects of human suffering. Others have argued (Costantini, Solano, Di Napoli, & Bosco, 1997) that "some areas of medicine, such as oncology and AIDS care, expose members of staff to higher work-related stress. The need to deal with dying and death, the feeling of helplessness, linked with the limits of medicine in these pathologies, the length of the disease, the need to maintain an empathic reaction with patients suffering or dying, the risk that empathy might lead to identification, are potentially stressful situations for caregivers" (p. 79).

Rinpoche and Shlim (2006) asserted that "doctors ... need to distance themselves from the pain, loneliness, and fear that many patients are suffering. If they identify too closely with their patients, they run the risk of emotional exhaustion. Emotional exhaustion can interfere with their ability to make clear decisions, so they try to maintain an objective distance, a distance that the patient interprets as not caring enough ... the only way they feel they can care more for patients is by not caring too much" (Rinpoche & Shlim, 2006, p. 4).

Too often, emotional involvement with the problems of their patients takes its toll on the health of physicians. Although they may enjoy better physical health than the general population, they have poorer psychological health, as shown by a high incidence of psychiatric disorders, drug and alcohol use, and suicide (Guthrie & Black, 1997). Schattner and Colman (1998) found that at any one time 13% of physicians were experiencing a severe psychiatric disturbance. The reported underlying stressors included threats of litigation, work overload, insufficient earnings, interactions with difficult patients, and administrative/paperwork demands.

Self-Destructive Behavior and Suicide

In keeping with commonly held perceptions, a high workload accompanied by corresponding levels of work-related stress is known to increase the risk of alcohol and drug

B. D. Kirkcaldy et al.
Stress and Its Impact on Psychosocial Well-Being Among Medical Professionals

107

abuse. Moreover, these factors can also cause problems in social relationships, serve to promote depression and anxiety, and even lead to suicide among doctors and associated healthcare professionals. Indeed, a report by the American Foundation for Suicide Prevention in 2004 (see Hampton, 2005) claimed that, on average, death by suicide was about 70% more likely among male physicians than among other professionals and 250–400% higher among female doctors. These increased risks of suicide seem logical if, as in other professions which demand long hours and considerable responsibility, there are significant potential rewards but also greater risks of experiencing burnout. The inherent pressures of stress and isolation increase the likelihood of the onset of depression, which may ultimately drive some people to take their own lives. Similar to the case of farmers, who often lead isolated lives and have access to guns, medical professionals (including doctors, nurses, pharmacists, therapists, and ward orderlies) have traditionally had high suicide rates and ready access to drugs.

Too frequently, psychiatric disturbances are sufficiently severe to precipitate suicide. Lindeman and co-workers (1996) compared the suicide rates of British physicians with those of the general population; figures were 1.1–3.4 times higher for male and 2.5–5.7 times higher for female doctors. Risks relative to other professionals were also 1.5–3.8 higher for male and 3.7–4.5 higher for female physicians. Likewise, suicide rates for physicians in the US were higher than in all other professional groups (males 70%, females 40% higher than the general population). Shernhammer and Colditz (2004) reviewed 25 US studies; suicide rates relative to the general population were 40% higher for males and 130% higher for females, although these authors cautioned that there was a possible publication bias.

A variety of mortality figures for doctors consistently suggest that they are at a higher risk of dying from such stress-related illnesses as suicide, cirrhosis, accidental poisoning, and accident in general (Registrar General, 1978). Moreover, suicide and suicide-related deaths are much higher again among nurses as well as physicians (Hawton & Vislisel, 1999). Others have reported higher levels of psychiatric illness among (male) doctors (Murray, 1977), borderline or depressive bouts (Caplan, 1994), sustained emotional distress among junior doctors (Cartwright, 1987), elevated job-related anxiety and depression (Belfer, 1989; Rucinski & Cybulska, 1985), and greater alcohol dependence (up to seven times more for doctors than controlled groups of similar social class) (Bissel, 1976; Brooke, Edwards, & Taylor, 1991). Allibone et al. (1981) found that a high proportion of medical doctors drink and smoke excessively. Health care is likely to entail risks, and these will differ to some extent dependent on the discipline or field of speciality, for example, common critical incidents in anesthesia (see Ennis & Vincent, 1990).

Sources of Stress and Perceived External Control

Conversely, it has been asserted that negative health frequently uncovered among healthcare providers and practitioners results more from organizational factors and working conditions. In other words, stress originates from strenuous workload, continuous time pressures, and difficulties associated with practice administration, "impairing" leisure and free-time and may cause spill-over problems in home and family life (Sutherland & Cooper, 1992).

In a Canadian study, Richardsen and Burke (1991) commented that "work pressures inherent in medical practise, together with disruptive events on the job may be stressful. Physicians are increasingly exposed to actual or threats of malpractice suits, and this is becoming an important job stressor that seems to have some relationship to job satisfaction .... After a malpractice suit, many physicians report feeling depressed and frustrated, they are less satisfied with their practise and start considering early retirement from the profession." They further add: "Doctors are often frustrated over loss of autonomy with stricter Medicare regulations, disillusioned over challenges to their competence by both professional boards and patients, and increasingly threatened with malpractice suits. Also, with patients becoming more knowledgeable consumers, informing themselves about medical problems, and asking second opinions, the need for physicians to keep up their own level of medical knowledge is increasing" (p. 1179).

Sutherland and Cooper (1993) examined predictors of mental ill-health and job dissatisfaction among a representative sample of almost one thousand British general practitioners. Three major stressors were identified: demands of the job and patients' expectations (e.g., fear of assault, adverse publicity by the media, and patients' complaints), role-related demands (e.g., conflicts between their task and role demands, role ambiguity, and implication of mistakes), and organizational climate/structure (the need for mundane administrative work, inadequate resources, low morale, staff shortages, lack of consultation, and communication). The extent of social support was a major determinant of job satisfaction. The authors suggested meeting these issues through a combination of individually focused interventions such as time management and assertiveness training, cognitive restructuring, and opportunities for physical activity or relaxation, plus organizationally oriented methods (see Sibbald, Enzer, Cooper, Rout, & Sutherland, 2000).

In a large-scale study of Dutch healthcare specialists, recorded levels of stress and job satisfaction bore more relation to the perception of working conditions than to either personal or organizational factors (Visser, Smets, Oort, & de Haes, 2003). More specifically, negative consequences of time pressures were important determining factors. Both the extent to which work was perceived to intrude into private life, and also the extent to which workload made one feel unable to work according to one's standards, contributed to the stressfulness of the job. The authors added that when stress was high and satisfaction was low, the risk for emotional exhaustion – the central aspect of burnout – increased considerably. Highlighting the effect that wider changes in society impacted on job stress, the authors uncovered specific stressors among the healthcare specialists including restriction of professional autonomy, job insecurity owing to mergers, and a fear of lawsuits.

Occupational Role: Generalists, Specialists, and Nurses

Given the variety of occupations and roles encompassed within and across the broad spectrum of the medical professions, researchers and authors have not been short on target

B. D. Kirkcaldy et al.
Stress and Its Impact on Psychosocial Well-Being Among Medical Professionals

109

groups to focus on. This has also encouraged a considerable number of comparative studies. A popular theme among researchers looking at issues relating to stress and well-being among medical professionals has been to examine differences between General Practitioners and those working in more specialist areas of medical practice. One study by Cooper, Rout, and Faragher (1989) found that among general practitioners, contrary to popular opinion, dealing with terminally ill patients was *not* a source of occupational stress, nor was the issue of technical skills. Their findings reported that job-related stress originated primarily through excessive job demands, practice administration and patients' expectations. It is worth considering that General Practitioners are perhaps less exposed to many of the more directly demanding situations than those in Specialist or Consultant roles. For example, terminal diagnoses are commonly communicated to patients by a specialist rather than a GP. Similarly, GPs may also have less input or direct involvement in palliative care.

In research specifically examining GP registrars, Chambers, Wall, and Campbell (1996) reported that the most potent sources of stress were family-job conflicts, patients' unrealistic expectations, disruption to social life, and working for the Membership of the Royal College of GPs (specifically in relation to addressing a highly demanding syllabus and a requirement to complete projects). These GP registrars were habitually imposed with additional burdens compared to established doctors, such as examination pressures, requirements of learning, conducting unfamiliar novel tasks in general practice, and stressors related to work on young family life.

The Canadian Health Care System experienced significant changes during the 1990s as provincial governments restructured, redesigned, and downsized to reduce costs and mitigate the effects of reduced funds from the federal government, with nurses having experienced the most turmoil, stress, and strain. More nurses lost their jobs than those in other categories of healthcare workers, or they were restructured. Work loads and complexity have increased significantly. Moreover, there was significantly more "casualization" of jobs and greater job insecurity among this professional group than others (O'Brien Pallas & Baumann, 1998). Sullivan, Kerr, and Ibrahim (1999) present a descriptive overview of job stress in healthcare workers using data from the first wave of the National Population Health Survey. Three occupational groupings were used: Group I (physicians, surgeons, dentists, veterinarians, pharmacists, dieticians, and nutritionists), Group II (registered nurses, nursing supervisors, physiotherapists, chiropractors, and medical laboratory technicians), and Group III (registered nursing assistants, orderlies, dental hygienists, and nursing attendants). Several variables were studied including psychological demands, decision latitude, job strain, social support and job satisfaction, job insecurity, physical exertion and daily activity, together with injury and back problems. Psychological demands included questions about hectic work and conflicting demands on the job. Decision latitude included learning new tasks, requirements for higher level skills related to job demands, freedom to decide how to do the job, nonrepetitive work, and the degree of latitude about what happens on the job. Higher levels of job stress were found in Groups II and III. Group II demonstrated the highest stress levels especially related to psychological demands, social support and job insecurity. Comparing this Group II with a group of similar status outside of health care, the registered nurse group demonstrated significantly higher levels of stress. Stressors differentiating health care Group II from their peers outside of health care included higher psychological demands of work, lower levels of decision authority, higher physical demand, heavier work, and lower levels of job satisfaction (Ontario Minstry of Health, 1999; Sullivan et al., 1999).

Job Stress and Work Satisfaction

The various components that contribute to comprehensive medical care all have an impact on a physician's job satisfaction. Kirkcaldy and Pope (1992) applied structural analysis to identify perceptions of "self" and "other" within a multidisciplinary medical hospital team. Physicians perceived themselves as separate from the psychological and therapeutic staff and patients' dependents. The patient was seen as falling within the network of the doctor's daily medical programs and, although the psychological requirements of the patients were acknowledged, the physician applied "emotional distancing" as a way of coping with his or her task. Meanwhile, the patients perceived the physician as more than a bodily healer, and expected a high level of personal care, psychological support, and offers of well-being. Ray and Baum (1985) had previously observed that doctors are frequently questioned on social, psychological, and ethical topics outside their domains of formal professional competency. Generally, physicians rely on their authority, without which it would be difficult to convince the patient to accept uncomfortable, distressing, painful, and possibly incomprehensible treatment. The invested authority may help the patient, too, bringing relief from a difficult decision-making process.

Pillay (2008) found perhaps unexpectedly that South African general practitioners were satisfied with the social and personal aspects of their work, but were likely to express dissatisfaction with the practice environment. Tension was experienced in complying with frequent patient requests and expectations such as the provision of medical reports, and absenteeism notes, and/or inappropriate demands for medication or surgery. Significant predictors of low work satisfaction included being female, working in large groups, more than 20 years of practice, treating a high proportion of insured patients and dealing with "incentives" designed to preserve healthcare resources. The greatest satisfaction was observed among those enjoying clinical freedom or with favorable perceptions of "managed" care, those remunerated on a fee-for-service basis and those working in small professional groups. The majority of Greek interns perceived their work as extremely stressful, and many reported a high degree of job dissatisfaction (Antoniou, Cooper, & Davidson, 2008). Working hours of the interns were long and conditions were difficult during night shifts. Hospitals commonly lacked air-conditioning and staff rest quarters were noisy. Opportunities for social interaction were limited, and superiors provided little support or sympathy. Male doctors were also irritated by frequent patient complaints about their treatment and the quality of their hospital stay. Finally, adverse media publicity was compounded by a fear of making mistakes, and there was overall dissatisfaction with the moral and economic aspects of their work.

Some have argued that there is a need and an opportunity to learn by focussing on areas of dissatisfaction in a physician's practice. Peterkin (2009) listed 10 major stressors for Canadian doctors: excessive workloads: frequent night calls; insufficient sleep (less than 3 hr some nights); uncompromising consultants; too much routine, tedious work, and record-keeping; high death rates among patients; scarce contact with fellow colleagues; inadequate sexual activity, and high peer competition/rivalry. Bogue and colleagues (2006) identified as causes of dissatisfaction efforts at cost containment; a limited quantity and quality of personal time; insufficient opportunities for research and teaching; utilization reviews (by hospitals); lack of autonomy; an inadequate income level; administrative responsibilities; a poor organizational climate; and an excessive workload. They also listed sources of job satisfaction: positive relationships with patients and colleagues; a successful resolution of family issues; opportunities for personal growth; freedom to provide quality care; availability of office and hospital resources, and the prestige of being a physician. They suggested that happiness among doctors focussed on their interactions with people, whether in their own families, in their organization or practice, and in providing "intelligent" care for their patients. Interviews with physicians who expressed the highest levels of satisfaction led to the recommendation of several interventions: design of a "healthy" work environment (allowing personal choice in practice structure and organization); exercising the body, enhancing diet and allowing adequate recuperation from potential stressors; promoting creative expression of the art of medicine; engagement with patients (improvement of personal listening skills, understanding and empowerment of patients); opportunities for travel (including cultural comparisons to assess the advantages of one's own medical care service); ensuring a clear demarcation between work and leisure/family time; and regulating emotional stress (identifying potential triggers and somatic cues).

The importance and relevance of support from management and colleagues, together with an availability and access to resources has been cited by researchers examining job satisfaction in the health professions (McMurray et al., 1997). Most specifically, if health specialists do not feel supported by colleagues and by the organization, their satisfaction level falls. In one specific US study, physicians who perceived greater control over the practice environment, who perceived that their work demands were reasonable, and who received more support from colleagues reported higher levels of satisfaction, greater commitment to their organization, and superior psychological well-being (Freeborn, 2001).

These various stressors and their resulting impact on satisfaction are not necessarily unique to doctors but have been commonly reported across other occupations within the health services. For instance, in a study of the largest group within most healthcare setting, nurses, Harris (1989) looked at four commonly perceived predominant dimensions of stress impacting job satisfaction including: difficulties in managing with the workload (especially problems of insufficient time to conduct nursing tasks whilst simultaneously having to perform clerical duties); interpersonal stress resulting from staff conflicts (as well as lack of involvement in decision-making processes, lack of social support, and poor communication); problems as a result of inadequate preparation for the role (lack of confidence in managerial role); and dealing with existential dilemmas (death and dying). Each represented factors that contributed to nurse dissatisfaction in the workplace. Many variables within each factor make achieving satisfaction for every individual a very complex task. Recognition of frustrations, such as turnover, lack of internal empowerment, burnout, and, elimination of external sources of stress can decrease dissatisfaction in the healthcare setting.

Overall, job satisfaction seems more likely when physicians, healthcare managers, administrators, and social and health policy makers learn to co-operate with each other. Nevertheless, many physicians still seek less involvement of healthcare organizations and administrators in the decision-making process. Unfortunately, relationships between medical and administrative staff are frequently burdened by "power and role" struggles (Gabe, Calnan, & Bury, 1991). In their daily tasks, doctors are required to adhere to the regulations imposed by their superiors as well as the time-intensive demands of administrative and organizational chores associated with economic constraints imposed by health insurance companies and hospital administrators. Constraints may include time limits for consultations and restrictions on the practitioner's decision making with regard to treatment options (Kirkcaldy, Brown, Furnham, & Trimpop, 2002). An additional "communication" pressure may be experienced, resulting from different priority ratings and personal stress-coping strategies. It seems clear that whereas a containment of the financial costs of health care is typically a central aim of administration, the "peripheral constraints" set by clinical management policies are often perceived as "irritating and random" by medical and allied personnel, and counter-productive to optimal patient treatment. Overall, the impression is often formed that physicians do not fully appreciate the economic limitations of any healthcare system; they have difficulty in reconciling the perceived needs of the individual patient with the impact of the proposed treatment upon the healthcare system as a whole. For the medical director and consultant physicians, the resulting role conflicts may cause them to become alienated from their personnel.

A study involving management level Swedish physicians (Jansson von Vulteé, Axelsson, & Arnetz, 2007) assessed the relationship between organizational settings and perceived well-being. The authors defined organizational setting as contact with top management, decision-making influence, clearly defined organization, and whether the physician was acting as a leader. Among the physicians, the perceived well-being was defined as social climate, work-related exhaustion, work satisfaction, influence, development ability, and supportive leadership. The results indicated that organizational support improved work satisfaction and mental energy, and decreased work-related exhaustion among physicians, culminating in a decreasing turnover rate among physicians. In addition to reducing work-related exhaustion, the importance of not only promoting, but moreover enhancing influence in decision-making processes was seen as a key mechanism by which organizational efficiency could be improved.

Working Hours

There has been increasing concern about the impact of long working hours on the physical and psychological health – especially among the medical profession – and this culminated in the European Directive of Working Time. Employers are concerned in whether there may be an optimal number of hours before productivity begins to decline and acute and chronic health problems arise (Kirkcaldy, Furnham, & Shephard, 2009).

Kirkcaldy, Levine, and Shephard (2000) examined the influence of working hours on the health of German managers. They found that those individuals working in excess of 48 hr per week were more likely to exhibit inferior psychological health and physical well-being. Moreover, the subscale "confidence level," which corresponded to the degree of expressed worry, was related to working hours. Persons working longer hours were more likely to worry than those working fewer hours. The authors concluded that prolonged working hours may be associated with a propensity to worry and express concern eliciting personal anxiety, but the direction of causality is uncertain. It is likely that incessant worry and long hours reinforce each other. Managers with longer working hours were more likely to display unique stress profiles as well as report greater workloads and more stress imposed by daily hassles. On the other hand, these "workaholics" reported less stress with respect to recognition (the degree they felt recognized for their achievements).

In a later study by Kirkcaldy and Siefen (2006) employees displaying longer working hours displayed poorer physical health, but no evidence of psychological ill-health or maladaptive stress. Such individuals were characterized by implementing a faster pace of life and showed more favorable attitudes towards exercise and medical treatment, whilst having below normal scores for health awareness and health consciousness. These findings are of interest because they suggest the possibility that there is scarce evidence of psychological ill-health due to lack of health awareness or denial, dissociation or isolation of affect. In an earlier study, Trimpop, Kirkcaldy, Athanasiou, and Cooper (2000) discovered that, among German veterinary surgeons, both working hours and perceived occupational stress were consistently related to specific accident behaviors. These findings lend credence to the idea that long working hours, characteristic of many forms of modern employment, have potentially debilitating effects.

Gender Differences

Given the considerable participation of both genders within and across the health professions, it is not surprising that research has often sought to examine the possibility of gender differences in the experience of job stress and its effects. Cooper et al. (1989) found that in general the four most important predictors of job stress were: work-home interface, demands of the job, patients' expectations, and practice administration. However, for women doctors heightened interference of the job with family life was the most significant predictor of stress, whilst for men it was the combined stressors of practice administration and job demands. Females experienced more stress than males from visiting during adverse weather conditions, a greater fear of assault on night visits, procuring a locum, a lack of emotional support at home, and dealing with friends or relatives as patients. A finding to emerge quite frequently from research is that the existence of a conflict between their work and personal lives seems to have been particularly stressful for female

GPs and doctors. Kirkcaldy and Siefen (1991) noted that relative to their female peers, male healthcare professionals in a large hospital were more inclined to report stress, complaining about relationships with their colleagues, and finding a greater adverse impact of job pressures in their family lives. However, this difference may reflect in part a sex difference in the choice of specialty, since female physicians tend to opt for those types of practice where more flexible time schedules are possible.

Richardsen and Burke (1991) carried out a large-scale study of Canadian physicians, and identified that the major sources of stress indicated by both female and male physicians were time pressures on the job, and major sources of satisfaction were relationships with patients and colleagues. However, significant sex differences were present in both demographic and situational variables as well as measures of occupational stress and attitudes about health care. A further study by Linzer et al. (2002) sought to determine the existence of sex differences in physician burnout in the Netherlands and in the United States. Their results showed that in the American sample women experienced more burnout than men, whereas in the Dutch sample no such disparity was observed. It also emerged that women in both countries described less work control than men, but that the effect size of the sex difference in the United States was more than twice that in the Netherlands. Furthermore, factors such as children, home support, and work-home interference were comparable between sexes in the United States. The authors concluded that the apparent gender parity in physician burnout in the Netherlands may be due to fewer work hours and greater work control of women compared to those in the United States.

Work-Related Accidents

Evidence has suggested that occupational stress and accidents are intimately interrelated. There is a growing literature that psychological factors are implicated in the incidence of personal injuries and accidents at work, and among these factors are job-related stress, inferior working climate, and work dissatisfaction (Kirkcaldy & Trimpop, 1997; Trimpop & Kirkcaldy, 1998). Moreover, they found that a variety of demographic variables were predictive of stress, including weekly working hours, age, distance from home to practice, gender, and duration of midday break. These in turn were implicated in the accident rate. Job stress, job dissatisfaction, and risk-taking attitudes were identified among the factors which determined work-related accidents.

In a cross-sectional survey of almost 8,000 US surgeons, 8.9% felt concerned over an error made during the last three months, and 70% of surgeons felt the error was at the individual, rather than system level. However, burnout and depression remained as independent predictors of errors. Frequency of overnight calls, methods of compensation, practice setting and number of hours worked were not associated with medical errors using multivariate analyses (Shanafelt et al., 2010).

B. D. Kirkcaldy et al.
Stress and Its Impact on Psychosocial Well-Being Among Medical Professionals

115

Theoretical Model

A number of psychological theories have been put forward to describe, predict and provide leverage for influencing psychosocial well-being as well as work results. One of the most influential has been the Job Characteristics Model (JCM) by Hackman and Oldham (1976, 1980). In its essence it states that job satisfaction, intrinsic work motivation, personal development, as well as absenteeism, turnover and productivity are a function of five core principles of work design. These are autonomy, skill variety, task identity, task significance, and feedback. Through several mediating psychological processes, involving feeling responsibility, importance, and knowledge of progress, Hackman and Oldham (1980) have argued (and later research has in part supported the notion) that the design of work influences work-related behaviors. There are important advantages in the JCM as a theoretical framework: Acknowledgment of the importance of workers' subjective experience of their job coupled with a recognition of differences among individuals – termed moderators – in the importance they place on situational factors of their work.

Kirkcaldy and Trimpop (1999) and Kirkcaldy et al. (2002) in a series of German surveys attempted to identify the moderating factors in a representative sample of members of healthcare practices who might be expected to place different degrees of importance on different situational aspects of work: physicians and auxiliary personnel. The following hypotheses arose from the above cited literature:

- Stress experiences will be higher for those who have little influence in organizational procedures.
- Job satisfaction will be higher for those individuals who have more skill and task variety.
- Individuals with a heavy work-family interface will experience more stress at work and more accidents. (It is plausible that gender differences exert a role here.)
- Individuals with higher and longer working hours will experience more stress and health problems.

In the last survey on a representative sample of medical practices across Germany, a questionnaire was disturbed to assess occupational stress and health outcome (including work satisfaction) measures as well as subjectively perceived perception of work (see Kirkcaldy & Trimpop, 1999). The first 1,000 completed questionnaire returned within the 3 month deadline were included in the analyses. The medical doctors average age was 47.6 years compared to the auxiliary personnel, 33.5 years ($t = -20.8$, $df = 900$, $p < .001$). They were likely to work longer hours (48.9 vs. 31.8 hr) compared to their auxiliary personnel ($t = -22.5$, $p < .001$). Of these medical doctors, 42.13% were specialists (including dental surgeons) and 57.87% were general practitioners (statistics are comparable to Daten des Gesundheitswesen, "Data of the German Health Ministry", 1999.).

Overall, 75% of the respondents were (highly) satisfied with the self-sufficiency and flexibility that their work brings them, and an almost equal proportion (77.1%) were satisfied with the intrinsic nature of their work. Three quarters (75.6%) reported excellent communication between personnel, with 63.5% positive about communication between medical staff and auxiliary personnel to resolve issues and challenges satisfactorily, with few complaining of adverse negative working climate (11.5%). The vast majority (72.9%) felt that they were offered the social support they required at home and within the family to cope with job-related difficulties. Affiliative support was also reported at the collegial level at work (68.4%).

With regard to occupational stress, the results were less clear. For example, although almost one third (30.0%) of respondents felt that their work was not particularly stressful, another third, 34.2%, did report that their work is stressful. And whilst almost 40% of individuals felt no pressures to arrive at work punctually, 38.8% felt that they experience tremendous pressure to arrive at work punctually.

Data Relating to Skill and Task Variety

It was assumed that generalists would experience higher satisfaction less stress and less health problems, due to their higher variety in their jobs. A comparison of specialists and general practitioners was performed and supported our assumptions. Also, we attributed the same differences to the employed staff, namely nurses of general practitioners and specialists (Table 1).

It appears that a main effect due to occupational status (doctor vs. auxiliary) was found for stress and participation (with no significant interactive term for occupational status × medical "domain"). Which specific work-related statements discriminated medical doctors (and dental surgeons) from their auxiliary personnel? The largest differences were observed with doctors "I find my work strenuous," Ma 3.74, Mp 2.72; $F(1, 863) = 163.70, p < .001$, "I have difficulties demarcating working and leisure/family domains" (Ma 2.75, Mp 1.96; $F = 85.54, p < .001$), "Whenever I get angry in at work, I find the necessary support within the family (and friends)" (Ma 4.04, Mp 4.09; $F = 34.07$, $p < .001$), "As a result of the working climate, I experience persistent pressures at work"

Table 1. Differences in stress and work satisfaction profiles of medical professionals and allied personnel for various work domains (bold print reflects highest group score and italics, lowest)

| | Dental surgeon | | GP | | Specialist | | | | |
	Pers.	MD	Pers.	MD	Pers.	MD	Domain (D)	Job (J) status	D × J
Stress	10.0	12.4	*9.6*	12.0	11.3	**12.8**	4.2*	41.5***	ns
Work climate	15.4	**15.9**	15.9	15.8	*14.5*	14.8	4.1*	ns	ns
Satisfaction	*19.5*	20.4	19.7	**20.5**	19.8	20.5	ns	5.8*	ns

*$p < .05$, ***$p < .0001$.

(Ma 2.19, Mp 1.78; $F = 25.12$, $p < .001$) and "When confronted with work-related problems, I get support from the co-workers within my practice" (Ma 3.62, Mp 3.96; $F = 17.64$, $p < .001$).

Data Relating to the Influence of the Work-Family Interface

It has frequently been found that a major impact on occupational stress (and possibly health and satisfaction at work) is the dual role/burden of parenthood and work, especially by women. In order to avoid the confounding effect of occupational status, MANOVA was computed looking at "number of dependent children" (defined as those under 10 years of age) and "gender" for doctors and medical consultants, and "Auxiliary personnel" separately. The three dependent variables were the job-related scales (participation, stress, and job satisfaction). No effects (main or interactive) were recorded for auxiliary personnel. The multivariate test was statistically significant, Pillai's trace = 0.98, $F(3, 231) = 4302.4$, $p < .001$. The differences were confined to a main effect attributable to "parenthood" on a autonomous, participative climate whereby doctors without dependent children (although not necessarily childless) evaluate a participatory climate more favorably than their counterparts who have "dependent" children (Mdep 14.61, Mnon-d 16.81; $F = 11.87$, $p < .001$). There were no gender differences in evaluation of working climate ($F = 0.10$, ns), nor for that matter an interaction Gender × Dependent ($F = 3.16$).

Although there was no significant main effect on occupational stress, the interaction Dependent children × Gender did emerge as statistically significant ($F = 4.62$, $p < .05$). Male doctors who had dependent children experienced greater job-related pressures than those without children, in contrast to women doctors. It emerged that women doctors with children experienced less work-related stress than those without children. One of the confounding factors here is whether the partner/spouse is at home managing the home, OR in a stressful and demanding jobs themselves. This is an example of a complex interaction confined to a particular occupational status, which would not have been witnessed in more simple linear analyses.

Moderators Predicting Absenteeism and Injury Rates

Finally, less than 1.4% of the sample reported days lost in the last year through work-related accidents, 1.6% due to traffic accidents, and a substantial 44% had been ill some days due to illness, taking an average of 3.5 days (with subjects varying from 0 to 150 days ill off work). For this reason, an attempt was made to account for the variance in days ill during the last year. Assuming background and psychological variable set are psychometrically and theoretical independent, an estimate of a total of c. 5% variance can be explained. The likelihood of being ill is greater if the person must travel further to work, is a healthcare auxiliary as opposed to a doctor/consultant (occupational status), and if the working atmosphere is perceived negatively and a resignatory attitude is adopted.

Four major predictors of absenteeism explained a significant amount of the variation in illness (psychological factors – external control and working climate; $R = 0.14$, adj. $R^2 = 0.02$, $F(1, 805) = 7.45$, $p < .001$); background factors – kilometers, and occupational status, $R = 0.22$, adj. $R^2 = 0.03$, $F(2, 549) = 14.39$, $p < .01$).

One of the core findings is that working climate consistently emerged as one of the (psychological) variables predictive for three of the four outcome variables (days off ill, work-related accidents, and satisfaction).

Data Relating to Hours of Work and Health Consequences

Step-wise linear regression analyses was computed incorporating all the demographic and job structural factors as independent variables in predicting occupational stress. Three potent predictors – occupational, onset of work, and working hours – emerged explaining 18% of the variance. Thus, it seems that people with longer working hours experience more stress and ill-health effects. Yet, overall, occupational status contributes more to stress than even weekly working hours (Table 2, cf. Kirkaldy & Trimpop, 1999).

Taken together, these hypotheses related to moderators – how one's role affects the importance one places on different situational factors – were generally supported. Individuals benefiting from greater levels of personal autonomy and influence displayed less absenteeism, experienced more job satisfaction, lower levels of stress, and reported fewer accidents. Furthermore, those who reported higher levels of participation, task variety and identity, as well as importance, experienced lower absenteeism. Finally, those with a heavier workload regarding hours of work showed more negative health effects than those who worked less or at more sociable times.

Contradictory findings in previous research on gender effects in physician satisfaction and stress studies may be attributable to the confounding effect of occupational status. With regard to gender differences, we did not establish meaningful variations that were not explained by the above named variables. Gender differences have emerged in previous stress research, with women often reporting higher levels of psychological distress and men often appearing more vulnerable to severe physical illness (Cooper & Baglioni, 1988). However, many of the findings have tended to be inconsistent for example,

Table 2. Determinants of job-related stress among health professionals

Stress	$R = 0.43$, $R^2 = 0.18$		$F(3, 527) = 39.36^{***}$
	β	t	p
Occupational status	+0.32	+6.49	.001***
Onset of work	−0.11	−2.70	.01**
Weekly working hours	+0.12	+2.30	.05*

*$p < .05$, **$p < .01$, ***$p < .001$.

B. D. Kirkcaldy et al.
Stress and Its Impact on Psychosocial Well-Being Among Medical Professionals

119

Kirkcaldy and Trimpop (1997) found that among veterinary and nursing personnel, males exhibited higher levels of occupational stress. In a study of social workers, Kirkcaldy, Thome, and Thomas (1989) were unable to find any significant gender differences in job-pressure and dissatisfaction profiles, with the exception of the scale, "career motivation" (marginally higher among males). Kirkcaldy and Siefen (1991) used the SBUS among health care and allied personnel in a child psychiatric clinic: Men reported greater occupational stress than women did. Furthermore, males displayed greater negative spill (lower recreation scores) than did women, even after the possible confounding effects of marital status, parenthood, and age were partialled out. They concluded that gender differences in such job-related scales probably reflected the working conditions of men and women confronted with dual pressures of work and family life. In a later large-scale survey (Kirkcaldy, Trimpop, & Cooper, 1997), observed that for a subsample-of nursing and allied personnel, males displayed higher job-related stress scores than females, but the position was actually reversed for the subsample of doctors and consultants.

If we consider the impact of having dependent children on work stress for men and women, some coherent findings emerge. Having dependent children is related to occupational stress, and this relationship is mediated by gender. The relationship itself is moderated by occupational status: More specifically, job stress is not related to parenthood or gender for auxiliary personnel. The position is different for healthcare doctors: Whereas male doctors report greater stress when they have dependent children (defined as less than 10 years of age) compared to those male doctors without (dependent) children, for female doctors the position is reversed, that is, female doctors exhibit substantially less job-related stress when they have dependent children than when they have no dependent children. Perhaps male doctors worry more, in part due to the substantial costs of having a family with small children, the physical exhaustion and emotional costs (Argyle, 1992). Alternatively, female doctors may focus more on the values of having children for example, primary group ties and affection, stimulation and fun, and expansion of self (Hofmann & Manis, 1982). This may in part be attributable to an increased likelihood for females to have spouses who are also working, hence they are likely to be financially more secure. Interestingly, female physicians generally show some of the characteristics commonly lacking in male doctors, seeing fewer patients per day, but investing more time in talking to individual patients. With women physicians taking more time with each patient and communicating more, one perception is that of increased quality and patient satisfaction.

Some interesting developmental trends were also observed. For example, occupational stress was found to decrease, as healthcare doctors became older, whereas the positive evaluation of working climate increased over age. This may reflect the more routine coping of healthcare tasks and the running of a clinical practice over time. In common with many situations, an increased confidence in one's role often develops as a result of experience, maturity, and stability. Moreover, the financial insecurities of getting a practice launched, and the inexperience of coping with unexpected work-related "episodes" begins to diminish. Perhaps not surprisingly, for auxiliary personnel, stress and working climate scarcely changed with age, but there was a gradual increase in job satisfaction with

increasing age, suggesting that the intrinsic elements of work satisfaction are most susceptible to change in the developmental career of healthcare personnel.

Finally, we found that doctors reported having significantly less time off sick compared
to the auxiliary employees. Possible explanations for this may include the ability of doctors to self-prescribe and self-medicate, or perhaps expose a personal and professional
reluctance on the part of some doctors to participate as patients to their peers (bad
patients?). The allied personnel exhibited a higher rate of work-related accidents, and
almost certainly coupled with this, took off more sick leave. Auxiliary personnel differed
in their attitudes towards risk-taking and safety at work, being less safety-conscious and
more "time-urgent," conceivably due to the time pressures and constraints imposed on
them.

Overall, we have seen that occupational status exerts a significant effect on the relationship between occupational stress and health outcome measures. While lots of effort
have been spent worrying about physicians, much less serious attention seems to be paid
to the auxiliary personnel. Further research should thus attempt to isolate and vary the
influential factors systematically under controlled conditions.

Implications

Our study which was set against the background, but within the context of contemporary
research showed that one possibility to influence psychophysical health at work is to
design work so that the opportunity to influence, the possibility to participate, and the task
variety are maximized. Health professionals would appear particularly susceptible to significant job demands exercising "little control over outcomes. Indeed the acts of psychological and physical caregiving require the dedication of personal resources which may be
reciprocated in minimal patient improvement or loss" (Munyon, Breaux, & Perrewe,
2009, p. 264). In common with other studies (Jansson von Vultee et al., 2007; Visser
et al., 2003) our study has highlighted the importance of providing and maintaining a supportive and positive working atmosphere for health professionals. Several ways of enhancing social relationships during work have been proposed by Argyle (1987) "including the
formation of natural co-operative work groups, improving supervisory skills, increasing
participation in decisions, creating contacts between workers and clients, and reducing status and pay differentials in the hierarchy" (p. 49). One constructive and practical step may
be to encourage the creation of a "pack" to promote both mutually supportive teamwork
and also support to individuals on both a professional, but also on a personal level. Similarly, the role of "mentors" or "buddies," popular in some Information Technology and
other industries may also be of practical benefit and reduce feelings of isolation and professional unease, as well as create cohesion and provide direction in healthcare settings.

Practical steps should aim to promote positive change within and across the medical
professions, specifically focusing on ways to increase personal control and create/enhance
participation in the workplace. For example, the creation of structured peer support services, which provide healthcare providers a safe and confidential environment to share

the emotional impact of adverse events and stressors, while serving as a foundation for open communication.

Similar suggestions have been offered by the Australian Medical Association (2006) in which they examined practical preventive and therapeutic options for physicians. Suggestions included: Maintaining a good relationship with a trusting fellow physician and developing a network of peers to allow "debriefing, support and mentorship," providing practitioners with relevant information on stress factors in their professional and personal lives, and offering peer assistance to those showing manifestations of stress. The Australian report also underlined the health importance of taking regular vacations, developing an awareness of personal nutrition and taking time out for family and lifestyle pursuits, whether as medical students or qualified practitioners.

From our own study it emerged that participation was seen to be related to lower accident rates, hence it would appear that a constructive step would be the inclusion of safety orientation and risk prevention (specific Health and Safety) training programs for all staff. This would require a relatively modest investment on the part of the employer, but would demonstrate a value and a commitment towards the well-being of staff.

An additional area where increased participation would promote a positive outcome would be with regard to absenteeism. As well as taking steps (through consultation and communication) to provide a more positive working climate, practical steps could be considered to reduce absenteeism by providing employees the chance to work nearer their home. Alternatively, where appropriate, stress management programs, or initiatives directed at tackling direct and indirect causes of employee absenteeism may prove beneficial.

Finally, irrespective of a health professional's gender, improving access to childcare could alleviate issues relating to the work-home interface. One possibility may be the creation of dedicated childcare co-ordinators at health authorities and hospitals, providing more flexible opening hours of hospital-based childcare services. Also, when required and appropriate, additional funding might be made available for childcare assistance.

Healthcare organizations may incur high costs due to a stressed, dissatisfied physician workforce. Moreover, the long-term implications not only for the well-being of healthcare workers, but also for the provision and quality of patient care should be apparent to all. Quite clearly, for the increasingly bureaucratic structures present in the reality of modern-day healthcare settings, the clinical work environment must be effectively managed. Targeted attempts have been made to reach this goal through organizational coaching procedures. To date, the initial results are promising (Trimpop & Kirkcaldy, 1999).

Many medical administrators and other senior medical consultants are experiencing increasing pressures related to their achieving specified administrative and financial goals ranging from maximum waiting times for admission or treatment of surgical conditions to the containment of budgetary shortfalls. They additionally face the rivalry that develops between competing medical specialities, and between doctors working in private practices compared with those employed within a medical institute. These tensions make it difficult to advocate a unified and effective strategy to ameliorate the stressors affecting the various physicians concerned. Herein lies a proposal that future research pays greater attention to these administrative and auxiliary personnel, groups that have previously been largely neglected compared to the experiences of "frontline" practitioners such as doctors and nurses.

However, across the wide spectrum there exists the need for further examination into specific details as to the exact mechanisms when, where and how different practices and different people working in them can be most effectively supported through specific job characteristics. What alternative instruments may be used to identify stress in health settings? An earlier attempt to identify subjective understanding of the "health and/or clinical" work context and to establish idiographic analysis of work stress was proposed by Kirkcaldy, Athanasou, and Trimpop (2000). Repertory grid analysis was applied to extract the underlying constructs that gave meaning to stress for each person. Results suggested idiosyncratic perceptions of the meaning of stress and diverse situational determinants. It was argued that current approaches to theorizing about stress in terms of general elements and common perceptions are challenged by these findings. In contrast to the findings of nomothetic research, a theoretical perspective evolving from the personal construction of the situation may be the significant determinant of anxiety and stressful reactions for each person.

Acknowledgment

Thanks go to the BGW (German Social Accident Insurance Institution for the Health and Welfare Services) for supporting much previous research on accident behavior among the medical and nursing professions. And to Beverly Simpson in Toronto for her comments as on earlier version of the manuscript.

References

A'Brook, M. (1990). The doctor's health. Psychosis and depression. *Practitioner, 234*, 992–993.

Agius, R., Blenkin, H., Deary, I., Zealley, H., & Wood, R. (1996). Survey of perceived stress and work demands of consultant doctors. *Occupational and Environmental Medicine, 53*, 217–224.

Allibone, A., Oakes, D., & Shannon, H. S. (1981). The health and health care of doctors. *Journal of the Royal College of General Practitioners, 31*, 728–734.

American Medical Association. (2004). *Physician characteristics and distribution in US.* Chicago, IL: AMA Press.

Antoniou, A. S., Cooper, C. L., & Davidson, M. J. (2008). A qualitative study investigating gender differences in primary work stressors and levels of job satisfaction in Greek junior doctors. *The Qualitative Report Volume, 13*, 456–473.

Argyle, M. (1987). *The psychology of happiness.* Methuen: London.

Argyle, M. (1992). *The social psychology of everyday life.* London, UK: Routledge.

Belfer, B. (1989). Stress and the medical practitioner. *Stress Health, 5*, 109–113.

Bissel, L., & Jones, R. W. (1976). The alcoholic practitioner: A survey. *American Journal of Psychiatry, 133*, 1142.

BMJ Editor. (2008). Healthy doctors – healthy practice. *British Medical Journal, 337*, 1121–1122.

Bogue, R. J., Gaueneri, J. G., Reed, M., Bradley, K., & Hughes, J. (2006). Secrets of physician satisfaction: Study identifies pressure points and reveals life practices of highly satisfied doctors. *The Physician Executive, 30*–33.

Brooke, D., Edwards, S. G., & Taylor, C. (1991). Addiction as an occupational hazard. *British Journal of Addiction, 86*, 1011–1016.

Caplan, R. P. (1994). Stress, anxiety and depression in hospital consultants, general practitioners, and senior health service managers. *British Medical Journal, 309*, 1261–1263.

Cartwright, L. K. (1987). Occupational stress in women physicians. In R. L. Payne & J. Firth-Cozens (Eds.), *Stress in the health professionals*. Chichester, UK: Wiley.

Chambers, R., Wall, D., & Campbell, I. (1996). Stresses, coping mechanisms and job satisfaction in general practitioner registrars. *British Journal of General Practice, 46*, 343–348.

Compton Interactive Encyclopaedia. (1995). *Women's history in America*. Retrieved from the Women International Centre Web Site: http://www.wic.org/misc/history.htm.

Constanti, A., Solano, L., Di Napoli, R., & Bosco, A. (1997). Relationship between hardiness and risk of burnout in a sample of 92 nurses working in oncology and AIDS wards. *Psychotherapy & Psychosomatics, 66*, 78–82.

Cooper, C. L., & Baglioni, A. J. Jr., (1988). A structural model approach toward the development of a theory of the link between stress and mental health. *British Journal of Medical Psychology, 61*, 87–102.

Cooper, C. L., Rout, U., & Faragher, B. (1989). Mental Health, job satisfaction, and job stress among general practitioners. *British Medical Journal, 298*, 366–370.

Daten des Gesundheitswesen. (1997). *Data of Health*. Statistical Office of the Ministry of Health, Vol. 91.

Elliott, G. R., & Eisdorfer, C. (1982). *Stress and human health*. New York, NY: Springer.

Ennis, M., & Vincent, C. A. (1990). Obstetric accidents: A review of 64 cases. *British Medical Journal, 300*, 1365–1367.

Felton, J. (1998). Burnout as a clinical entity – its importance in health care workers. *Occupational Medicine, 48*, 237–250.

Firth-Cozens, J. (2003). Doctors, their wellbeing, and their stress. *British Medical Journal, 326*, 670–671.

Forum Gesundheitspolitik. (2009). *Die Frauenanteil den Ärzten steigt: Ist dadurch die sprechende Medizin im Kommen?* Retrieved from http://www.forum-gesundheitspolitik.de/artikel/artikel. pl?artikel=0628.

Freeborn, D. (2001). Satisfaction, commitment, and psychological well-being among HMO physicians. *The Western Journal of Medicine, 174*, 13–18.

Fuchs, E. (2008). *Physicians, medical students struggle with mental illness and suicide*. Association of American Medical Colleges. Retrieved from http:/www.aamc.org/newsroom/reporter/dec08/ mentalillness.htm

Fung, K. (2007). *Why are we at risk?* Department of Psychiatry, University of Alberta.

Gabe, J., Calnan, M., & Bury, M. (1991). *The sociology of the health service*. London, UK: Routledge.

Gefken, T. (2008). *Arzt- Traumberuf oder Knochenjob?* [Doctor – ideal job or hard graff?]. Hamburg: Ergebnisse einer Umfrage der Ärztekämmer Hamburg und frischerAppelt.

Guthrie, E., & Black, D. (1997). Psychiatric disorder, stress and burnout. *Advances in Psychiatric Treatment, 3*, 275–281.

Hackman, J. R., & Oldham, G. R. (1976). Motivation through the design of work: Test of a theory. *Organizational Behavior and Human Performance, 16*, 250–279.

Hackman, J. R., & Oldham, G. R. (1980). *Work redesign*. Reading, MA: Addison-Wesley.

Hampton, T. (2005). Experts address risk of physician suicide. *The Journal of the American Medical Association, 294*, 1189–1191.

Harris, P. E. (1989). The nurse stress index. *Work and Stress, 3*, 335–346.

Hawton, K., & Vislisel, L. (1999). Suicide in nurses. *Suicide and life-threatening behaviour, 29*, 86–95.

Hofmann, L. W., & Manis, J. P. (1982). The value of children in the United States. In F. I. Nye (Ed.), *Family relationships. Rewards and Costs* (pp. 143–170). Beverley Hills, London, and Delhi: Sage.

Jansson von Vultee, P., Axelsson, R., & Arnetz, B. (2007). The impact of organizational settings on physician wellbeing. *International Journal of Healthcare Quality Assurance, 20*, 506–515.

Kaiser, R., Kohler, S., Popovic, M., & Stilwe, U. (2005). Rambaoll – Gutachten. Datenbasis noch unbefriedigend – Empfehlung für die Politik. [Case report. Data base as dissatisfactory – suggestions for politics]. *Deutscheaerzteblatt, 102*, 34–35.

Kirkcaldy, B. D., Athanasou, J., & Trimpop, R. (2000). The idiosyncratic construction of stress: Examples from medical work settings. *Stress Medicine, 16*, 315–326.

Kirkcaldy, B. D., Brown, J., Furnham, A., & Trimpop, R. (2002). Job stress and dissatisfaction: Comparing male and female medical practitioners and auxiliary personnel. *European Review of Applied Psychology, 52*, 51–61.

Kirkcaldy, B. D., Furnham, A., & Shephard, R. J. (2009). The impact of working hours and working patterns on physical and psychological health. In C. L. Cooper & S. Cartwright (Eds.), *The Oxford Handbook of organizational well being* (pp. 303–330). Oxford: Oxford University Press.

Kirkcaldy, B. D., Levine, R., & Shephard, R. J. (2000). The impact of working hours on physical and psychological health of German managers. *European Review of Applied Psychology, 50*, 443–449.

Kirkcaldy, B. D., & Pope, M. (1992). A structural analysis of a psycho-oncology unit. *European Work and Organisational Psychologist, 2*, 33–51.

Kirkcaldy, B. D., & Siefen, R. G. (1991). Occupational stress among medical health professionals. *Social Psychiatry and Psychiatric Epidemiology, 26*, 238–244.

Kirkcaldy, B. D., & Siefen, G. (2006). The influence of gender and ethnic origin on health awareness, stress and physical and psychological well-being. ICSOMH, Unpublished Manuscript.

Kirkcaldy, B.D., Thome, E., & Thomas, W. (1990). Job satisfaction amongst psychosocial workers. *Personality and Individual Differences, 10*, 191–196.

Kirkcaldy, B. D., & Trimpop, R. (1997). Organisatorische und individuelle Faktoren im Arbeits- und Verkehrsunfallgeschehen in Tierarztpraxen [Organizatory and individual differences in work and traffic accidents in veterinary surgeon practises]. *Intermediate Research Report.* Hamburg: BGW. ISSN 1434-1344.

Kirkcaldy, B. D., & Trimpop, R. (1999). *Stress, Verkehrs- und Arbeitsunfallpräventionen in Arzt- und Zahnarztpraxen durch der Einsatz von Printmedien.* Hamburg, Germany: BGW.

Kirkcaldy, B. D., Trimpop, R., & Cooper, C. L. (1997). Working hours, job stress, work satisfaction and accident rates among medical practitioners, consultants and allied personnel. *International Journal of Stress Management, 4*, 79–87.

Köhler, S., Napp, L., & Kaiser, R. (2003). Arztin–Traumberuf oder Alptraum [Female doctor – a dream career or a nightmare]. Landeskammer Hessen. Hess: Ärzteblatt, *12*, 631–633.

Lindemann, S., Laara, G., Hakko, H., & Lonnqvist, J. (1996). A systematic review of gender, specific suicide mortality in medical doctors. *British Journal of Psychiatry, 168*, 274–279.

Linzer, M., McMurray, J., Visser, M., Oort, F., Smets, E., & de Haes, H. (2002). Sex differences in physician burnout in the United States and The Netherlands. *Journal of the American Medical Women's Association, 57*, 191–193.

McCranie, E. W., & Brandsma, J. M. (1988). Personality antecedents of burnout among middle-aged physicians. *Journal of Behavioural Medicine, 11*, 30–36.

McMurray, J. E., Williams, E., Schwartz, M. D., Douglas, J., Van Kirk, J., Konrad, T. R., . . . Career Satisfaction Group (CSSG). (1997). Physician job satisfaction: Developing a model using qualitative data. *Journal of General Internal Medicine, 12*, 711–714.

Munyon, T. P., Breaux, D. M., & Perrewe, P. L. (2009). Implications of burnout for health professionals. In G. Chrousos, C. Cooper, M. Eysenck, C. Spielberger, & Stamatios-Anthoniou. (Eds.), *Handbook of managerial behaviour and occupational health* (pp. 328–344). Cheltenham UK: Edward Elgar.

Murray, R. M. (1977). Psychiatric illness in male doctors and controls: An analysis of Scottish inpatient data. *British Journal of Psychiatry, 131*, 1–10.

O'Brien Pallas, L., & Baumann, A. (1998). *The state of nursing practice in Ontario: The issues, challenges and needs.* Toronto: Nursing Effectiveness, Utilization Outcomes Research Unit, University of Toronto-McMaster University.

Ontario Ministry of Health. (1999). *Good nursing, good health: An Investment for the 21st century. Report of the nursing Task Force. Queen's Park.* Ontario: Ontario Ministry of Health.

Peterkin, A. (2009). *Resident health: Risks and challenges* [PowerPoint slides]. Retrieved from http://hsl.mcmaster.ca/medicine/unit6/allanpeterkin.ppt.

Pillay, R. (2008). Work satisfaction of medical doctors in the South African private health sector. *Journal of Health Organisation and Management, 22*, 254–268.

Ray, C., & Baum, M. (1985). *Psychological aspects of early breast cancer.* New York, NY: Springer.

Registrar General. (1978). *Decennial supplement for England and Wales.* London, UK: HMSO.

Richardsen, A. M., & Burke, R. J. (1991). Occupational stress and job satisfaction among middle-aged physicians: Sex differences. *Social Sciences and Medicine, 33*, 1179–1187.

Rinpoche, C. D., & Shlim, D. R. (2006). *Medicine and compassion. A Tibetan Lama's guidance for caregivers.* Massachusetts: Wisdome.

Rose, M. (2005). *Subjective well-being and the job satisfaction Premium of British Women Employers.* Sociol. Associ., Philadelphia: Paper at Amer.

Royal College of Physicians. (2006). *Briefly on women in medicine.* Retrieved from http://www.rcplondon.ac.uk/college/statements/briefing_womenmed.asp.

Rucinski, T., & Cybullska, E. (1985). Mentally ill doctors. *British Journal of Hospital Medicine, 43*, 90–94.

Schattner, P. I., & Colman, G. S. (1998). The stress of metropolitan general practices. *Medical Journal of Australia, 169*, 133–137.

Shanafelt, T. D., Balch, C. M., Bechamps, G., Russell, T., Dyrbye, L., Satele, D., . . . Freischlag, J. (2010). Burnout and medical errors among American surgeons. *Annals of Surgery, 251*, 995–1000.

Shernhammer, E. S., & Colditz, G. A. (2004). Suicide rates among physicians: A quantitative and gender assessment (meta-analysis). *American Journal of Psychiatry, 161*, 2295–2302.

Sibbald, B., Enzer, I., Cooper, C., Rout, U., & Sutherland, V. (2000). GP job satisfaction in 1987, 1990 and 1998: Lessons for the future? *Family Practice, 17*, 364–71.

Sullivan, T., Kerr, M., & Ibrahim, S. A. (1999). Job stress in heath care work. *Hospital Quarterly, 2*, 34–40.

Sutherland, V. J., & Cooper, C. L. (1992). Job stress, satisfaction, and mental health among general practitioners before and after introduction of new contact. *British Medical Journal, 304*, 1545–1548.

Sutherland, V. J., & Cooper, C. L. (1993). Identifying distress among general practitioners: Predictors of psychological ill-health and job dissatisfaction. *Social Science and Medicine, 37*, 575–581.

Symons, L., & Persuade, R. (1995). Stress among doctors. *British Medical Journal, 310*, 742.

Trimpop, R., & Kirkcaldy, B. D. (1998). Stress indicators among medical personnel: A comparison of the "old" and "new" Länder. *Journal of Managerial Psychology, 13*, 22–27.

Trimpop, R., & Kirkcaldy, B. D. (1999). Organisationale Faktoren integrativer Arbeits-, Verkehrs- und Gesundheitsschutzarbeit [Organisation factors in integrative work, traffic and health protection domain]. In Gesellschaft für Arbeitswissenschaft (Ed.), *Arbeitsschutz. Managementsysteme.*

Risiken oder Chancen [Work Safety, Management Systems. Risks and Chances] (pp. 39–44). Dortmund, Germany: Gesellschaft für Arbeitswissenschaft.

Trimpop, R. T., Kirkcaldy, B. D., Athanasiou, J., & Cooper, C. L. (2000). Individual differences in working hours, work perceptions and accident rates in veterinary surgeons. *Work and Stress, 14,* 181–188.

Visser, M., Smets, E., Oort, F., & de Haes, H. (2003). Stress, satisfaction and burnout among Dutch medical specialists. *Canadian Medical Association Journal, 168,* 271–275.

Wong, J. (2008). Doctors and stress. *The Hong Kong Medical Diary, 13,* 4–7.

World Health Organization. (2006). *The World Health Report 2006 – Working together for health.* Geneva.

Selecting a Medical Practitioner

Adrian F. Furnham

University College London, UK

To a large extent people choose their professionals: be they accountants, lawyers, hairdressers, or babysitters. They make that choice based on a wide variety of criteria from personal chemistry to cost, as well as reputation, convenience, or personal recommendation.

The choice of medical practitioners is often more complicated. In some countries choice is restricted while in others it is quite the opposite. Much depends on the countries national health system. Some countries have public and private medicine. Those with money can choose. Even within the public health system doctors often work in practices or units and patients have some degree of choice. Thus women can ask specifically for a woman doctor, and patients can ask for a doctor of their own ethnic, religious, and linguistic group. These choices include General Practitioners (Physicians) as well as Specialist Consultants.

This chapter is concerned with patient choice and what patients look for in a doctor. It explores the medical consultation from the patient's perspective and considers the academic literature on patient choice.

The Medical Consultation

The medical consultation is an integral part of patient diagnosis and recovery. Kleinman (1980) defined the consultation as a transaction between lay and professional explanatory models with the patient and doctor exchanging information in order to reach a satisfactory outcome for both parties. Medical consultations have been shown to have very significant repercussions for patients' immediate and long-term health outcomes (Pendleton & Hasler, 1983). This occurs for various reasons: Poor consultation could lead to the patient not following medical advice; the patient may feel unwilling to visit the practitioner again; the practitioner coming to the wrong diagnosis due to the fact they have not elicited all the information from the patient leading to the wrong treatment, and so on. Patient compliance, now called adherence, is most strongly related to their satisfaction with the consultation. Satisfaction with consultants is probably the strongest predictor of a patient requesting a particular doctor.

Smith and Hoppe (1991) stated that the ideal medical interview for both, doctor and patient, integrates the *patient-centered* and *physician-centered* approaches so that the patient leads in areas where they are the expert, for example, symptoms, concerns, preferences, and the physician leads in areas of their expertise, for example, diagnosis and treatments. This model is consistent with what other researchers have also put forward. Roter and Hall (1988) referred to this relationship as "mutuality."

A number of the studies have demonstrated that doctor-patient communication can influence patient satisfaction with care, recall and understanding of medical information, how the patients cope with disease, their quality of life, and even their state of health (Ong, De Haes, Hoos, & Lammes, 1995). The majority of complaints which arise in orthodox medicine do so because of communication difficulties rather than practitioner negligence (Lloyd & Bor, 2004).

A standard research procedure to measure consultation satisfaction is to have patients fill in a patient satisfaction questionnaire after they come out of a consultation (Kaplan et al., 1995). These scores can be related to what happened in the consultation (as audio or video-recorded and analyzed) as well as patients "recovery" data. For example, Marvel, Epstein, Flowers, and Beckham (1999) recorded a large sample of doctor-patient interactions in a primary care setting and found that in 72% of consultations the patient did not complete talking about their concern(s). In all 35% of cases this was due to the doctors not making any solicitation of the patients' agenda and 65% of non-completed patient concerns were due to the physician redirecting and focusing the interaction. They found the average length of time before a patient was "redirected," or in other words interrupted, was 23.1 s. It has been found that patients have on average three major sociomedical concerns per visit to a GP and that they will leave the most important concern until last (Kaplan, Gandek, Greenfield, Rogers, & Ware, 1995; Stewart, Brown, Levenstein, McCracken, & McWhinney, 1986) meaning in these instances where the doctor is redirecting the most important information will never be elicited.

Arborelius and Bremberg (1992) conducted a study in Sweden that asked the question "What can doctors do to achieve a successful consultation?" It was found that the differentiating features of a positive consultation were that GP and patient were in agreement about the *reason* for the consultation and the GP had *inquired* about the patients' ideas and concerns. The time for explanation was much longer in the positive consultations compared to the negative ones.

Patients' expectations also have an impact on how they experience that consultation. Zebiene et al. (2004) found predictably that there was higher satisfaction among patients who have more expectations met. The most frequently reported expectations were "getting information" and "understanding and explanation" of the health problem. They also found that different expectations carried different influences on patient satisfaction and the most important expectations to be met were "understanding and explanation" followed by "emotional support" while "getting information" was less important.

Wensing, Jung, Mainz, Olesen, and Grol (1998) conducted a systematic review of the literature on patients' needs and priorities. Based on 19 studies the most important features for patients were: *humanness*, meaning respect and personal interest for the patient as an individual, was the aspect rated highest, followed by *competence/accuracy, patients' involvement in decisions, time for care, other aspects of availability/accessibility, informativeness* and *exploring patients needs*. The patients' top priority reflected a preference for a psychotherapeutic approach to the consultation followed by medical ability.

Little et al. (2001) attempted to identify patient's preferences for a patient-centered consultation in general practice using pre-consultation and post-consultation questionnaires. The aspects they placed most importance on were "communication, partnership, and health promotion." They also found that the patients who felt more unwell and worried, had a high incidence of anxiety and depression. Middle aged patients were more likely than older patients to strongly want good communication. This may be because older individuals are used to the traditional approach of the doctor having all the authority in the consultation and being a figure who is above them in the hierarchy of the interaction. None of these studies show counter-intuitive results except for the fact that many seem to rate communication skills over diagnostic ability.

A number of studies into patients' preferences have also focused on decision making. McKinstry (2000) found that patients vary in their preference for how much they are involved in the decision making process in a consultation. Those patients who presented with physical problems preferred a directed approach, older patients (over 61 years) also preferred a directed approach, but those in higher social class groups preferred a shared approach. Ford, Schofield, and Hope (2003) found that patients who preferred doctors to make their decisions for them (35%) were more likely to have their preferences met (64%), compared to patients who wanted to share decisions (47%) of which 52% had their preferences met, 18% wanted to make decisions of their own and 41% has this preference met. Suarez-Almazor's (2004) review of doctor-patient communication concluded that patients' expectations are not always fulfilled: Patients' desires are for increased participation in the consultation and an increase in information sharing from the practitioner. Patients who receive patient-centered care have a greater likelihood of having their symptoms resolved and being more pleased with their care.

Vincent and Furnham (1996) investigated the reasons individuals start using Complementary Medicine (CM) because they believed it was the fact that CM practitioners were judged to have better consultations that they were often chosen in the first place. They identified four principle factors one of which was the experience of poor communication with orthodox practitioners. This suggests the patients are dissatisfied with the consultations they receive from orthodox practitioners and see the complementary practitioner-patient relationship as more positive.

The use of CM reflects how patients are now consumers of health care, each patient having their own preference of how they want to be treated, both in terms of communication style and medical remedy. The consultation is a large part of the popularity of CM (Vincent & Furnham, 1997); but are the components of a CM consultation important and valued by everyone? Or is one of the reasons non-users are non-users because they do not value these components? Or perhaps they have not been in a situation where they needed a more patient-centered consultation? Comparisons of users and nonusers of CM have looked at beliefs about health and disease in general and found numerous important differences.

Communicative Competence

Until recently, little or no attempt was made to train doctors to communicate more effectively with their patients. It was, and for some still is, assumed that this skill or set of skills is no more than common sense, which, anyway, will be acquired or improved by practitioners "on the job" with increasing experience. Yet it has not been denied that these skills may be directly related to such things as diagnosis and patient compliance (Furnham, King, & Pendleton, 1980).

Over the past 20 years there has been considerable interest in social-skills training and research (Argyle, 1981; Furnham, 1983, 1985). The underlying message of this approach is that the ability to communicate efficiently and effectively is a skill that can (and must) be taught and learnt. Many individual skills make up social competence, which is thought of as the ability to produce the desired effects in other people in social situations. Much of the research in this field has concentrated on groups who, for one reason or another, are perceived as not possessing these skills such as mental health patients (schizophrenics and neurotics), addicts (particularly alcoholics), criminal offenders (recidivists and delinquents), disturbed adolescents, and people with disabilities.

However, a number of researchers have pointed to the importance of these skills for professionals such as doctors, lawyers, and teachers, whose day-to-day lives involve communication with many different individuals. In a comprehensive and scholarly review on doctor-patient communication, Pendleton (1983) has shown how the doctors' skills and consultative style can have considerable effects on the immediate, intermediate and long-term outcomes of patient health.

McGuire (1986) has attempted to specify the range of communication or social skills that doctors need, but which they do not appear to acquire during professional training. First and foremost are history-taking skills, which are so clearly relevant in diagnosis. McGuire (1986) reviewed numerous studies on junior, and experienced, hospital doctors and general practitioners, and showed that there is a consistent lack of certain key, history-taking skills that are not compensated for, or acquired with, greater experience or post-graduate training. He argued that doctors lack skills of exposition in the giving of information and advice to patients. The reasons why these crucially important skills are not acquired are:

1. The time-honored apprenticeship method is inappropriate, both because the models are not very good and also because social and psychological aspects are ignored.
2. Doctors are assumed to possess these skills despite the considerable evidence that they do not.
3. Doctors cannot acquire these skills, believing that they cannot be learnt – either one has them or not.
4. The use of these skills will only create problems in that practicing them would lead to patients disclosing difficult-to-handle problems.

5. The skills are assumed to have no important effect on care despite the considerable evidence to the contrary.

He believed that these five objections are misplaced and that it is necessary to develop more effective skill-training methods for doctors that would identify deficiencies, measure performance, and provide feedback.

McGuire (1986) has documented the sort of key communication skills that all doctors need: those of eliciting patient problems (information gathering), establishing patient responses (exploring how patients have responded to diagnosis, explanations, and treatment), correcting misconceptions that patients may hold about their illness, and monitoring the impact of treatment. He argued that some people may suggest that because medical training has changed and improved over the last 20 years or so, such training is unnecessary. Yet the contemporary research reviewed leads on "to conclude that a strong case for feedback-training in interviewing skills can still be made, indeed it could be argued that it is even stronger than when the original work began" (p. 159). However, certain critical issues remain, such as the validity and general effectiveness of training.

An interest in communication or interpersonal-skills courses for medical students or, indeed, qualified doctors, has attracted evaluative research. Despite the use of different methods, nearly all studies have demonstrated the benefits of these courses (Alroy, Ber, & Kramer, 1984; Shepherd & Hammand, 1984). Yet as Schofield (1983) has recognized, communication-skills courses need to be arranged for trainers (established doctors engaged in teaching those newly qualified) and trainees. Furthermore, because of the sensitivity of feedback on performance, certain specific rules have to be laid down for effective and acceptable feedback as well as a consideration of ethical issues.

Despite the importance, relevance and efficacy of communication-skills training it appears that in many countries the medical profession as a whole, and general practice in particular, have not laid down any criteria or rules for the training or assessment of communicative competence in doctors.

Patient's Perspectives on Clinical Competence

Various organizations and individuals have attempted to help clients/patients assess the clinical competence of their doctors. In the case of individuals, they have frequently become dissatisfied with the professional advice that they have been given. Those interested in particular illness like breast cancer believe encouraging patient assessment may be a very effective and efficient way of maintaining regular checks on clinical competence.

Various books and pamphlets are available on patients' rights (Faulder, 1985). King, Pendleton, and Tate (1985) have written a useful handbook for the layman/patient titled "A family guide to dealing with your GP." In this book there is a section on clinical competence that has four sections: accessibility, clinical competence, communication skills, and values, which are divided into two subdivisions, the practice and the doctor him/herself. After the relevant chapter, the authors provide a questionnaire, which is simple and straightforward, but useful for patients to use in assessment. The 19 items used to assess the GP by the patient are set out as follows (Table 1).

This questionnaire is, no doubt, not meant to be exhaustive or psychometrically sophisticated. It is simply meant to aid patients considering four aspects of competence in their doctor. This may indeed influence who they choose (and avoid) as a doctor.

There are, of course, numerous dangers in using this as an assessment device. Firstly, there are various constraints on the individual doctor and practice (i.e., size, location, and demography of catchment), about which individual doctors can do little. Secondly, it is important to know various salient features about the clients (demographic and psychographic details as well as medical history) in order to establish which subgroups find which features of general competence more, or less, important. For instance, if there are reliable sex, age, or ethnic differences in what patients expect of their doctor, the

Table 1. A check-list for patients

Your doctor	
A. Accessibility. (Can you get to see her/him?)	
1. Does s/he provide enough surgeries?	Yes No
2. Can you usually see *your* doctor within two days?	Yes No
3. Can you get to speak to *your* doctor on the telephone?	Yes No
4. Will your doctor do home visits?	Yes No
5. Are her/his appointments at least five minutes long?	Yes No
B. Clinical competence. (Does s/he know her/his stuff?)	
1. Is your doctor a Member or Fellow of the Royal College of General Practitioners?	Yes No
2. Does your doctor examine you thoroughly from time to time?	Yes No
3. Are you always given a prescription? (You probably should not be)	Yes No
4. Is your doctor mean with antibiotics and tranquilizers?	Yes No
C. Communications. (Can you talk to her/him?)	
1. Does your doctor listen?	Yes No
2. Does your doctor make you feel rushed?	Yes No
3. Is your doctor often interrupted?	Yes No
4. Does your doctor ask what you think about your problem?	Yes No
5. Does your doctor ask what you are worried about?	Yes No
6. Does your doctor give you plenty of information?	Yes No
7. Does your doctor let you decide with her/him how your problem should be handled?	Yes No
D. Professional values. (What does s/he regard as important?)	
1. Is your doctor interested in you as a person?	Yes No
2. Is your doctor enthusiastic about health?	Yes No
3. Is your doctor involved in health matters in the community?	Yes No

responses one may get on such questionnaires probably reflect more about the patient profile than the doctor's competence.

Few professionals would wish to have their competence evaluated exclusively by their clients. Nevertheless, patients' perspectives on clinical competence can add a great deal to an objective assessment of a doctor's general competence to practice medicine.

Preferences for Medical Doctors

For obvious reasons patients express strong preferences for particular medical practitioners. This is partly because of their fundamental concerns about their health but also because of the intimate and sensitive nature of consultation conversations and examinations.

Where patients do have informed choice they certainly exercise it. The research questions that have been most frequently posed concern *what particular doctor characteristics* seem most closely related to particular choices and what is the interaction between patient and doctor characteristics.

Studies have looked at factors affecting patient preferences (Braman & Gomez, 2004; Heaton & Marquez, 1990), patient satisfaction (Derose, Hays, McCaffrey, & Baker, 2001), willingness to disclose information and discuss symptoms (Young, 1979), and general aspects of the physician-patient relationship (Elstad, 1994; Weisman & Teitelbaum, 1985).

Several important variables with reference to gender preferences, including general health and treatment of specific conditions (Heaton & Marquez, 1990; Nichols, 1987), practitioner ethnicity and language ability (Ahmad, Kernohan, & Baker, 1989), practitioner style (Bertakis, Helms, Callahan, Azari, & Robbins, 1995), and even physical attractiveness (Young, 1979) have been examined.

Female patients prefer female doctors. It has been demonstrated by numerous researchers since the 1960s (Hopkins, 1967) and in various parts of the world (Ahmad, Hansa, Rawlins, & Stewart, 2002; Brink-Muinen, Bakker, & Bensing, 1994; Elstad, 1994) that for general health issues (Graffy, 1990, Phillips & Brooks, 1998) and, especially intimate symptoms, female patients tend to show a clear preference for female practitioners (Brink-Muinen et al., 1994; Nichols, 1987; Waller, 1998; Young, 1979).

Preferences are often attributed to commonly held views such as "female doctors spend more time with their patients in consultation," "female doctors are more understanding" or "female doctors tend to involve the patient more in medical decisions" (Brink-Muinen et al., 1995; Elstad, 1994; Weisman & Teitelbaum, 1985).

Overall, both male and female patients show a preference for same-sex practitioners in order to reduce potential embarrassment in intimate examinations (Ahmad et al., 2002; Elstad, 1994; Heaton & Marquez, 1990; Kerssens, Bensing, & Abdela, 1997; Plunkett, Kohli, & Milad, 2002; Waller, 1998).

Factors other than gender, like doctor attractiveness, experience and age have also received research attention. Young (1979) found that patients were more willing to disclose symptoms to physically attractive physicians. It should be noted that female patient preferences for female doctors are moderated by other variables, such as doctor experience (Plunkett et al., 2002), patient age, and education (Bertakis et al., 1995; Brink-Muinen et al., 1994). One survey showed that younger women were more likely than their older counterparts to favor female general practitioners (Brink-Muinen et al., 1994).

There has been little research into patient preferences for practitioner age. Most patients value medical experience (Plunkett et al., 2002), which is confounded with age. Interesting questions that have not yet been addressed include whether age preferences are different for GPs versus consultants and whether people tend to prefer doctors of an age similar to their own.

Patients (particularly women) tend to prefer doctors from the same ethnic background as their own and with whom they can communicate in their native language (Ahmad et al., 1989, 2002; Kapphahn et al., 1999). Ahmad et al. (1989) studied Caucasian, Pakistani, and Indian patients attending a general practice in Bradford who were seeing either an Asian man (fluent in Urdu, Hindi, Punjabi, and English) or a Caucasian woman. They found that 80% of the Asian doctor's patients were Pakistani or Indian, whilst over two thirds of the Caucasian doctor's female patients were Caucasian. Even though 62% of Pakistani women patients reported that they would object to being examined by a male doctor, the majority of them actually chose to consult the male Asian doctor. Ahmad et al. concluded "the linguistic and broad cultural concordance between the patient and the general practitioner was more important in the choice of doctor than the sex of the general practitioner" (p. 153).

Ahmad et al. (2002) found differences between Canadian women of European descent and their counterparts of South-Asian descent in terms of their preferences for family physicians. In particular, the former showed a preference for female physicians in life-threatening cases, whereas the latter showed a preference for female physicians in cases involving overall health care, general ailments, and gynecological issues.

It has been found in various studies (Ahmad et al., 2002; Kerssens et al., 1997; Young, 1979) that the degree to which doctor gender affects patient preferences depends on the type of health care being sought. Kerssens et al. (1997) investigated patient preferences for doctor gender across 13 different medical specialties, including surgeons, neurologists, psychiatrists, and social workers. Gender preferences were weak for instrumental health professionals like surgeons and anesthetists, but stronger for specialists who treat intimate and psychosocial health problems, such as gynecologists and GPs. Participants who expressed gender preferences cited the same reasons for their preference, irrespective of whether it was for a male or a female GP. Thus, participants favored male or female GPs because they made them feel at ease and were approachable and open.

Furnham, Petrides, and Temple (2006) asked a sample of 395 white, native English-speaking adults to rate eight medical doctors (general practitioners and consultants), representing all permutations of the following three attributes: age (< 35 vs. > 50), training location (UK vs. Asia), and gender. Approximately half the participants were allocated in a group with a condition involving an intimate type of health problem and the rest in a group with a nonintimate condition. Participants showed a preference for UK-trained doctors, although it was unclear whether this was due to the homogeneous composition of the sample. There were significant two-way interactions involving patient gender and donor gender in the first case and doctor age and training location in the second.

On the whole, Furnham et al.'s (2006) study's findings replicate findings from postal surveys (Nichols, 1987), "on-site" surveys (Ahmad et al., 1989, 2002), and interviews (Ford et al., 2003). However, women patients did not show a stronger preference for women doctors as reported elsewhere (Graffy, 1990). Male patients showed a stronger preference for male doctors (GPs) than female patients did for female doctors. They argued that it may be that this reflects a change in the sex ratio of doctors. Because the ratio has changed, males are perhaps becoming increasingly sensitive to the fact they may not be able to see a male doctor and therefore express a stronger preference.

Furnham et al. (2006) found male participants showed stronger preferences for male GPs than female participants did for female GPs, though they both favored their own sex as predicted. Female, but not male, GPs were rated higher by participants allocated the nonintimate condition than those allocated the intimate condition. In a related finding, Ahmad et al. (2002) found that female patient preferences for female, as opposed to male, doctors were much stronger for intimate health problems (gynecological, family, emotional issues, etc.) than for less intimate problems (flu, stomach ache, etc.). Males rated GPs trained in Asia higher than females did, though there was no such difference for UK-trained GPs.

Furnham et al. (2006) noted that the fact that there were fewer statistically significant effects for the consultant ratings (compared with the GP ratings) may be because patients believe, with some justification, that they have less choice when it comes to consultants and feel grateful to be able to see any qualified specialist. Nevertheless, it should be noted that the overall pattern of results was generally similar for GPs and consultants.

There remains more work to be done on doctor preference. There are probably main effects for the doctor, the patient, and the problem they are presenting with, but also interactions between these three variables.

Preferences for Psychological Counselors

What of those who seek "talking cures"? Overall it appears that clients prefer counselors, like doctors, of their own sex, age, and ethnicity. There is a fairly consistent literature focusing on schoolchildren, university students, and adults, showing that all prefer counselors of their own ethnic backgrounds. This appears to be more strongly the case for Black, for example, rather than White Americans (Abbott, Tollefson, & McDermott, 1982; Haviland, Horswill, O'Connell, & Dynneson, 1983; Wolkon, Moriwaki, & Williams, 1973). More generally, this same-ethnicity preference has been established all over the world from Malaysia to New Zealand (e.g., Atkinson, Wampold, Lowe, &

Ahn, 1998; Littrell, Hashim, & Scheiding, 1989; Turner & Manthei, 1986; but see Ang & Yeo, 2004).

There is also some evidence that clients of all sorts prefer same-sex counselors (Haviland et al., 1983; Littrell & Littrell, 1982). Although some studies show that clients discount the importance of sex on questionnaire-based studies of preference, there does appear to be a same-sex preference when more explicit measures of preference are used (Ang & Yeo, 2004; Littrell et al., 1989; Turner & Manthei, 1986). Specifically, women and younger patients show stronger same-sex and age preferences than men or older clients (Cooper, 2006). However, a wide range of potential confounding variables may influence these preferences, such as the client's age, experience of counseling, and the presenting problem (see Furnham et al., 2006; Turner & Manthei, 1986; Woodstock, Margavio, & Cotter, 2006).

Recently Furnham and Swami (2008) asked a representative British sample of 257 adults to indicate their preferences for eight psychological counselors differentiated by sex, age, and training location. A five-way mixed analysis of variance (participant sex and age as within variables, and counselor sex, age, ethnicity as between variables) indicated a significant main effect for only counselors' ethnicity. There were also sex and age interactions showing evidence of a matching hypothesis: participants preferred counselors of their own sex and age.

They noted that there was strong evidence for a similarity, or matching, effect. Specifically, they found a strong interaction between counselor sex and participant sex, indicating a sex-matched preference. There was also a counselor age by participant age interaction, again in the direction of age-matched preferences. Also there was a significant main effect for only one counselor variable (ethnicity). These results are discussed in greater detail below.

The finding that only counselor ethnicity showed a significant effect was no doubt due to the fact that the large majority of participants were Britons of Caucasian descent. These participants likely showed a preference for British (or more accurately, perceived British) counselors who were locally trained. Neither the age nor sex of the hypothetical counselor showed significant main effects. Thus, female counselors were not preferred over males, or the middle-aged over the young. However, there was evidence of a similarity, or matching effect. Specifically, participants appeared to show a preference for counselors who were of the same sex and age as themselves.

When people seek out counselors and psychotherapists they know they might end up in many sessions "baring their soul" and discussing many highly intimate and sensitive issues. The same is true of executive coaches. Hence the choice is very important, although this is a rather unexplored field.

Preferences for Dentists

What work that does exist has tended to focus on dental practitioners' preferences for patients (Brennan & Spencer, 2006) or the influence of dentists' personalities or communication styles on practitioner-patient interactions (e.g., Street, 1989). Where patient preferences for dentists have been explicitly examined, the literature suggests little evidence of either sex- (AIHW, 2002; Stokes, Pack, & Spears, 1992) or racial-concordance (Bender, 2007; Hardie, Ransford, & Zernick, 1995). In contrast, one Australian survey did suggest a strong preference for younger and locally trained dentists (AIHW, 2002).

More recently Furnham and Swami (2009) asked a representative British sample of 257 adults to complete a questionnaire in which they indicated their preference for eight dentists stratified by sex, age, and training location. These data were analyzed in relation to participants' own sex and age, the latter stratified by a median split. A mixed analysis of variance indicated two main effects: A preference for younger (rather than older) dentists and dentists trained in Britain (rather than in Asia). There was also a significant two-way interaction between dentist age and training location: for the British-trained there was a preference for younger dentists, whereas for the Asian-trained there was a preference for older dentists.

The results showed that participants had a general preference for younger dentists and dentists trained in Britain. This is consistent with a previous survey of dental preferences (AIHW, 2002) and may reflect a proclivity for practitioners who are equipped with the most up-to-date techniques. For instance, participants may be aware of advances in dental surgery, which in turn feed into a preference for younger dentists who are trained in such techniques. The results showed that participants preferred locally trained dentists, which may reflect a preference for practitioners who share a similar cultural background with participants. This, in turn, may increase the likelihood of patient-practitioner understanding and empathy (e.g., Ahmad et al., 1989).

Clearly as dentistry becomes more sophisticated and cosmetic work is sought after, more research needs to be done in this area.

Lessons From Alternative and CM

One fundamentally important but neglected area of research is the doctor-patient encounter and more particularly how it differs between orthodox medicine OM) and CAM (complementary and alternative) practitioners. This may be part of the reason for the attractiveness of CAM. Taylor (1985) argued that scientific medicine sees the human body as a machine, like any other, which needs servicing. Patients, who are described as cases, should not distract the doctor by their unique personal feelings and experiences. Thus the orthodox doctor is teacher and facilitator, while the alternative practitioner is therapist. Taylor (1985) concluded that too many people have become accustomed to the sort of medicine which "relies on magic bullets administered by harassed physicians who cannot distinguish us one from another as we flow from waiting room to examination room to billing office" (p. 197).

Conventional medicine concentrates on sickness and alternative medicine concentrates on wellness. CAM practitioners seem to characterize orthodox medical practices as technological and aggressive and their own as natural and noninvasive.

The rise and fall of different healing systems is contingent in large part on the changing nature of the medical encounter in the traditional 6–8 min clinical consultation. When medicine can promise neither relief nor cure, the quality of the individual doctor-patient relationship is paramount. The consumer movement, the women's movement, and the more general demand for participation all focused on the medical consultation, but some traditional medical schools and practicing doctors have resisted populist demands and the pressure for democratization and customer service. Not only has medicine resisted change, but for many there has been a perceptible deterioration of the medical encounter in terms of "quality time" for the patient. Patients have neither a "voice option" in the medical encounter, nor an "exit option" to leave. Changing doctors, getting second opinions, and paying for insurance are very difficult particularly for older and less educated people; hence patients have to confront the many problematic aspects of the relationship with a conventional medical doctor.

What the modern Western patient (of all ages) wants, and appears not to be getting, is to be treated with individual respect; not to have to endure crowded waiting rooms, or be patronized. Being processed as a "case" not a person is a common complaint among many patients. Patients want to be treated as educated consumers, yet find they are still being met by a wall of clinical autonomy and a refusal to share information. Patients resent being faced by doctors who claim to have nothing to offer and do nothing, either because in their view treatments do not work or because the best policy is judged to be to do nothing. Many patients now want a consumer contract with equal responsibilities. Many patients complain that doctors do not trust them to make appropriate decisions about their health care (Furnham, 2003).

Thus for Taylor (1985) medicine is basically a professional relationship. The fate of CAM is determined not so much by the proven efficacy of its methods, but rather by orthodox practitioners being either unwilling or unable to deliver what the modern patient wants.

It is possible to compare and contrast the stereotypic CAM and OM consultation (Table 2) (Furnham, 2003). Sixteen differences are noted many of which suggest the CAM consultation would be more attractive to patients particularly the elderly: They get more time, with a more sympathetic doctor, who appears to have tremendous faith in his or her speciality. It is readily acknowledged that the table encourages stereotypes and is not empirically based.

It may be argued that the idea of comparison is essentially flawed for what is essentially an analysis of variance problem. That is that the variation is consultations *within* either OM or CM is of necessity greater than the variation *between* them. It concerns whether one can legitimately talk about any typical or average consultation. Thus it is inevitable and expected that an aromatherapist's consultation differs widely from that a homeopath. Similarly an osteopath will do quite different history taking and treatment from an iridologist. The same is true for conventional medicine: Consider how a psychiatrist and an orthopedic surgeon operate. Consider for instance that the nature of the patient's problem means that there may well be significant similarities between branches of CAM and OM in the treatment by osteopath and orthopedic surgeon.

Table 2. The stereotype CAM and OM consultation. A compare and contrast exercise

	CAM	OM
Time	More	Less
Touch	More	Less
Money	More	Less
History taking	Holistic	Specific
	Affective	Behavioral
Language	Healing	Cure
	Holistic	Dualistic
	Subjective	Objective
	Personal story	Case history
	Wellness	Illness
Patient role	Consumer	Sick role
Decision making	Shared/consumer	Doctor/paternalistic
Bedside manner	Charismatic	Cool
	Empathic	Professional
Sex ratio/role	F = M; feminine	M > F; masculine
Time spent talking	Patient > or = to practitioner	Practitioner > patient
Style	Authoritative	Authoritarian
	Supportive	Information/advice giving
	Counseling	
Confidence in methodology/ outcome	Very high	High
Client relationship	Long term	Short term
Consulting rooms	Counseling	Clinical
Practitioner history	Second profession	First profession
Ideology	Strong	Moderate
	Left wing	Middle way

There are two further problems which make comparisons problematic. The first is that there may be within each CAM or OM specialty different "schools of thought" which results in different types (styles) of consultations. Secondly and inevitably there is the issue of individual differences of practitioner (their personality, biography, education, and experience). In this sense it is difficult to suggest that there is ever such a thing as a typical consultation. However, despite these acknowledged problems it may be that it is the medical encounter which "sells" the treatment best. There is considerable research to suggest that patient compliance is best predicted by the patient evaluation of the consultation. Certainly the consultation may account for why patients stay with, and/or leave, a particular practitioner for a specific problem (Furnham, 2003).

Wyatt and Furnham (2010) investigated the question of whether users and nonusers of CM wanted different things from the consultation. They gave nearly 200 people a 58-item questionnaire that asked how important, or not, various aspects of the consultation were. The aspects rated of highest importance by participants were: "Practitioner giving you their full attention," "Practitioner presenting the diagnosis in an understandable way," "Feel you are being listened to by the practitioner," "Practitioner giving detailed explanation of your condition/diagnosis at the end of the consultation," and "Practitioner discussing treatment options with you." These aspects are concerned with attention and listening, and a focus on the patient, but also information giving is rated equally important. The statement rated of lowest of importance included a number of practitioner attributes, "the race of the practitioner," "the gender of the practitioner," "the age of the practitioner" but also "practitioner questioning you about your general values and beliefs in life" (Table 3).

Females placed more importance on the practitioner explaining diagnoses and discussing treatments with high patient involvement. Older, less educated, and more religious individuals were found to place higher importance on practitioners' appearance and attributes, including race, age, gender, and dress sense.

Wyatt and Furnham (2010) revealed that the majority of individuals place highest importance on the practitioner giving them their full attention and listening, and giving them full information they can understand. The high preference for information giving supports previous findings (Beisecker, 1990; Blanchard, Labrecque, Ruckdeschel, & Blanchard, 1988; Zebiene et al., 2004) although this study found it to be right at the top for importance whereas others (Wensing et al., 1998) had it lower down on the preference list after "competency" and "patient involvement in decisions." The practitioner being attentive and listening to the patient are aspects of a consultation which have shown up repeatedly in research, they are typical features of a patient-centred approach. Participants placed lowest importance on the practitioner's attributes including the race, gender, and age of the practitioner, and also the practitioner questioning them about their general values and beliefs in life.

Interestingly, users and nonusers of CM do not differ in their views of a consultation, possibly reflecting the changing preferences of society. The majority of the public now favor an egalitarian relationship with their practitioner and patients have taken on the role of consumers desiring information and someone to listen to them.

This recent study demonstrated that users and non-users of CM place the same importance on patient-centred aspects of a consultation. This is probably because of the shift in society away from physician-centred consultations and firmly on the patient in orthodox medical encounters, taking the same stance as the complementary medical egalitarian relationship as a means to a more successful consultation for both patient and doctor. The public is now approaching health care as another consumer product where they are forming expectations of how they should be treated. Every patient is distinct and practitioners have to be sensitive to their individual differences; the patients' age, education, gender, personality, beliefs, and their perception of the state of their health will all affect how they want to be approached. Despite these differences, across complementary and orthodox medical users all individuals on the whole want the same thing from their practitioner in a

Table 3. A factor analysis of the 58 questions showing five clear factors

Factors	Statement
Practitioner listening and talking time	Practitioner allowing you to tell your story in your own words
	Practitioner discussing the effect of your symptoms on your quality of life
	Time for a detailed discussion of your problems
	Practitioner summarizing what you have told them after you have finished presenting your list of symptoms
	Practitioner listening to all the information even if you thing it is irrelevant
	Practitioner displaying open-mindedness and considering every possibility rather than the most obvious
Appearance/atmosphere of consultation room/ practitioners display of warmth	Relaxing atmosphere in the consultation room
	Cleanliness of the consultation room
	Tidiness of the consultation room
	Practitioner displaying a warm personality
	Practitioner displaying sensitivity
Practitioner giving information and discussing treatments	Practitioner giving detailed explanation of your condition/diagnosis at the end of the consultation
	Practitioner giving you their full attention
	Practitioner discussing treatment options with you
	High level of participation by you in making treatment decisions
Practitioners' appearance and attributes	The gender of the practitioner
	The dress sense of the practitioner (e.g., smart and casual)
	The age of the practitioner
	The race of the practitioner
	First language of the practitioner
Topics questioned by practitioner	Practitioner questioning you about your diet
	Practitioner questioning you about your lifestyle
	Practitioner questioning you about your general values and beliefs in life

consultation; the practitioner to listen to what they have to say and provide them with information in answer to their problems.

Conclusion

When people seek out professionals they usually have a number of criteria they use. These include professional competence as well as communication skills. However there are many other factors of relevance. For instance consider the criteria that people are advised to consider when seeking out a business coach. These include confidentiality; clarity of communication and the ability to listen carefully; and understanding of the client's and the coachee's (the person being coached) needs. The best coaches manage to combine sensitivity with strength of character that enables them to challenge the coachee effectively. These are questions/issues which the would-be coach is encouraged to ask. They seem equally applicable to those in the medical world:

Training: Has the coach/practitioner undergone formal, independently accredited training or qualified in the use of therapies and tests? Do they have relevant qualifications in psychology/the speciality which indicates a deeper level of knowledge about human behavior? Is there evidence of continuing professional development – courses, reading professional journals, and current business awareness?

Experience: What is the coach's/practitioners background? Are they familiar with how business works? Do they have experience at a senior level?

Style and chemistry: Does the coach/practitioner inspire a sense of trust, motivation or positive energy in the coachee? If they do, there is a good chance that the relationship will yield dividends. Is the coach's/practitioners style broadly in line with yours or is it too flamboyant/conservative?

Intellectual framework: What is the theoretical framework for coaching? If the coach only has a background in psychotherapy, pop psychology or sport, chances are they will not be delivering business coaching. The coach must indicate how he/she works and outline a program: Boundaries of the relationship must be discussed and agreed before work begins and a clear statement reached about confidentiality and timeframes for achieving goals.

Measuring success: A professional coach will give some indication of how the success (or not) of the program will be measured. This can be difficult because the process is very personal, but companies should insist on performance goals. Another option is to collect feedback from colleagues before and after the coaching program.

Supervision: Does the coach/practitioner have formal supervision for his or her caseload? Supervision supports a coach/practitioner and assists learning. It also helps them maintain perspective, preventing them getting lost in their own judgments, organizational politics, or the coachee's "reality."

Self-awareness: Why is the coach coaching or the practitioner practicing? To help others or to help themselves? Answers to this question will give a good insight into the coach's level of self-awareness. Remember, if they are not aware of their own make-up they are unlikely to be able to understand or help anyone else.

What is perhaps most interesting in this area of the choice of professional is how few differences there are between the criteria for choosing any sort of profession be it a doctor or a dentist, a counselor or a coach. Inevitably there will be individual differences associated with culture, demography, gender, and personality that mean certain selection criteria are emphasized over others.

References

Abbott, K., Tollefson, N., & McDermott, D. (1982). Counsellor race as a factor in counsellor preference. *Journal of College Student Personnel, 23*, 36–40.

Ahmad, F., Hansa, G., Rawlins, J., & Stewart, D. E. (2002). Preferences for gender of family physician among Canadian European-descent and South-Asian immigrant women. *Family Practice, 19*, 146–153.

Ahmad, W. I. U., Kernohan, E. E. M., & Baker, M. R. (1989). Patients' choice of general practitioner: Influence of patients' fluency in English and the ethnicity and sex of the doctor. *Journal of the Royal College of General Practitioners, 39*, 153–155.

AIHW Dental Statistics and Research Unit. (2002). *Public perceptions of dentistry: Stimulus or barrier to better oral health? (AIHW Cat. No. DEN 96)*. Adelaide: AIHW Dental Statistics and Research Unit.

Alroy, G., Ber, R., & Kramer, D. (1984). An evaluation of the short-term effects of an interpersonal skills course. *Medical Education, 18*, 85–98.

Ang, R., & Yeo, L. (2004). Asian secondary school students' help seeking behaviour and preferences for counsellor characteristics. *Pastoral Care, 12*, 40–48.

Arborelius, E., & Bremberg, S. (1992). What doctors do to achieve a successful consultation? *Family Practice, 9*, 61–66.

Argyle M. (Ed.), (1981). *Social skills and health*. London, UK: Methuen.

Atkinson, D., Wampold, B., Lowe, S., & Ahn, H. (1998). Asian American preferences for counsellor characteristics. *Counselling Psychologist, 26*, 101–123.

Beisecker, A., & Beisecker, T. (1990). Patient information seeking behaviour when communicating with doctors. *Medical Care, 28*, 19–28.

Bender, D. J. (2007). Patients preference for a racially or gender-concordant student dentist. *Journal of Dental Education, 71*, 726–745.

Bertakis, K. L., Helms, L. J., Callahan, E. J., Azari, R., & Robbins, J. A. (1995). The influence of gender on physician practice style. *Medical Care, 33*, 407–416.

Blanchard, C., Labrecque, M., Ruckdeschel, J., & Blanchard, E. (1988). Information and decision making preferences of hospitalized adult cancer patients. *Social Science and Medicine, 27*, 1139–1145.

Braman, A. C., & Gomez, R. (2004). Patient personality predicts preference for relationships with doctors. *Personality and Individual Differences, 37*, 815–826.

Brennan, D., & Spencer, A. (2006). Dentists preferences for patients. *International Journal of Behavioural Medicine, 13*, 69–79.

Brink-Muinen, A. V. D., Bakker, D. H. D., & Bensing, J. M. (1994). Consultations for women's health problems: Factors influencing women's choice of sex of general practitioner. *British Journal of General Practitioners, 44*, 205–210.

Cooper, M. (2006). Scottish secondary school students' preferences for location, format of counselling and sex of counsellor. *School of Psychology International, 27*, 627–638.

Derose, K. P., Hays, R. D., McCaffrey, D. E., & Baker, D. W. (2001). Does physician gender affect satisfaction of men and women visiting the emergency department? *Journal of General Internal Medicine, 16*, 218–226.

Elstad, J. I. (1994). Women's priorities regarding physician behaviour and their preference for a female physician. *Women and Health, 21*, 1–19.

Faulder, C. (1985). *Whose body is it?* London, UK: Virago.

Ford, S., Schofield, T., & Hope, T. (2003). What are the ingredients for a successful evidence-based patient's choice consultation? *Social Science and Medicine, 56*, 589–602.

Furnham, A. (1983). Research in social skills training. In R. Ellis & D. Whittington (Eds.), *New directions in social skills training* (pp. 266–293). London, UK: Croom Helm.

Furnham, A. (1985). Social skills training: A European perspective. In L. L'Abate & M. Milan (Eds.), *Handbook of social skills training and research*. New York, NY: Wiley.

Furnham, A. (2003). Why do the elderly use complementary and alternative medicine? In P. Chernaick & N. Chernaick (Eds.), *Alternative medicine for the elderly* (pp. 9–25). Berlin, Germany: Springer.

Furnham, A., King, D., & Pendleton, D. (1980). Establishing rapport: Interaction effects and occupational therapy. *British Journal of Occupational Therapy, 43*, 322–325.

Furnham, A., Petrides, K., & Temple, J. (2006). Patient preferences for medical doctors. *British Journal of Health Psychology, 11*, 439–449.

Furnham, A., & Swami, V. (2008). Patient preferences for psychological counsellors: Evidence of a similarity effect. *Counseling Psychology Quarterly, 21*, 361–370.

Furnham, A., & Swami, V. (2009). Patient preferences for dentists. *Psychology Health and Medicine, 14*, 143–149.

Graffy, J. (1990). Patient choice in a practice with men and women general practitioners. *British Journal of General Practice, 40*, 13–15.

Hardie, R., Ransford, E., & Zernick, J. (1995). Dental patients' perceptions in a multi-ethnic environment. *Journal of the California Dental Association, 23*, 77–80.

Haviland, M., Horswill, R., O'Connell, J., & Dynneson, V. (1983). Native American college students' preferences for counsellor race and sex and the likelihood of their use of a counselling centre. *Journal of Counseling Psychology, 30*, 267–270.

Heaton, C. J., & Marquez, J. T. (1990). Patient preference for physician gender in the male genital/ rectal exam. *Family Practice Research Journal, 10*, 105–115.

Hopkins, E. (1967). The study of patients' choice of doctor in an urban practice. *Journal of Royal College of General Practitioners, 14*, 282.

Kaplan, S. H., Gandek, B., Greenfield, S., Rogers, W., & Ware, J. E. (1995). Patient and visit characteristics related to physicians' participatory decision-making style: Results from the Medical Outcomes Study. *Medical Care, 33*, 1176–1187.

Kapphahn, C. J., Wilson, K. M., & Klein, J. D. (1999). Adolescent girls' and boys' preferences for provider gender and confidentiality in their health care. *Journal of Adolescent Health, 25*, 131–142.

Kerssens, J. J., Bensing, J. M., & Abdela, M. G. (1997). Patient preference for genders of health professionals. *Social Science and Medicine, 44*, 1531–1540.

King, J., Pendleton, D., & Tate, P. (1985). *Making the most of your doctor: A family guide to dealing with your GP*. London: Methuen.

Kleinman, A. (1980). *Patients and healers in the context of culture*. Berkeley, CA: University of California Press.

Little, P., Everitt, H., Williamson, I., Warner, G., Moore, M., Gould, . . . Payne, S. (2001). Preferences of patients for patient centred approach to consultation in primary care: observational study. *British Medical Journal, 322*, 468–472.

Littrell, J., Hashim, A., & Scheiding, S. (1989). Malaysian students' preferences for counsellors. *International Journal of the Advancement of Counselling, 12*, 181–190.

Littrell, J., & Littrell, M. (1982). Counsellor-client matching on ethnicity, gender and language. *North American Journal of Psychology, 4*, 367–380.

Lloyd, M., & Bor, R. (2004). *Communication skills in medicine* (2nd ed.). London, UK: Churchill Livingstone.

Marvel, M., Epstein, R., Flowers, K., & Beckham, H. (1999). Soliciting the patient's agenda. *Journal of the American Medical Association, 281*, 283–287.

McGuire, P. (1986). Social skills training for professionals. In C. Hollin & P. Trower (Eds.), *Handbook of social skills training* (pp. 143–165). Oxford, UK: Pergamon.

McKinstry, B. (2000). Do patients wish to be involved in decision making in the consultation? A cross sectional survey with video vignettes. *British Medical Journal, 321*, 867–871.

Nichols, S. (1987). Women's preferences for sex of a doctor: A postal survey. *Journal of the Royal College of General Practitioners, 37*, 540–543.

Ong, L., De Haes, C., Hoos, A., & Lammes, F. (1995). Doctor-patient communication: A review of the literature. *Social Science and Medicine, 40*, 903–918.

Pendleton, D. & Hasler, J. (Eds.), (1983). *Doctor-patient communication*. London, UK: Academic Press.

Phillips, D., & Brooks, F. (1998). Women patients' preferences for female or male GPs. *Family Practice, 15*, 543–547.

Plunkett, B. A., Kohli, P., & Milad, M. P. (2002). The importance of physician gender in the selection of an obstetrician or a gynecologist. *American Journal of Obstetrics and Gynaecology, 185*, 926–928.

Roter, D., Hall, J., & Katz, N. (1988). Patient physician communication: A descriptive summary of the literature. *Patient Education and Counselling, 12*, 99.

Schofield, T. (1983). The application of the study of communication skills in training for general practice. In D. Pendleton & J. Hasler (Eds.), *Doctor-patient communication*. (pp. 259–271). London, UK: Academic Press.

Shepherd, D., & Hammond, P. (1984). Self-Assessment of specific skills of medical undergraduates using immediate feedback through closed-circuit television. *Medical Education, 18*, 80–84.

Smith, R. C., & Hoppe, R. B. (1991). The patient's story: Integrating the patient- and physician-centred approaches to interviewing. *Annals of Internal Medicine, 115*, 470.

Stewart, M., Brown, J., Levenstein, J., McCracken, E., & McWhinney, I. R. (1986). The patient-centred clinical method, changes in residents' performance over two months of training. *Family Practice, 3*, 164–167.

Stokes, J., Pack, A., & Spears, G. (1992). A comparison of patients' perception of dental care offered by male and female dentists in New Zealand. *International Dental Journal, 42*, 217–222.

Street, R. (1989). Patients' satisfaction with dentists' communicative style. *Health Communication, 1*, 137–154.

Suarez-Almazor, M. (2004). Patient-physician communication. *Current Opinion in Rheumatology, 16*, 91–95.

Taylor, R. (1985). Alternative medicine and the medical encounter in Britain and the United States. In W. Salmon (Ed.), *Alternative medicine: Popular policy and perspectives*. London, UK: Tavistock.

Turner, G., & Manthei, R. (1986). Students' expressed and actual preferences for counsellors race and sex. *International Journal for the Advancement of Counselling, 9*, 351–362.

Vincent, C., & Furnham, A. (1996). Why do patients turn to complementary medicine? An empirical study. *British Journal of Clinical Psychology, 35*, 37–48.

Vincent, C., & Furnham, A. (1997). *Complementary medicine: A research perspective*. Chichester, UK: Wiley.

Waller, K. (1998). Women doctors for women patients? *British Journal of Medical Psychology, 61*, 125–135.

Weisman, C. S., & Teitelbaum, M. A. (1985). Physician gender and the physician patient relationship: Recent evidence and relevant questions. *Social Science and Medicine, 20*, 1119–1127.

Wensing, M., Jung, H. P., Mainz, J., Olesen, F., & Grol, R. (1998). A systematic review of the literature on patient priorities for general practice care. Part 1: Description of the research domain. *Social Science and Medicine, 47*, 1573–1588.

Wolkon, G., Moriwaki, S., & Williams, K. (1973). Race and social class as factors in the orientation towards psychotherapy. *Journal of Counselling Psychology, 20*, 312–316.

Woodstock, S., Margavio, C., & Cotter, L. (2006). Gender and race matching preferences for HIV post-test counselling in an African-American sample. *AIDS Care, 18*, 49–53.

Wyatt, B., & Furnham, A. (2010). The medical consultation: What do users and non-users of CAM value. *Focus on Alternative and Complementary Therapies, 15*, 88–96.

Young, J. W. (1979). Symptom disclosure to male and female physicians: Effects of sex, physical attractiveness, and symptom type. *Journal of Behavioural Medicine, 2*, 159–169.

Zebiene, E., Razgauskas, E., Basys, V., Baubiniene, A., Gurevicius, R., Padaiga, Z., & Svab, I. (2004). Meeting patient's expectations in primary care consultations in Lithuania. *International Journal of Qualitative Health Care, 16*, 83–89.

Training the Trainers

Dinesh Bhugra[1] and Gurvinder Kalra[2]

[1]Health Service and Population Research Department, Institute of Psychiatry,
King's College London, UK
[2]Department of Psychiatry, Lokmanya Tilak Municipal Medical College and Lokmanya Tilak
Municipal General Hospital, Sion, Mumbai, India

The practice of psychiatry and medicine does not occur in a vacuum and it is strongly influenced by the society and culture in which it is practiced. It is inevitable that society will determine resources in training and salaries. Professionalism is about primacy of patient welfare, managing resources effectively, ethical practice, and altruistic service. In recent years, there have been many challenges to professionalism in the USA and the UK. These are related to various medical scandals in the UK, Health Maintenance Organisation (HMO) interference in patterns of offering treatment, and various other factors thus affecting healthcare regulation. Instilling professionalism and leadership skills at an early stage in medical training in general and psychiatric training in particular is crucial not only for better care but also for acceptance by patients and families. Doctors are still by far the most trusted group, certainly in the UK, with overwhelming public support, but this trust has to be earned and cannot be taken for granted. It is the responsibility of senior consultants who teach the next generation of professionals and also play a part in delivering of health services to healthcare consumers. Training is at the heart of learning by experience. Learning best takes place when there is a comfortable environment with peers, individual commitment and involvement with the planning of the actual learning process, control of the learning process, an awareness of learning needs, support, and opportunity for feedback and reflection. In this chapter we explore not only the attributes of professionalism and leadership but also the role of training, and its components are described along with various tools for trainers and the implications of different approaches. Training of the trainers is important for a number of reasons. These include giving a scientific grounding in principles of learning and training but also highlighting responsibility and providing peer support in order to deliver the foundation for the future of psychiatric training and practice. Trainers are individuals who have taken on the responsibility of training, whether the trainees are junior doctors or other professionals who may play different roles in the team. The importance of training the trainers lies in not simply homogenizing the training but the process makes trainers aware of their own weaknesses and strengths so that the best can be achieved.

In these rapidly changing times educators and mentors have to learn how to best nurture the sensitivities, insights, and skills of the trainees so that they are able to address the ethical aspects of their work each day (Roberts, 2009).

Psychiatry: A Specialty

The authors of this chapter, being psychiatrists themselves, focus their examples on the psychiatric profession but all these concepts are applicable to other specialties in medicine, too. Psychiatry as a specialty has evolved over the years from being an analytic medicine to being a therapeutic specialty. Until the 19th century, the specialists were known as alienists and the focus was on containment so training was the model of apprenticeship which had its advantages and disadvantages. Advantages were close proximity and learning by observation and following the examples. The key disadvantage was a strong likelihood of learning poor practice and having no other models to compare with if the individual worked with only one mentor. This started to change toward the beginning of the last century in the UK at least. As a medical specialty psychiatry makes an effort to understand the psyche of man, not only from an analytical perspective but also from biological and social perspectives. The role of a psychiatrist has changed dramatically in the last few decades and the psychiatric services have simultaneously evolved along with these changing roles. The psychiatrist as a professional has evolved from being a passive listener to an active leader, and the psychiatric practice has evolved from the mental asylums and analytic couch to the modern day consultation liaison services and services over the Internet. At the same time, the specialty has seen the development of various subspecialties, including child and adolescent psychiatry and psychiatry of old age and that of learning disability, addiction psychiatry, and forensic psychiatry, to mention just a few. These rapid changes in the field along with an expansion in our knowledge base, technology advances, and the associated changes in service delivery have challenged our assumptions of training in the subject. It is inevitable that with increased specialization the skill-set changes. With newer technological advancements, old certainties and patterns are giving way to more personalized and individualized training.

The specialty of psychiatry differs from other medical specialties in that it takes an in-depth analytic and holistic view of the patient. It seems to be the only specialty that sees how the past affects the future and how an attempt can be made to change the future or at least a change in perspective toward the future. It would not be wrong to say that everything is psychiatry and nothing is also psychiatry, which means that psychiatry deals with nothingness and also deals with everythingness [sic]. Dealing with uncertainty and ambiguity are at the heart of psychiatric practice and these qualities need to be highlighted and trainees encouraged to identify their responses and ability to deal with these. To teach such varied dimensions in the subject, the trainers have to keep coming up with newer and more innovative methods of teaching that will keep put the interest of the trainee in the subject. The values of excellence, self-sacrifice, and accountability are at the heart of every profession, and they serve as the foundation of public trust in medicine (Roberts & Dyer, 2004) and form the basis of our privilege to enter into the lives of our patients in such a deeply personal and distinct way (Roberts, 2009). The relationship between the trainer and the trainee is almost never

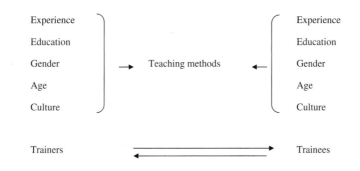

Figure 1. Inter-relationship between trainees and trainer.

equal. The trainer by virtue of their experience and other factors, including knowledge, will have a degree of power over the trainee as illustrated in Figure 1.

The Psychiatric Trainer

The psychiatrist, let us assume that she/he is a consultant, will have to connect with the patients at a personal level on certain occasions. These consultations can give rise to varied issues like transference from the patient's side and counter-transference from the consultant's side. Psychiatric consultants may have to fulfill multiple roles apart from being a clinician (who treats the patients in distress), a teacher (who teaches undergraduates, postgraduates, and other professionals), a manager (managing time, teams, and resources efficiently and effectively), and a professional (see Figure 2). The trainer may have to act as an efficient trainer for the psychiatric trainees in addition to acting as a mentor to them and an advocate to the general public. The word "trainer" in this chapter is used to describe trainers, supervisors and others supporting the learning and assessment of the trainee doctors.

The Canadian Medical Education Directives for Specialists (CanMEDS) model proposed by the Royal College of Physicians and Surgeons of Canada (RCPSC) espouses these multiple roles that a physician has to play (see Figure 2). This model, created by the RCPSC in 1996, discusses certain key competencies that are needed for medical education and practice which ultimately lead to an improvement in patient care (About CanMEDS, 2007). It has been effectively used in certain other specialty education worldwide (Chou, Cole, McLaughlin, & Lockyer, 2008) like surgery (Frank & Langer, 2003) and dermatology (Freiman, Natsheh, Barankin, & Shear, 2006). A similar model was later proposed by the Accreditation Council of Graduate Medical Education (ACGME) Outcomes Project that suggested six desirable competencies in physicians. However, the ACGME has also devised tools of assessment methods for educators to teach and evaluate various core competencies (Macneily, 2007), something which was

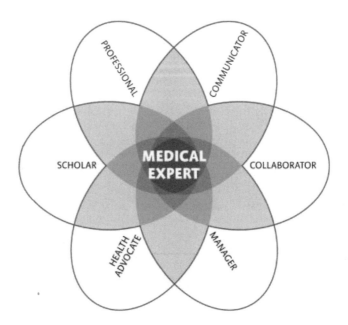

Figure 2. The CanMEDS model.

lacking in the CanMEDS. Nevertheless, the general goal of both projects was to foster the necessity of the broader roles that a physician has to play, beyond just being a medical expert.

The CanMEDS model has been used by the Royal College of Psychiatrists in the UK in describing the role of the psychiatrist (RCPsych, 2010). We deploy this model to illustrate the role of the trainer in psychiatric training. It is helpful to have a description of the various components of the CanMEDS model in understanding the roles and responsibilities.

Medical Expert

At the heart of psychiatric practice is the role of the psychiatrist as a doctor because of their medical training. Here we must emphasize that medical training and the term used in this context is much broader than simply using an organic or physical-medical model. Here medicine also includes social and anthropological factors. Being a medical expert means that the psychiatric consultant has to have sufficient clinical knowledge and skills to perform appropriate assessments of patients and when to use various preventive and therapeutic interventions effectively. They must also be capable of recognizing the limits of their expertise and should not refrain from seeking appropriate and timely consultation from other health professionals. The CanMEDS model encourages optimal, ethical, and patient-centered medical care.

Communicator

The ability to communicate is the primary factor that distinguishes humans from animals and it is the ability to communicate well that distinguishes one individual from another. Communication skills are perhaps the most important in psychiatry. The psychiatric consultant ought to have sufficient communication and interpersonal skills, and should be able to understand not only what is being said but also what is *not* being said. The communication skills of consultants go a long way in helping them to establish sufficient rapport with the patients and their families, which acts as a foundation for the doctor-patient relationship. These skills help the consultant to elicit and synthesize all the relevant information from patients and their families to reach a diagnosis and also accurately convey the relevant information and explanations to them for effective management. It is important to note that the messages conveyed to the patients and their families have to be clear and free of any jargon. Better communication skills also help in maintaining better interpersonal relationships between team members, who in the long run form the face of the institution and reflect the work culture of that particular institution. Good communication skills are also required for public education and informing the media.

Collaborator (Team Player)

Being able to collaborate with different disciplines in the medical field is an everyday necessity for psychiatrists working in multi-disciplinary teams, which form the backbone of the patient management systems. The psychiatric consultant should be able to collaborate and effectively participate in these inter-professional healthcare teams, and, at times, may also be required to effectively work with other professionals to prevent, negotiate, and resolve inter-professional conflict that may arise anytime during the course of working together. This collaboration and close working is also significant for the psychiatrists in their relationships with managers, politicians, and various policy makers.

Manager

As mentioned above the psychiatrist as the trainer must be capable of effectively managing the organization and the staff, their own time, the allocated resources, and thus enhance the effectiveness of their organization. Being an effective manager also includes the ability to allocate the limited healthcare resources appropriately and in a balanced way to the healthcare consumers. Good management is directed toward coordinating activities in order to get a job done efficiently and effectively thereby producing order and consistency in the therapeutic processes that occur.

Health Advocate

Although the health needs of individual patients form the core of what the clinical practice is about, the health needs of the community at large cannot and must not be ignored. The psychiatrist therefore should be able to identify the various determinants of health of the populations that they serve. They should take initiatives in leading various advocacy groups and help in promoting the health of the population. This is important for the simple reason that doctors are the people who have the potential to influence the general public (Northouse, 2009), due to the position that they hold. They have the capacity or potential to influence and affect the beliefs, attitudes, and courses of action of others.

Scholar

The knowledge base in the entire medical field is ever-increasing. In order to be updated about the recent advances in the field, one has to keep up-to-date with journals or through conferences and continuing medical education programs. This updated knowledge can be then used to facilitate the learning of patients and their families, students, resident trainees, other health professionals involved in the healthcare teams, the public and others, as appropriate. The consultants should not only stay limited at being the end-users of these updates, but should also contribute to the creation, dissemination, and translation of new medical knowledge and practices.

Professional

The ability to make sound decisions with full professionalism defines the truly good doctor (Feudtner & Christakis, 1994; Inui, 2003). Teaching professionalism through formal curricula is important in helping develop new generations of compassionate and responsible physicians (Schwartz, Kotwicki, & McDonald, 2009) and psychiatrists. The psychiatrist should be aware of the appropriate personal and interpersonal behaviors and should be able to deliver the highest quality care with compassion. He/she should be fully aware of the locally prevalent sociocultural and ethicolegal issues and also respect patient's confidentiality, which is one of the core concepts of professionalism (Graham, 2006). Awareness of the privileges and limits of one's role as physician, as well as recognition and respect for the patient as a human being are all central to an ethical medical and psychiatric practice (Lapid, Moutier, Dunn, Hammond, & Roberts, 2009).

These roles are relevant for the trainees to be aware of and the trainers must enable the trainees to develop these skills. They must be willing to learn these in the training period and beyond so that these skills serve as the standards of practice for their long-term career. Professionalism is not guaranteed by simply issuing a graduation or post-graduation degree. For many years acquisition of professional values occurred largely informally during the residency training, but these are no longer sufficient and efficient to help the students deal with the increasingly complex ethical questions that arise in the day-to-day clinical practice these days (Swick, Szenas, Danoff, & Whitcomb, 1999). Training in ethics and professionalism is a fundamental component of residency education, but there is little information to guide any curricula on the same (Civaner, Sarikaya, & Balcioglu, 2009; Goold & Stern, 2006). Ethics education is gradually being recognized as a solution to many of the professional challenges in medicine. Today's patient is more updated and well informed and ready to openly question the honesty, integrity, and management of their treating psychiatrist. This makes it all the more important for ethics education to be made a part of the undergraduate and graduate training programs, and this has been demonstrated by Roberts, Warner, Hammond, Geppert, and Heinrich (2005) who emphasize the importance of ethics education directed at practical real-world dilemmas and ethically important professional developmental issues for the physicians in training. Diverse methods can be used in this endeavor, such as individual clinical supervision and mentoring, consultation with experts, didactic and small group learning, and formal education (Christakis & Feudtner, 1993). Braunack-Mayer (2001) warns that the ethics curricula should cover the day-to-day moral struggles faced by early career psychiatrists and not concentrate on rarely encountered situations.

Apart from the CanMEDS key competencies, there are other characteristics that make a good psychiatrist. We believe these to be increasingly important.

Mentor

Mentoring can be simply defined as the process in which one person (the mentor) encourages and nurtures the development of another person (mentee) during the course of one's career, leading to the development of a relationship between the two whether it is short-term or long-term. As mentoring is a two-way process, as is any therapeutic intervention, when carried out properly it also allows for the development of the mentor.

Academic mentorship is a complex relationship and a professional development strategy that enables budding and developing professionals to take advantage of the skills and expertise of the experienced and senior members for their own professional growth (Wang, 2001). Some of the mentoring functions aim at the mentees' academic growth and others at personal growth. It has been suggested that for some individuals influential mentors were second in importance only to education as a factor in their career success (International Executive's Profile, 1990). A mentor serves as role model, counselor, and advocate for an understudy or protégé (Pellegrini, 2006). Various studies have demonstrated the importance of mentoring in the career development of resident trainees (Donovan,

2009, 2010). Trainees themselves perceive mentoring as important and it has been suggested that these mentorship programs should be incorporated in the residency training programs (Flint, Jahangir, Browner, & Mehta, 2009; Gurgel, Schiff, Flint, Miller, Zahtz, Smith, Fried, & Smith, 2010). Residents with mentors, residents in mentoring programs, and residents who selected their own mentors had higher satisfaction with their training environment than those who did not have any formal mentoring program (Flint et al., 2009). In psychiatric training, Lis, Wood, Petkova, and Shatkin (2009) pointed out that having a clearly defined mentor was associated with twice the odds for feeling well-prepared to practice psychiatry upon graduation compared with those who did not have a clearly defined mentor. In specialties like surgery, mentored surgical residency graduates were likely to enter the same specialty and practice type as their mentor (McCord, McDonald, Sippel, Leverson, Mahvi, & Weber, 2009).

Mentoring plays a critical role in setting a standard and a model for all those individuals who want to be involved in research (Fuller, 2000) and continues to evolve as a service in the psychiatric profession. It has been rightly said that mentors have the ability to inspire confidence in others, push them to their limits, and continue to develop them to their greatest potential (Schrubbe, 2004). They are the people who can see more in the mentee than the mentee can see in themselves. They thus have the ability to guide the mentees to identify their strengths, abilities, and potentials for growth and create a vision and development plan in which the mentee has a clear stake. An effective mentor facilitates the development of independence, self-confidence, job satisfaction, upward mobility, and decision-making and problem-solving skills in the understudy or protégé (Gordon, 2000) but also avoids the development of dependence. Successful mentoring of resident physicians has been linked to several beneficial outcomes for trainees, such as increased research productivity, enhanced career satisfaction, and increased retention in academics (Donovan, 2010). On the other hand, a lack of mentors has been shown to be related to the trainees losing interest in pursuing a career in academic training (Reck, Stratman, Vogel, & Mukesh, 2006). It is interesting to know that female residents may have a greater difficulty in establishing mentoring relationships than male residents and thus have specific mentoring needs that need to be addressed (Donovan, 2010). These factors may be related to gender roles and gender role expectations but also to a number of other factors, such as lack of time, less than full-time training, to mention among a few.

Residency programs should consider establishing formal mentorship programs and encourage residents to select their own mentors (Flint et al., 2009). The mentees should actively involve themselves in the development of mentoring programs in their institutions. An equally proactive attitude from the mentor's side is also required for a successful mentorship program. Mentors should be sincere in their dealings with mentees, be able to listen actively and patiently, understanding the mentees' needs and should treat the mentee as an equal, willing to learn from them and not just teach and guide the mentee. Maintaining a nonjudgmental attitude in approach towards the mentee's problems and life-situations is also important as much as being flexible enough to be able to shift roles while dealing with the mentee. Successful mentoring also requires commitment and interpersonal skills of both the mentor and the mentee apart from a facilitating environment at academic institutions (Sambunjak, Straus, & Marusic, 2010). Barriers to mentoring can result from personal factors (related to both the mentor and the mentee), relational difficulties and institutional and administrative barriers. For the training in mentoring to work both the mentor and the mentee have to have the time, institutional support, and adequate resources to ensure that training and support take place.

Psychological Mindedness

Of the various characteristics, a good psychiatrist needs to be psychologically minded. Psychological mindedness is the understanding of the patient's and the trainee's subjective responses, the ability to take an objective approach to behavior, to make an empathic contact with the patient and to have an understanding of the self, including an understanding of psychiatric signs and symptoms. Psychological mindedness can be basically seen as an umbrella concept involving an interest in and an ability to extract and make sense of psychological information (thoughts, feelings, and behaviors) from a situation. This term is commonly used in clinical settings to describe patients, trainees, and staff and is usually regarded as a positive attribute. It is different from intelligence, although an intelligent person is often thought to possess high psychological mindedness, which may not always be the case. The term has been used interchangeably with other concepts like insight, introspection, self-awareness, self-reflection, and the capacity for self-observation and has been viewed as a motive, ability, expectancy, an attributional style, and an interest (McCallum & Piper, 1997) or simply as reading between the lines (Dollinger, 1997). The very nature of psychiatric practice demands that the psychiatric consultants think about basic motives, distortions, and inner experiences of others (Daw & Joseph, 2010).

For psychiatric trainers who are teachers, psychological mindedness is not the only condition for being a good teacher; apart from subject knowledge and sound technical training, social awareness, and moral consciousness are also crucial (Hanifin & Appel, 2010). Psychological mindedness can be taught using a number of strategies such as vignettes, clinical supervision, and role play.

Leadership

The last few decades have seen various organizations and institutions turning from the traditional hierarchical structures to the currently prevalent team structures. Even the teams have evolved to become multi-disciplinary health teams, consisting of healthcare members from different disciplines working together toward the optimal care of a patient. These teams work best with a team leader, who, once chosen, has to fulfill certain administrative roles apart from the clinical ones. The clinician who moves from a mainly clinical role and responsibility to a mainly administrative role must be aware of the simple fact that there are certain similarities and differences in the two roles and skills; leadership sometimes differs from management and at others is embedded in it. By virtue of their training and experience of using bio-psychosocial models, psychiatrists are well placed in understanding a broader perspective and group dynamics. Thus they can be aware of behaviors that may be facilitating and productive or others that may be impeding to these roles (Daniels & Daniels, 1989). The psychiatrist can act as an effective team leader in various multi-disciplinary health teams in the hospitals. There is a possibility that psychiatrist-led health teams may help in destigmatizing mental health treatment, since the psychiatrist can be a positive educator of the public, other professionals, and stakeholders, as well as of team members regarding mental illnesses and their treatment, and also provide an effective liaison with other specialties. Overall, a psychiatrist in the position of a leader in a hospital healthcare team should lead to the humanizing of health care by addressing both psychological and physical needs of the patients at one time and in one location. Leadership skills can be learnt but there also needs to be an inherent interest.

Leadership, a highly sought after and highly valued commodity (Northouse, 2009) is now required at all levels in a hospital, from a single departmental level to various inter-departmental collaborative efforts. Kotter (1996) rightly describes leadership as the engine that drives change and there is no doubt that this quality is indeed a key part of a doctors' professional work, regardless of the specialty. As mentioned above, although manager and leader may seem to be similar, Kotter (1990) argues that these are two distinct constructs. Whereas management produces order and consistency and means accomplishing activities and mastering routines, good leadership produces change and movement and specifically means influencing others and creating visions for change; nevertheless both are essential to prosper (Bennis & Nanus, 1985; Kotter, 1990). Bennis and Nanus (1985) made this distinction clear by quoting: "Managers are people who do things right and leaders are people who do the right things" (p. 221). However, there also seems to be quite some overlap between the two; when managers are involved in influencing a group to meet its goals, they are in effect involved in leadership. Similarly when leaders are involved in planning, organizing, and controlling, they are in fact acting as managers.

Leadership is an influence process that influences a group of individuals to achieve a common goal (Northouse, 2009). One can look at leadership from the *trait* perspective, which suggests that some individuals may have certain innate characteristics that make them born leaders, thus making leadership a set of properties possessed by different people in differing degrees (Jago, 1982). Some of these characteristics include physical factors like height, or personality features like extraversion (Bryman, 1992). Another perspective to look at leadership is the process perspective (Northouse, 2009), which suggests that leadership is a phenomenon residing in the context of the interactions between leaders and the followers. The process can be observed in various leader behaviors (Jago, 1982). This view suggests that leadership is a process that can be learned and thus is available to everyone as compared to the restricted view taken by the trait approach. Some of the positive communication behaviors that account for successful leadership include being firm but not rigid, seeking others' opinions and getting them involved in the decision-making processes for the organization, and initiating new ideas (Fisher, 1974). Apart from these communication skills, certain personality factors may help in becoming good leaders. Individuals who are more dominant, more intelligent, and more confident about their own performance are more likely to become leaders in their own groups (Smith & Foti, 1998).

People may be leaders because of their formal positions in an organization, like the department heads, while there may be others who become leaders because of the way other people respond to them. The leadership skills can be acquired during the undergraduate or the post-graduate training period, which is the basic training period and will enable all future healthcare providers to contribute to the effective delivery of health care for patients through their roles as team members, and, at the same time, will also prepare them for their future employment and practice. Great leadership is required at all levels to deliver standard healthcare services to patients and communities. Good leaders bring special assets to various organizations and improve the services, changing the way people think about what is possible (Northouse, 2009) and what can be made possible.

The National Health Services (NHS) in the UK provides a range of interventions to help build leadership capability and capacity across the NHS. The Enhancing Engagement in Medical Leadership Project develops and promotes medical leadership and engagement across the UK in conjunction with the Academy of Medical Royal Colleges and helps create organizational cultures where doctors seek to be more engaged in management and leadership of health services and nonmedical leaders genuinely seek their involvement to improve services for patients across the UK. The Medical Leadership Competency Framework (MLCF) is a part of this Medical Leadership Project and describes the leadership competencies doctors need in order to become more actively involved in the planning, delivery, and transformation of health services through their day-to-day practice. The MLCF addresses five domains pertinent to leadership in clinical settings with delivery of the health services at the center of the five domains, thus forming the leadership wheel (Figure 3). These five domains include: demonstrating personal qualities, working with others, managing services, improving services, and setting directions (Medical Leadership Competency Framework, 2009) and are described here in brief.

(a) *Demonstrating personal qualities*

Doctors who are effective leaders need to depend on their own values and abilities to deliver high standards of care. The doctors should be competent in managing themselves and also take into account the needs of others. The former is possible only if the level of self-awareness is high. The doctor should be ready to learn through experience and feedback, which will ultimately lead to personal development and improve the personal qualities.

(b) *Working with others*

Team work may come as a part and parcel of being a healthcare provider. Thus doctors get a chance to show leadership by working with others in these teams, wherein they have to learn to build and develop relationships by listening and showing understanding, supporting others, and gaining the trust of others. The efficiency of the doctor is visible in the ability to develop networks by working with colleagues, patients, and other healthcare consumers and their representatives.

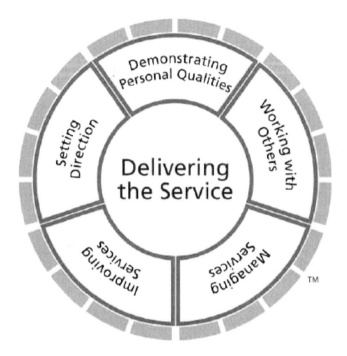

Figure 3. The medical leadership competency framework.

(c) *Managing services*

Doctors should be able to exhibit competence in managing services and this has been discussed earlier in describing their roles as effective managers. There should be proper planning and use of available resources to get the maximum outcome.

(d) *Improving services*

Along with managing services, there should be a constant attempt at encouraging improvement and innovation by creating a climate of continuous service improvement. Effective managers and leaders can facilitate this transformation with ease.

(e) *Setting direction*

Doctors should be able to identify the contexts for change required in the progress of the organization and be aware of the range of factors to be considered for the same. In making such progress, the leading physician is the one who sets the direction for the team.

All these skills can be learnt again using a number of strategies, from didactic lectures to experiential work and shadowing. In addition, the trainers must be aware of their own strengths and weaknesses so that they can be used in teaching these skills.

Emotional Intelligence

The term emotional intelligence (EI) is defined as a subset of social intelligence that involves the ability to monitor one's own and others' feelings and emotions, to discriminate among them and to use this information to guide one's thinking and actions (Salovey & Mayer, 1990). Again this and other traits described are also the desirable attributes in all medical doctors. Researchers have hypothesized about the possible links between a high EI and leadership (Caruso, Mayer, & Salovey, 2002; George, 2000) and suggested that there is a positive relation between EI and leadership effectiveness (Kerr, Garvin, Heaton, & Boyle, 2006; Rosete & Ciarrochi, 2005; Wong & Law, 2002). The concept of EI gains more importance in the light of the emerging team-work culture in the institutional set-ups, wherein understanding and dealing with other team members' emotions becomes important.

Other desirable qualities in psychiatrists are altruism, accountability, responsibility, humanistic qualities, and empathy. Self-confidence is another trait that helps one to be an effective service provider and it may also further leadership qualities. It is the ability to be certain about one's competencies and skills and includes a sense of self-esteem and self-assurance, the belief that one can indeed make a difference.

The Training Environment

Cruess (2006) described the principles for educating trainees and pointed out that institutional support, environment processes using experiential learning and role modeling, along with the individual's personality traits, such as cognitive base, are important factors in creating the learning environment and also getting trainees to be more aware of issues related to learning. Furthermore, he notes that narrative medicine, communication, and spirituality can be used in teaching professionalism. Thus, professionalism can be taught but the trainers must be aware of their own needs of learning and disseminating training. Ratanawongsa, Bolen, Howell, Kern, Sisson, & Larriviere (2006) identified a lack of time and increased workload as significant barriers in teaching professionalism. Trainers must have the time and space to create an environment in which the training of professional values can take place. These authors also indicate that role modeling and role play can be significant factors in learning these values. Therefore, trainers must also be good at using these strategies in engaging trainees.

In identifying core values of the profession, Page (2006) emphasizes that greed, misrepresentation, abuse of power and position are unacceptable. Joyner and Vernulkonda (2007) urge that knowledge, skills, and a sense of service are important components of professionalism and can be taught. Professional values can be measured (Stern, 2004) and thus can be taught.

It has been argued that by virtue of their expertise in the areas of culture, the ability to deliver comprehensive health care, and their communication skills, psychiatrists are best placed to provide teaching and education (Talbott & Mallott, 2006). Using portfolios, patient case histories and other means, professionalism can be taught (Goldie, Dowie, Cotton, & Morrison, 2007). There is no doubt that, as professionals, we carry a major responsibility to teach and train in professionalism (Bhugra, 2010).

In an editorial, Bhugra and Gupta (2010) point out that the role of the medical professional as a healer has shifted considerably as a result of changes in society, in the funding of health care, and in the attitudes and expectations of the public. Emotional intelligence in their physicians is a key expectation of patients and their families. The components of emotional intelligence include self-awareness, self-regulation, self-motivation, and social skills and social awareness (Wagner, 2006). Social skills and social awareness can be taught, but what about self-awareness and self-motivation?

There are various phases in learning (Bloom, 1985). From the introduction of activities to an extended period of preparation to full-time commitment to improving practice on to training reaching beyond the knowledge of the teachers, these phases mean that in any group learning will not be homogenous. Bhugra and Gupta (2010) point out, professionalism combines both theoretical constructs and practical components. Thus the trainers must be aware of the theoretical constructs and their impact on learning and practice. They also need to ensure that trainers can employ theoretical constructs in improving their practical learning.

Levenson, Atkinson, and Shepherd (2010) observe that problem-based learning in medical schools aims to encourage a group of undergraduates to collaborate in order to provide reasoned possible solutions to a posed question or scenario to which there may not be a single correct answer, and discussion of clinical issues may raise ethical and nonclinical matters. This approach uses greater student cognitive involvement resulting in better retention. Using problem-based learning means that trainers may need to move away from traditional teaching techniques and models. Learning about professionalism and resulting assessment will require multiple levels of examination of skills, values, and attitudes.

The Training Process

The training of future mental health professionals must develop to ensure that psychiatric practice meets almost all the needs of the modern evolving societies.

Along with the characteristics of the trainer, one also has to understand the various characteristics of the trainee. Each individual has a different style of teaching and learning so the skills required cannot be the same for everyone. In any group of people, including psychiatric trainees, there will be people with different personality types and learning styles. It is important to understand how the personality type of a particular trainee fits with his or her specialty choice and the training process. There is a possibility that the trainee's personality type will affect the comfort of the trainee with certain psychiatric trainers and not with others. The trainee's personality type also affects the understanding and dealing of certain conditions and patients by the trainee. Certain aspects of the specialty may be easily understood by the trainee and others may not be.

Different individuals have different ways of taking in and processing information, which means that everyone has different learning styles (Felder & Spurlin, 2005). Based on this, a learning style model was formulated by Felder and Silverman (1988), which suggested different learning styles such as active/reflective learning, sensing/intuitive learning, visual/verbal learning, and sequential/global learning. It is important that trainers themselves explore newer ways of training and supervising the students, and to monitor their work. The basic purpose of training is introducing information. At the same time the introduction of basic skills are necessary to deal with the patient effectively. The ultimate purpose of ongoing training and supervision is to improve the ability of trainers to provide accurate information and confidently influence their students in a positive way. An attempt should be made by the trainers in order to achieve a balance of various instructional methods being used to teach the trainees.

Active learners actively do something and learn things, for example, by discussing or applying or explaining it to others. Reflective learners tend to think and reflect on the activity and then learn it. Active learners are more interested in group learning while the reflective ones prefer learning alone. Sensing learners are more into learning facts, memorizing things, and solving problems by well-established methods. Intuitive learners, on the other hand, are more into discovering possibilities and relationships and are more innovative as compared to sensors. They are better at grasping new concepts and dislike repetitions or memorization and routine calculations. Visual learners learn by seeing pictures, flowcharts, films, and demonstrations, while verbal learners learn through written and spoken explanations. Sequential learners understand processes in logical stepwise paths, each step following the previous one. Global learners tend to learn in large jumps, absorbing material almost randomly without seeing connections, and then suddenly "getting it." Global learners may be able to solve complex problems in novel ways but once they have done it, they may not be able to explain how they did it (see Felder & Silverman, 1988).

One of the major challenges to trainers and trainees alike is in dealing with diversity. Americano and Bhugra (2010) emphasize that competence in diversity is central to the successful relationship between clinician and patient. The perceived and real power differential between the doctor (who may be seen to have a significant amount of power based on knowledge and expertise) and the patient (who may be totally reliant on the doctor in making clinical decisions for the patient) is caused by a number of factors. However, with the spread of knowledge and ease of access to such knowledge through the Internet and other sources, the power differential is beginning to change. Paralleling this differential is the relationship between teacher and student, where such a power discrepancy may exist. The concepts of diversity and equality are socially constructed (Americano & Bhugra, 2010) and their role in delivery and acceptance of health care is significant, though often overlooked.

Diversity itself can be used in a group in ascertaining performance and behavior which can be employed in learning about a patient's cultural values, strengths, and weaknesses. Trainers, therefore, need to be cognizant of the impact of cultural factors and diversity itself. Americano and Bhugra (2010) argue that there are five essential elements that contribute to a system's ability to become more competent in diversity. These include valuing diversity, self-assessment on diversity, awareness of dynamics when two cultures come in contact with each other, ensuring that institutions take ownership of the diversity values, and making appropriate changes in policy and action. The trainer has to be aware of the context of these competencies and also have the skills to transmit these values and knowledge to the trainees. Personal attributes of empathy, understanding similarities and differences across cultures, flexibility and openness, willingness to work, train, and learn about diversity are all important in training. Disability itself in the patient, trainer or trainee raises interesting questions and there remains a major need both in healthcare delivery and in training to take it into account.

Training takes place in different clinical and nonclinical settings. Various models are utilized for training. Training in diversity and disability can be delivered directly by trainers or under supervision by students and trainees themselves, using personal experiences, case vignettes, experiential role play, etc. Working across healthcare disciplines may work, too. An important principle for diversity training has to be an awareness of and availability of a structured framework. Existing available and potential resources will dictate what components can be utilized in this structure. Americano and Bhugra (2010) further suggest a number of models using different resources and strategies for training in diversity.

Conclusions

Trainees learn various aspects of medicine and aspects of professionalism using a number of strategies and techniques. On the other hand, trainers need to be aware of changing aspects of society and patient expectations. Trainers, knowingly or otherwise, will use their gender, age, education, training, and experience at various levels in their teaching and interaction with trainees. A relationship between learning styles and teaching methods, on the one hand, and methods of assessment and feedback, on the other, is at the heart of training. Trainee feedback is crucial in modifying methods of training as well as contents. However, trainers need to be open minded to deal with fair criticism. It is likely that increasingly trainees will own their training and be able to vocalize their training needs. Trainers will need to get into a dialog in order to deliver appropriate and accessible training. Lastly, the various models and concepts discussed in this chapter are not necessarily limited to the psychiatric domain and can be applied to any medicine subspecialty.

References

About CanMEDS. (2007). Royal College of Physicians and Surgeons of Canada. CanMEDs Framework. Retrieved October 24, 2010, from http://rcpsc.medical.org/canmeds/about_e.php.

Americano, A., & Bhugra, D. (2010). Dealing with diversity. In T. Swanick (Ed.), *Understanding medical education: Evidence, theory and practice*. London, UK: Association for the Study of Medical Education.

Bennis, W. G., & Nanus, B. (1985). *Leaders: The strategies for taking charge*. New York, NY: Harper & Row.

Bhugra, D. (2010). Teaching professionalism in psychiatry. *International Journal of Social Psychiatry, 56*, 323–325.

Bhugra, D., & Gupta, S. (2010). Teaching and learning professional values. *Asia-Pacific Psychiatry, 2*, 65–67.

Bloom, B. S. (1985). Generalizations about talent development. In R. S. Bloom (Ed.), *Developing talent in young people* (pp. 507–549). New York, NY: Ballantine.

Braunack-Mayer, A. J. (2001). What makes a problem an ethical problem? An empirical perspective on the nature of ethical problems in general practice. *Journal of Medical Ethics, 27*, 98–103.

Bryman, A. (1992). *Charisma and leadership in organizations.* London, UK: Sage.

Caruso, D. R., Mayer, J. D., & Salovey, P. (2002). Emotional intelligence and emotional leadership. In R. E. Riggio, S. E. Murphy, & F. J. Pirozzolo (Eds.), *Multiple intelligences and leadership* (pp. 55–74). Mahwah, NJ: Erlbaum.

Chou, S., Cole, G., McLaughlin, K., & Lockyer, J. (2008). CanMEDS evaluation in Canadian postgraduate training programmes: Tools used and programme director satisfaction. *Medical Education, 42*, 879–886.

Christakis, D. A., & Feudtner, C. (1993). Ethics in a short white coat: The ethical dilemmas that medical students confront. *Academic Medicine, 68*, 249–254.

Civaner, M., Sarikaya, O., & Balcioglu, H. (2009). Medical ethics in residency training. *Anadolu Kardiyoloji Dergisi* [The Anatolian Journal of Cardiology], *9*, 132–138 [in Turkish].

Cruess, R. L. (2006). Teaching professionalism. *Clinical Orthopaedics and Related Research, 449*, 177–185.

Daniels, A. S., & Daniels, R. S. (1989). The psychiatrist as administrator and organizational leader: An application of social psychiatry. *Social Psychiatry and Psychiatric Epidemiology, 24*, 295–300.

Daw, B., & Joseph, S. (2010). Psychological mindedness and therapist attributes. *Counselling and Psychotherapy Research, 10*, 233–236.

Dollinger, S. J. (1997). Psychological mindedness as "Reading between the Lines". In M. McCallum & W. E. Piper (Eds.), *Psychological mindedness: A contemporary understanding.* Mahwah, NJ: Erlbaum.

Donovan, A. (2010). Views of radiology program directors on the role of mentorship in the training of radiology residents. *AJR American Journal of Roentgenology, 194*, 704–708.

Donovan, J. C. (2009). A survey of dermatology residency program directors' views on mentorship. *Dermatology Online Journal, 15*, 1.

Felder, R. M., & Silverman, L. K. (1988). Learning and teaching styles in engineering education. *Engineering Education, 78*, 674–681.

Felder, R. M., & Spurlin, J. (2005). Applications, reliability and validity of the index of learning styles. *International Journal of Engineering Education, 21*, 103–112.

Feudtner, C., & Christakis, D. A. (1994). Making the rounds: The ethical development of medical students in the context of clinical rotations. *Hastings Center Report, 24*, 6–12.

Fisher, B. A. (1974). *Small group decision making: Communication and the group process.* New York, NY: McGraw Hill.

Flint, J. H., Jahangir, A. A., Browner, B. D., & Mehta, S. (2009). The value of mentorship in orthopaedic surgery resident education: The residents' perspective. *The Journal of Bone and Joint Surgery American, 91*, 1017–1022.

Frank, J. R., & Langer, B. (2003). Collaboration, communication, management, and advocacy: Teaching surgeons new skills through the CanMEDS Project. *World Journal of Surgery, 27*, 972–978.

Freiman, A., Natsheh, A., Barankin, B., & Shear, N. H. (2006). Dermatology postgraduate training in Canada: CanMEDS competencies. *Dermatology Online Journal, 12*, 6.

Fuller, S. S. (2000). Enabling, empowering, inspiring: Research and mentorship through the years. *Bulletin of the Medical Library Association, 88*, 1–10.

George, J. M. (2000). Emotions and leadership: The role of emotional intelligence. *Human Relations, 53*, 1027–1055.

Goldie, J., Dowie, A., Cotton, P., & Morrison, J. (2007). Teaching professionalism in the early years of a medical curriculum: A qualitative study. *Medical Education, 41*, 610–617.

Goold, S. D., & Stern, D. T. (2006). Ethics and professionalism: What does a resident need to learn? *The American Journal of Bioethics, 6*, 9–17.

Gordon, P. A. (2000). The road to success with a mentor. *Journal of Vascular Nursing, 18*, 30–33.

Graham, H. J. (2006). Patient confidentiality: Implications for teaching in undergraduate medical education. *Clinical Anatomy, 19*, 448–455.

Gurgel, R. K., Schiff, B. A., Flint, J. H., Miller, R. A., Zahtz, G. D., Smith, R. V., Fried, M. P., & Smith, R. J. (2010). Mentoring in otolaryngology training programs. *Otolaryngology – Head and Neck Surgery, 142*, 487–492.

Hanifin, E., & Appel, S. (2010). Transference and psychological-mindedness in teachers. Retrieved October 22, 2010, from http://ajte.education.ecu.edu.au/ISSUES/PDF/252/Hanifin.pdf.

International Executive's Profile. (1990). A decade of change in corporate leadership. New York, NY: Korn/Ferry International and UCLA Anderson Graduate School of Management.

Inui, T. S. (2003). Flag in the wind: Educating for professionalism in medicine. Association of American Medical Colleges.

Jago, A. G. (1982). Leadership: Perspectives in theory and research. *Management Science, 28*, 315–336.

Joyner, B. D., & Vemulakonda, V. M. (2007). Improving professionalism: Making the implicit more explicit. *Journal of Urology, 177*, 2289–2293.

Kerr, R., Garvin, J., Heaton, N., & Boyle, E. (2006). Emotional intelligence and leadership effectiveness. *Leadership & Organization Development Journal, 27*, 265–279.

Kotter, J. (1990). *A force for change: How leadership differs from management.* New York, NY: Free Press.

Kotter, J. (1996). *Leading change.* Boston, MA: HBS Press.

Lapid, M., Moutier, C., Dunn, L., Hammond, K. G., & Roberts, L. W. (2009). Professionalism and ethics education on relationships and boundaries: Psychiatric residents' training preferences. *Academic Psychiatry, 33*, 461–469.

Levenson, R., Atkinson, S., & Shepherd, S. (2010). *Understanding the doctors of tomorrow.* London, UK: King's Fund.

Lis, L. D., Wood, W. C., Petkova, E., & Shatkin, J. (2009). Mentoring in psychiatric residency programs: A survey of chief residents. *Academic Psychiatry, 33*, 307–312.

MacNeily, A. E. (2007). CanMEDS: Time to teach the teachers. *Canadian Urological Association Journal, 1*, 370.

McCallum, M., & Piper, W. E. (1997). *Psychological mindedness: A contemporary understanding.* New Jersey, NJ: Erlbaum.

McCord, J. H., McDonald, R., Sippel, R. S., Leverson, G., Mahvi, D. M., & Weber, S. M. (2009). Surgical career choices: The vital impact of mentoring. *Journal of Surgical Research, 155*, 136–141.

Medical Leadership Competency Framework. (2009). Retrieved October 28, 2010, from http://www.institute.nhs.uk/assessment_tool/general/medical_leadership_competency_framework_-_homepage.html.

Northouse, P. G. (2009). *Leadership: theory and practice* (5th ed.). Thousand Oaks, CA: Sage.

Page, D. W. (2006). Professionalism and team care in the clinical setting. *Clinical Anatomy, 19*, 468–472.

Pellegrini, V. D., Jr. (2006). Mentoring during residency education: A unique challenge for the surgeon? *Clinical Orthopaedics and Related Research, 449*, 143–148.

Ratanawongsa, N., Bolen, S., Howell, E. E., Kern, D. E., Sisson, S. D., & Larriviere, D. (2006). Residents' perception of professionalism in training and practice: Barriers, promoters and duty hour requirements. *Journal of General Internal Medicine, 21*, 758–763.

Reck, S. J., Stratman, E. J., Vogel, C., & Mukesh, B. N. (2006). Assessment of residents' loss of interest in academic careers and identification of correctable factors. *Archives of Dermatology, 142*, 855–858.

Roberts, L. W. (2009). Professionalism in psychiatry: A very special collection. *Academic Psychiatry, 33*, 429–430.

Roberts, L. W., & Dyer, A. R. (2004). *Ethics in mental health care*. Washington, DC: American Psychiatric Publishing.

Roberts, L. W., Warner, T. D., Hammond, K. A., Geppert, C. M., & Heinrich, T. (2005). Becoming a good doctor: Perceived need for ethics training focused on practical and professional developmental topics. *Academic Psychiatry, 29*, 301–309.

Rosete, D., & Ciarrochi, J. (2005). Emotional intelligence and its relationship to workplace performance outcomes of leadership effectiveness. *Leadership and Organization Development Journal, 26*, 388–399.

Royal College of Psychiatrists. (2010). Role of the consultant psychiatrist: Leadership and excellence in mental health services. Occasional Paper OP74. London, UK: Royal College of Psychiatrists.

Salovey, P., & Mayer, J. D. (1990). Emotional intelligence. *Imagination, Cognition and Personality, 9*, 185–211.

Sambunjak, D., Straus, S. E., & Marusic, A. (2010). A systematic review of qualitative research on the meaning and characteristics of mentoring in academic medicine. *Journal of General Internal Medicine, 25*, 72–78.

Schrubbe, K. F. (2004). Mentorship: A critical component for professional growth and academic success. *Journal of Dental Education, 68*, 324–328.

Schwartz, A. C., Kotwicki, R. J., & McDonald, W. M. (2009). Developing a modern standard to define and assess professionalism in trainees. *Academic Psychiatry, 33*, 442–450.

Smith, J. A., & Foti, R. J. (1998). A pattern approach to the study of leader emergence. *Leadership Quarterly, 9*, 147–160.

Stern, D. T. (2004). *Measuring medical professionalism*. New York, NY: Oxford University Press.

Swick, H. M., Szenas, P., Danoff, D., & Whitcomb, M. E. (1999). Teaching professionalism in undergraduate medical education. *JAMA, 282*, 830–832.

Talbott, J. A., & Mallott, D. B. (2006). Professionalism, medical humanism and clinical bioethics: The new wave – does psychiatry have a role? *Journal of Psychiatric Practice, 12*, 384–390.

Wagner, P. J. (2006). Does high EI (Emotional Intelligence) make better doctors? *Virtual Mentor (American Medical Association Journal of Ethics), 8*, 477–479.

Wang, H. (2001). Academic mentorship: An effective professional development strategy for medical reference librarians. *Medical Reference Services Quarterly, 20*, 23–31.

Wong, C., & Law, K. S. (2002). The effects of leader and follower emotional intelligence on performance and attitude: An exploratory study. *Leadership Quarterly, 13*, 243–274.

Cultural and Individual Differences: Aspects in Patient Care

Patient Involvement in Medical Management

Factors that Affect Involvement and Implications for Clinical Practice

Rachel Davis and Charles Vincent

Clinical Safety Research Unit, Department of Surgery and Cancer, Imperial College London, UK

Over the years (in the last decade in particular) there has been a noticeable shift from the traditional paternalistic delivery of healthcare to a healthcare system which aims to be more patient-centric and that strongly promotes the involvement of the patient. Empowering patients to take an active role in their own healthcare has been nationally and internationally identified as a key factor in the drive to improve health services for the patient. Involving patients has many potential benefits such as increasing patient satisfaction, facilitating recovery and improving health outcomes, enhancing the quality and efficiency of care received, and helping to reduce healthcare costs. Patients may primarily be involved in improving the quality and safety of their own care, or be more widely involved in efforts to improve the wider healthcare system.

Given these benefits one might assume that all patients (when possible) should be involved in their healthcare. However, while this may seem straightforward, on closer inspection, it is by no means an easy task to address. The degree to which patients will want to be involved will vary enormously from patient to patient and will be influenced by a wide range of factors. Furthermore the nature and extent of patient involvement varies widely in different clinical settings. A single chapter cannot possibly encompass this diversity and our intention is therefore to present and discuss some critical issues which are relevant to patient involvement in any setting. We first consider some of the different ways patients may be involved in their care. Second, we highlight some of the many factors that influence patient involvement. Finally we consider how patient involvement may be encouraged and the wider implications for practice.

How Can Patients Be Involved?

There are many opportunities for patient involvement in the primary, secondary, and tertiary-care setting. However for any patient to effectively participate in any health-related behavior three essential ingredients are required: (1) knowledge, (2) ability, and (3) willingness (see Box 1).

Box 1. The three essential ingredients for patient involvement

- *Knowledge*: Patients must be knowledgable on how to participate – we cannot expect patients to participate if they do not understand how to do this.
- *Ability*: Patients have to be able to participate; this ability is derived in part from the patient's knowledge but is also largely affected by the patient's physical and cognitive capacity.
- *Willingness*: Patients have to want to participate.

For now however, assuming that patients are knowledgeable, able, and willing to participate – how can they be involved? Here we discuss some of the key opportunities.

Helping to Reach a Diagnosis

Patients can help doctors to reach a diagnosis of their problem by providing information about their current symptoms and details of their medical history (Vincent & Coulter, 2002). Patients can also help to reduce errors in diagnosis by getting staff to double check test results. This could help to reduce testing errors where tests results are false positives or false negatives (see Box 2 for examples).

Box 2. How patients can prevent errors related to a false negative or false positive test result

False negative: A doctor misinterprets an X-ray of a small fracture on a patients arm and concludes that there is no fracture when in fact the fracture has just been missed. The patient asks the doctor to double check the X-ray and the fracture is discovered and the patient subsequently treated.

False positive: A diabetic patient has a blood sugar finger prick test to check their blood sugar levels. The patient ate a cake prior to the test (traces of which were left on their finger) which meant when the nurse took the patient's blood the results came back as the blood sugar levels being falsely elevated. The patient notified the nurse they had eaten a sugary food and the nurse repeated the test – this time the patient's blood sugar levels were in the normal range for the patient.

It is particularly important for patients to request a repeat test for pathology tests for any serious diagnosis that results in significant treatment, such as organ removal for cancer. While within any healthcare system quality assurance steps are taken to avert laboratory errors, no system is infallible and system flaws or human mistakes can occur with test results.

Choosing a Treatment Provider

Patients can, if given the requisite information, make important choices regarding their treatment provider for a particular problem. For example in the United Kingdom the government have introduced their "Choose and Book" scheme. This is a national service that allows patients a choice of place, date, and time for their first hospital or clinic appointment. Patients who require hospital treatment are provided with the choice of different hospitals in England funded by the NHS (including NHS hospitals and some independent hospitals) where they can undergo the treatment. Patients are more likely to be more satisfied with the service because they will experience increased personal control and will get to choose a provider most suitable to their individual needs. In addition to increasing patient satisfaction, providing patients with a choice of healthcare provider could also have potential benefits in terms of reducing susceptibility to iatrogenic harm (Vincent & Coulter, 2002).

For several years now patients in a number of countries (e.g., France, Germany, Belgium, Australia, and United States) have been offered, at least in part, the opportunity to choose their provider (Goddard & Hobden, 2003). For example, in the United States the Leapfrog Group has developed an online database of quality and safety information for US hospitals (http://www.leapfroggroup.org/). The Leapfrog Group advises patients to choose hospitals and doctors that perform high numbers of the procedure they require, as this is positively associated with patients' health outcomes. In Britain, the commercial provider Dr. Foster also produces official information on mortality and morbidity rates of individual clinicians or hospitals for British hospitals (www.nhs.uk/www.drfoster.co.uk).

Sharing Decisions About Treatments

One of the most frequent sources of patient dissatisfaction is failures in communication about illness and treatment options (Ha & Longnecker, 2010). In the present day most patients expect to be provided with information about their condition and treatment options available. In situations where more than one treatment modality is available some patients will also want to take this one step further by helping to choose the treatment option. Patients should be provided with information on the risks and benefits to each treatment in order to make an informed decision about the treatment most suitable to their needs. This is beneficial to the patient for two key reasons. First, if the patient is involved in the treatment decision making process they are likely to be happier with the course of treatment prescribed (Cockburn & Pit, 1997; Coulter, 2005), this in turn, can improve adherence to medical and treatment recommendations (Mullen, 1997). Second, providing information to patients on the risks and benefits of procedures can enable patients to opt for less risky procedures. For example, research shows patients who are fully informed about the risks (and benefits) of prostate specific antigen (PSA) screening for prostate cancer are less likely to have the test (Volk, Cass, & Spann, 1999; Wagner, Barrett, Barry, Barlow, & Fowler, 1995). Among other issues, PSA testing identifies cancers that may never become problematic and treatment side effects can result in various risks including erectile dysfunction and incontinence (http://www.mayoclinic.com/health/psa-test).

Identifying and Reporting Treatment Complications or Errors

Patients can help to ameliorate the outcomes of treatment complications or errors by reporting if they believe there is a problem. There have been some impressive examples of how patients have played a valuable role in alerting staff to errors or problems in their care (Unruh & Pratt, 2007). For example patients receiving treatment in an outpatient oncology clinic reported how they were able to detect a number of problems in their care (see Box 3). One patient alerted staff to a procedural error in which their intravenous drip delivering their chemotherapy medication finished earlier than usual. When brought to the staff's attention it emerged that the patient had been given twice the concentration of chemotherapy in half the recommended time. The patient played a fundamental role in mitigating the effects of the error by notifying staff so that prompt action could be taken.

In addition, to patients "real-time" reports of treatment complications, patients can also provide retrospective accounts. One context in particular where this is particularly important is in the reporting of adverse drug reactions. Research in this area indicates that patients have the potential to contribute to the understanding of the nature and prevalence of particular reactions to a variety of different drugs (Egberts, Smulders, de Koning, Meyboom, & Leufkens, 1996; van den Bemt et al., 1999).

In Britain a scheme is now in operation on the Medicines and Healthcare products Regulatory Agency (MHRA) website, called the "Yellow Card Scheme." The scheme, run by the MHRA and the Commission on Human Medicines, is used to collect information from anybody – health professionals and the general public or patients. Patients can report through the "yellow card scheme" if they think a medicine or herbal remedy has caused an undesirable side effect or an adverse reaction (http://yellowcard.mhra.gov.uk/). This is particularly important when the patient is taking a "black triangle" – a new drug monitored by the Committee on Safety for Medicine for which the full extent of (rare) side effects is unknown.

Participating in Infection Control Initiatives

There has been considerable attention paid to the problem of healthcare acquired infections (HAI's), especially within the last 10 years. For example in England alone 9,000 people in hospital were recorded as dying in 2007 from methicillin resistant *Staphylococcus aureus* (MRSA) or *Clostridium difficile* (Office for National Statistics, 2008). The etiology of HAIs is complex; however we know that poor hand hygiene among healthcare staff can play a salient role. A series of small studies in both the United States and United Kingdom have shown that patients could increase handwashing compliance among healthcare staff by asking doctors or nurses involved in their care if they have washed their hands before treating them (McGuckin, Taylor, Martin, Porten, & Salcido, 2004; McGuckin et al., 1999; McGuckin et al., 2001).

In recent years many campaigns and interventions have been introduced aimed at increasing the patients' role in infection control initiatives. For example, in the UK the National Patient Safety Agency has introduced the "Clean Your Hands Campaign," part of which aims to empower patients to question staff on their hand hygiene behaviors.

Box 3. Preventing errors in an outpatient oncology clinic: The patients contribution

Detecting procedural errors
Here the patient noticed that their intravenous drip had finished more quickly than it should have. The patient alerted a member of staff:
"It's obvious. The nurse said that it would take 20 minutes, but I noticed it started beeping after only 8 minutes. I thought to myself, that's not right, and I told someone. I found out there had been a confusion and I had been given 100 ml bag instead of a 50 ml bag." (p. S238)

Coordinating treatment tasks
Here, unbeknown to the clinician the patient was receiving radiation therapy in a different department alongside their other treatment. The staff had informed the patient not to apply any adhesive to the area of skin that was being irradiated:
"Hmm, you know, because of my radiation I have been told I am not supposed to have a dressing there." (p. S239)

Maintaining continuity of care
Here a patient made sure they took action to educate unfamiliar staff about their health situation:
"You know, I came into the infusion clinic and I would have to say to a new nurse: 'Can you also listen to my lungs?' I need to keep track of this because I have Hodgkins and as part of the treatment for this I had to have my spleen taken out. I have to be really careful because of this as I am at greater risk of pneumonia and other thing." (p. S239)
Adapted from Unruh and Pratt (2007).

Practising Effective Self-Management

Perhaps one of the most important ways that patients can be involved in order to facilitate their health outcomes is by practicing effective self-management strategies – taking medication(s) at the right time of day in the right dose and in the correct manner (with food for example). If patients do not adhere to their treatment regimen the costs to the patient can be far-reaching resulting in a missed opportunity for treatment gain, which if their condition worsens can result in decline in quality of life, admission into hospital, and sometimes even death (Clifford, Garfield, Eliasson, & Barber, 2010; Ho, Magid, Masoudi, McClure, & Rumsfeld, 2006; Yang et al., 2009).

In recent years technological developments have also enabled patients to participate in care practices that were previously conducted by doctors or nurses. One of the main bodies of evidence relates to patients self-monitoring of anticoagulation therapy (Heneghan et al., 2006). Research shows that patients undertaking self-management remained in the therapeutic range for the same time or longer than patients under usual care and that the incidence rate of adverse effects was the same as or less for patients under usual care (de Sola-Morales & Elorza, 2005; Odegaard, 2004; Siebenhofer, Berghold, & Sawicki, 2004).

Shaping the Design and Improvement of Services

While patients can influence the quality of the care they themselves receive on an "individual" level (e.g., by providing feedback to healthcare staff), patients are likely to have much more impact if they work together on a "collective" level. Patients can do this by joining organizations or patient groups that operate on a local, national, or international level.

One organization that has successfully brought patient involvement into all aspects of their healthcare management is the Dana Farber Cancer Centre in the US. The Centre has demonstrated on numerous occasions how by giving patients the opportunity to provide feedback on their healthcare experiences, significant improvements in the delivery of services can be observed. For example, the Centre sought feedback on the care experience for patients that were being treated for neutropenia (a reduction in white blood cells occurring in many diseases). By doing this the admission process was completely transformed (Vincent & Coulter, 2002). Telephone screening and direct admission to appropriate wards was introduced – prior to this patients had been subjected to long, wearying waits in Accident and Emergency departments; this had delayed the start of their treatment, increasing the risk of infections and other complications.

Patients can also help to facilitate safer delivery of healthcare by forming groups or organizations aimed at educating the public about patient safety and how they can be involved in reducing their susceptibility to medical errors. For example, in Britain MRSA Action UK was founded by a group of people who had contracted MRSA or lost loved ones due to MRSA. The organization aims to educate the public and increase awareness about healthcare associated infections (HAIs) and to provide a support and advocacy service to patients (and their families) affected by HAIs (http://www.mrsaactionuk.net/).

Patients as Educators

Patients can also serve as educators to other patients, using their own experiences to help other patients cope with their illness. The most notable exemplar is the "Expert Patient"

(EPP), introduced in the 1970s with Kate Lorig's patient education program in California for patients with arthritis (http://patienteducation.stanford.edu/programs/). In 1994 the program was introduced to the UK. The Long Term Medical Conditions Alliance funded the setting up of lay-led self-management programs for chronic conditions such as diabetes, heart disease, arthritis, and asthma.

In 1999, "The Expert Patient: A New Approach to Chronic Disease Management for the 21st Century" was published and the Expert Patient Programme (EPP) began (Department of Health, 2001). Lay people with experience of managing their illness were offered training so that they could deliver training to other patients on how to manage their illness most effectively. In more recent years the Chronic Disease Management Program has used the experience of the EPP to inform the development of a number of self-management options within the primary care setting, such as anxiety and/or depression and schizophrenia.

How Willing Are Patients to Be Involved?

In the previous section we have presented a number of ways that patients can participate in their own healthcare. However while there are clear benefits to patient involvement, we also need to ask whether patients really want to be involved? This is by no means an easy question to answer.

When patients visit a doctor in a general practice do they go with the intention of simply being "cured" or do they want to know about their illness and the chosen method of treatment? One could reasonably assume that most patients would want to know about their illness – however, some patients will expect more information than others. Equally, for some patients "being involved" could just mean "being informed" whereas other patients will actually want to be involved in any treatment decisions made and adopt more control in managing their illness.

There are a number of factors that affect these preferences – here we discuss some of the key factors.

Patient Knowledge, Beliefs, and Coping Style

Researchers for many years have examined the role of patients' health beliefs in the uptake (or lack thereof) in different behaviors. With any given behavior, the degree to which patients believe they should participate and the relative importance they place on such involvement will undoubtedly influence their behavior. Many theories and models have been proposed, largely originating from the health psychology paradigm that address the relationship between knowledge and beliefs and intentions to participate and/or actual behavior. Two of the key models used extensively for understanding patients' health behaviors and for developing patient education programs and interventions are the Theory of Planned Behavior and the Health Belief Model (Ajzen, 1985; Becker, 1974). Using these models a number of different beliefs have been shown to shape patients behaviors:

- *Normative beliefs*: Beliefs about "important" others attitudes towards the behavior and motivation to comply with these attitudes (e.g., "*my parents think I should give up smoking; it is important to me that I do what my parents think I should do*").
- *Behavioral beliefs*: Beliefs about the outcomes of behavior and evaluations of these outcomes (e.g., "*if I give up smoking this will improve my health; improving my health is beneficial to me*").
- *Control beliefs*: Patient's confidence and capabilities in taking on an active role (e.g., "*I feel confident I can give up smoking; I am in control of whether I can give up smoking*").
- *Perceived susceptibility*: Whether the patient feels they are susceptible to a particular illness or problem (e.g., "*my chances of getting lung cancer are high*").
- *Perceived severity*: Whether the patient thinks the illness is severe (e.g., "*lung cancer is a serious illness*").
- *Perceived costs*: The costs involved in carrying out behavior (e.g., "*if I give up smoking I will become agitated*").
- *Perceived benefits*: The benefits involved in carrying out behavior (e.g., "*if I give up smoking I will save money*").

In addition, to the above, several other factors have been shown to influence patients' beliefs. Perhaps one of the most important is trust. Research has shown a clear correlation between patients trust in their physician and their attitudes towards involvement in treatment decision making. Patients that have low levels of trust are more likely to prefer autonomous roles whereas patients that prefer passive roles are more likely to have high levels of trust (Kraetschmer, Sharpe, Urowitz, & Dever, 2004).

Health Literacy

Health literacy is fundamental to patient engagement. If patients do not have the capacity to obtain and assimilate basic health information they will not be able to look after themselves effectively or make appropriate health decisions. Inadequate health literacy can have far-reaching consequences and has been associated to many negative consequences including (but not limited to): Poorer health status, greater risk of hospitalization, lower adherence to treatment regimens, low ability in terms of communicating with healthcare professionals about their needs and preferences, greater numbers of treatment errors, and less knowledge of health-promoting behaviors (Ad Hoc Committee on Health Literacy, 1999; Institute of Medicine, 2004; Sihota & Lennard, 2004). A further discussion on health literacy is also provided in this book in Eysenck's chapter on "Cognitive Psychology's Contributions to Medical Care."

Experience of Illness

Preliminary findings indicate that severity of illness may influence patient involvement, although there is not a clear direction in relationship. For example, some research indicates that patients with less severe conditions such as mild hypertension or minor upper-respiratory tract infections are more willing to participate in their care than patients with severe diabetes, heart disease, or cancer (Arora & McHorney, 2000). In the same way, asymptomatic HIV patients prefer more involvement than symptomatic patients (Catalan et al., 1994). Conversely however, research on women with ovarian cancer exemplified that, regardless of age, women with more serious prognosis or metastases were more willing to get involved than those with better prognoses (Stewart et al., 2000).

These equivocal findings could suggest that rather than illness severity per se affecting patient involvement, a number of other factors related to illness severity may mediate patients' willingness – these include the manifestation of illness symptoms; how the symptoms affect functionality; the type of treatment plan for the illness and opportunity for involvement this allows, and; the likely impact of patient involvement on health outcomes (Davis, Sevdalis, Jacklin, & Vincent, 2007).

Prior experience of an illness could affect patients' preferences for involvement. A study on patients who have had a recent myocardial infarction (MI), angioplasty, or coronary artery bypass graft reported that these patients want more involvement on decisions concerning acute MI than patients that have no history of heart disease (Mansell, Poses, Kazis, & Duefield, 2000).

Patients' involvement preferences may also change over time and through the course of an illness depending on the patients presenting symptoms. For example, patients that are further progressed in their illness may have limited functionality (e.g., they may be bedridden, need to be fed and bathed); this may, depending on the type of behavior required, inhibit patients' involvement levels.

The Attitude and Beliefs of Healthcare Professionals

The knowledge and beliefs of healthcare professionals (and subsequent behaviors) can strongly influence patients' opportunities for involvement. For example, midwives' beliefs can influence patients' decisions to opt for antenatal HIV testing. This same research also reported that midwifes may withhold information from the patient (e.g., leaflets) if it was not concordant with their beliefs, this in turn, could reduce the potential for patient participation (O'Cathain, Walters, Nicholl, Thomas, & Kirkham, 2002).

Patients learn health-related behaviors, particularly by way of operant conditioning, which highlights the use of consequences to modify the occurrence and form of behavior (Thorndike, 1901). Behavior is influenced by three consequences:

1) *Reinforcement*: Positive outcomes of a behavior reinforce the behavior.
2) *Extinction*: If the consequences that maintain behavior are eliminated, the response tendency gradually weakens.

3) *Punishment*: If behavior brings an unpleasant consequence the behavior tends to be suppressed.

In the previous section one of the ways we suggested patients could participate is by helping to increase hand washing compliance among healthcare staff. Preliminary data indicates though that when patients have asked a doctor or nurse if they have washed their hands they have not always been greeted with a positive response. For example, in one study one patient said: "*when I asked the doctor if they had washed their hands they looked at me like I had two heads*"; another patient said: "*when I asked a nurse the nurse laughed at me*" (McGuckin et al., 2001, p. 225). Patients are unlikely to repeat this behavior in the future if they believe they will be greeted with a similar response. Equally however, if the patient is given praise by a doctor for asking the question (e.g., positively reinforced) they are more likely to repeat the behavior.

The Healthcare Setting and the Medical Context

The setting of healthcare delivery (i.e., primary, secondary, or tertiary) in which healthcare is delivered may affect patients' preferences for involvement. For example some patients may experience greater difficulty communicating with hospital staff than with their GPs due to lack of familiarity with the medical setting.

The nature of the behavior will influence patients' willingness to participate. Patients are more willing to participate in behaviors that are long-standing recommendations or have been normalized into current medical practice. For example, a hospital patient informing a doctor of their drug allergies (if any) would be considered a necessary behavior by all – patients and clinicians alike. However, a hospital patient asking a doctor to check they are being given the right medicine before administration may be considered offensive (by both) and also a considerable extension of the patients' role.

In addition, the extent to which patient's cognitive and emotional resources are required to perform the behavior will exert an effect. Consider for example, a hospital patient who notifies a nurse they have not received their medication when they should have. In order for the patient to do this they would have to be well aware of their personal medication regimen, be vigilant over a period of days, and get involved into a potentially challenging interaction with a (typically busy) member of staff. Now consider a hospital patient who informs a nurse that the wrong telephone number has been recorded in their medical records – this would be easier to engage in because it requires lower levels of knowledge and vigilance.

Encouraging Patient Involvement

Given the wide ranging benefits of patient involvement a vast array of patient-focussed interventions aimed at educating patients and encouraging involvement have been introduced over the years. However, there is no exact formula – different things will work for different patients. We cannot cover all the literature in this chapter. Instead we provide a brief overview of some of the key strategies that have been employed which could help to facilitate patients' involvement in their healthcare management.

Providing Clear Information and Advice

On average patients may forget half of what a doctor tells them within five minutes of leaving the consultation (Kitching, 1990). Written information, such as patient information leaflets can, if appropriate to the patients' needs, be a valuable adjunct to information delivered verbally by the doctor. The patient information leaflet remains the most widely used method of conveying information. Good written information can aid recall of advice, improve compliance to treatment, reduce anxiety about treatment, inform patients about their treatment and encourage patient participation (Coulter & Ellins, 2006).

In addition to written information, due to technological advances health information is now increasingly made available on the internet. Patients can receive information and advice from support groups, virtual health communities and participate in e-health commerce. Research suggests that internet based educational programs can help to encourage positive behavioral change and provide social support for patients. Online health services (e.g., in cancer) can also have positive effects on self-efficacy and empower patients to make health-related decisions and improve confidence in the doctor-patient encounter (Eysenbach, 2003).

Other strategies to provide clear advice to increase understanding and encourage involvement have also been employed. For instance, a number of studies show patients find it extremely valuable when they are provided with recordings of their medical consultation (audiotapes). Many patients reported better recall of information and were more satisfied with the information they received (Pitkethly, MacGillivray, & Ryan, 2008; Scott, Entwistle, Sowden, & Watt, 2001). Videos can also help to increase patient participation in health-related behaviors. For example by encouraging question asking, raising concerns, and increasing the extent to which patients feel comfortable and confident in participating in different health-related behaviors (Anthony et al., 2005; Gagliano, 1988; Krenzischek, Wilson, & Poole, 2001; Roth-isigkeit et al., 2002).

There are a number of issues that should be borne in mind when providing health-related information to patients irrespective of the medium of delivery:

- *Information needs*: Patients' information needs are highly diverse and shaped by a number of factors (e.g., demographics, preferences and circumstances, and style of coping). Information that is personalized to patients' individual preferences and personal characteristics is more likely to encourage involvement and result in better outcomes. It is also important to provide patients with the right amount of information. Providing too much could cause "cognitive overload" and overwhelm the patient.

- *Accessibility*: Providing patients with accurate, evidence-based information in a timely manner is an essential part of their treatment. The way in which information is delivered and at what time point can, in terms of encouraging involvement, be as important as the information itself.
- *Quality*: Information needs to be accurate, complete, and (if written) readable, and esthetically appealing to the patient.
- *Comprehensibility*: Information must be presented in such a way that it is easy for the patient to understand. The extent to which patients may understand health information may vary during the course of their illness with some patients becoming familiar with specific medical terminology and the meaning of it.
- *Usefulness*: The information needs to be relevant to the patient and help to improve patients' ability to assimilate health information so they can make appropriate decisions.

Healthcare Professionals Providing Support and Encouragement

Patient involvement is largely a function of patients' interactions with healthcare professionals. With this in mind, in order to achieve effective and sustainable outcomes for the active involvement of the patient, it is important to foster a working partnership between patients and healthcare professionals. This requires that patient involvement be perceived by all (e.g., nurses, doctors, and patients) as beneficial to the medical encounter.

Patients, particularly those that are more inclined to remain passive, need extra encouragement to participate. Some patients feel that they need to be granted permission to participate. Doctors or nurses directly telling patients "it is ok" to be involved and actively encouraging such involvement can increase patients' participation levels and adherence to long-term treatment modalities. In particular healthcare professionals could potentially help to increase patient involvement in behaviors that are less normalized in current medical practice; these are behaviors that patients are least willing to participate in – for example, a hospital patient asking a doctor or nurse if they have washed their hands (Davis, Koutantji, & Vincent, 2008).

In addition, it has been established that medical staff can create better relationships with patients if they gain knowledge on patients' subjective theories and evaluations of their illness. Doing this enables patients to feel that their concerns and needs are being taken more seriously and patient participation can be increased (Kirkcaldy et al., 2007).

Prompts

Any patient that wants to participate needs information on what to do, when, and where and how to do it. In some cases providing this information, for example, in a written information leaflet or through verbal discussion with a doctor, will be enough to encourage involvement. In other situations, other strategies including visual prompts or reminders may need to be employed. For instance, healthcare professionals can encourage patients to write down any questions or concerns they may have and bring them to their medical appointment. When patients have a structured set of questions to ask their doctor this can promote doctor-patient communication and encourage patients to ask questions (Clayton et al., 2003).

Another method of encouraging patient participation that has shown some promise, particularly in relation to adherence to medication regimens, is texting patients to remind them to take their medication at the correct time. For example, an initiative called "On-cue compliance" which was set up in South Africa (and now being run in Belgium, parts of the UK and elsewhere) has shown that this can serve as a reminder for patients who may otherwise forget to take their medication.

Decision Aids

Decision aids can improve patients' knowledge of their treatment options and outcomes, reduce decisional conflict, facilitate information recall, lead to greater involvement and help to increase agreement between the doctor and patient regarding decisions made (O'Connor & Edwards, 2001).

Decision aids can therefore be particularly useful in situations when more than one treatment option is available. Equally decision aids can be valuable when there is an uncertain balance of benefits and harms of a particular treatment or procedure because of gaps in supporting evidence. A good example here relates to prostate cancer screening (which we have already discussed earlier on in this chapter). There is a lack of evidence that PSA screening for prostate cancer actually decreases mortality due to the disease. Moreover, it is not clear whether the risks outweigh the benefits – for example, the PSA test may detect small cancers that would never become life threatening – this situation called "over diagnosis" can put men at an increased risk of complications due to treatment (http://www.cancer.gov/cancertopics/factsheet/Detection/PSA).

Seeing the Patient as a Partner in Care

In addition to the above examples, considering the patient as an important part of the healthcare team can help to drive standards to delivering more patient-centered care and foster an environment where patients can be actively involved. A major barrier to patient empowerment and, in turn, patient involvement is professional defensiveness and resistance to move away from the paternalistic viewpoint that the "doctor knows best."

Doctors or nurses may also be culturally averse to increasing patient involvement due to fears relating to the negative psychological impact that discussions of risks may have on the patient (Bishop, Kirwan, & Windsor, 1996). Interestingly however, research tends to indicate quite the opposite – providing more information to patients or involving them in

decisions can help to reduce patient anxieties (Kenny et al., 1998). Given this many organizations are actively involved now in encouraging healthcare professionals to adopt a
more patient-centered consulting style. For example, in the United Kingdom the General
Medical Council's guidance on undergraduate medical education states that graduates
must have knowledge and understanding of the principles of good communication, must
be aware of how to take into account the patient's preferences when considering treatment
options and should involve patients when designing self-management plans (General
Medical Council, 2003).

Key Messages

There are a number of implications for practice in terms of encouraging patients to be
involved in their healthcare. While we cannot discuss all of these here, before ending this
chapter we want to summarize what we believe are some of the key take home messages.

Given the number of factors that can affect patients' involvement preferences interventions adopting a "one size fits all" approach are likely to be less successful in facilitating
involvement than those that are tailored to the specific needs of the patient.

Interventions need to meet the informational needs and requirements of the patient.
Patients should always be given clear information on how to manage their treatment
and what to expect in terms of the recovery process from their illness. In addition,
resources, including information sheets, medication leaflets, consent forms and internet
health materials need to be written with the average reading level in mind. Involving
patients in the design stage and evaluation of information resources can be a useful
way of ensuring they meet specific preferences of the patient(s) in question.

Information also needs to be accessible to patients. Consideration needs to be paid to
the individual circumstances of the patient. For example, while many patients may seek
information about their health issues on the internet or join web-based interactive support
groups this will not be appropriate for all patients. Internet and access and use is more
prevalent among younger, more affluent and advantaged groups.

Empowerment should be a key feature of any intervention aimed at the patient so that
their sense of personal control and capabilities in performing the behavior is increased. If
patients feel confident and able (i.e., have high levels of self-efficacy) in participating in
their healthcare, this is likely to have a direct impact on patients' actual engagement in the
behaviors.

Clinicians can encourage patients to exchange health-related information by adopting a
patient-centered consulting style. Patients are much more likely to speak up and voice their
concerns if they think their doctor genuinely wants to hear what they have to say and is
sympathetic to their needs.

Doctors should address patients anxieties (irrational or rational) associated with the
uncertainties in decisions which impact on life and death and/or general quality of life.
In order for the patient to get the best out of the clinical encounter the patient needs to

be able to express clearly what they think their problem is and any anxieties they may have about this. The doctor needs to address these anxieties and describe the intended course of "treatment" action in a way that the patient understands it.

Interpersonal interventions that target both patients and healthcare professionals may show more promising findings in terms of encouraging patient involvement, than interventions aimed at patients alone. Healthcare professionals' attitudes and beliefs can play a significant part in facilitating or inhibiting patients' involvement levels. Both parties should be educated on the importance of patient involvement and encouraged to work together to effectively achieve this.

References

Ad Hoc Committee on Health Literacy. (1999). Health literacy: Report of the Council on Science Affairs, American Medical Association. *Journal of American Medical Association, 281*, 552–557.

Ajzen, I. (1985). From intention to actions: A theory of planned behaviour. In J. Kuhl & J. Beckman (Eds.), *Action-control: From cognition to behaviour* (pp. 11–39). Heidelberg, Germany: Springer.

Anthony, R., Miranda, F., Mawji, Z., Cerimele, R., Davis, R., & Lawrence, S. (2005). The LVHHN Patient safety video: Patients as partners in safe care delivery. *Joint Commission Journal on Quality and Patient Safety, 10*, 566–572.

Arora, N. K., & McHorney, C. A. (2000). Patient preferences for medical decision making: Who really wants to participate? *Medical Care, 38*, 335–412.

Becker, M. H. (1974). The health belief model and personal health behaviour. *Health Education Monographs, 2*, 324–508.

Bishop, P., Kirwan, J., & Windsor, K. (1996). *The ARC patient literature evaluation project.* Chesterfield, UK: The Arthritis and Rheumatism Council.

Catalan, J., Brener, N., Andrews, H., Day, A., Cullum, S., Hooker, M., & Gazzrd, B. (1994). Whose health is it? Views about decision-making and information-seeking from people with HIV infections and their professional carers. *AIDS Care, 6*, 349–356.

Clayton, J., Butow, P., Tattersall, M., Chye, R., Noel, M., Davis, J. M., & Glare, P. (2003). Asking questions can help: Development and preliminary evaluation of a question prompt list for palliative care patients. *British Journal of Cancer, 89*, 2069–2077.

Clifford, S., Garfield, S., Eliasson, L., & Barber, N. (2010). Medication adherence and community pharmacy: A review of education, policy and research in England. *Pharmacy Practice, 8*, 77–88.

Cockburn, J., & Pit, S. (1997). Prescribing behaviour in clinical practice: Patients' expectations and doctors' perceptions of patients' expectations. *British Medical Journal, 315*, 520–523.

Coulter, A. (2005). What do patients and the public want from primary care? *British Medical Journal, 331*, 1199–1201.

Coulter, A., & Ellins, J. (2006). *Patient-focused interventions: A review of the evidence.* London, UK: Picker Institute Europe/Health Foundation.

Davis, R., Koutantji, M., & Vincent, C. (2008). How willing are patients to question healthcare staff on issues related to the quality and safety of their healthcare? An exploratory study. *Quality and Safety in Health Care, 17*, 90–96.

Davis, R., Sevdalis, N., Jacklin, R., & Vincent, C. (2007). Patient involvement in safety: What factors influence patient participation and engagement? *Health Expectations, 10*, 259–267.

Department of Health. (2001). *The expert patient: A new approach to chronic disease management for the 21st century.* London, UK: DOH.

De Sola-morales, S. O., & Elorza Ricart, J. M. (2005). Portable coagulometers: A systematic review of the evidence on self-management of oral anticoagulant treatment. *Medicina Clinica (Barc), 124,* 321–325.

Egberts, T., Smulders, M., de Koning, F., Meyboom, R., & Leufkens, H. (1996). Can adverse drug reactions be detected earlier? A comparison of reports by patients and professionals. *British Medical Journal, 313,* 530–531.

Eysenbach, G. (2003). The impact of the internet on cancer outcomes. *CA: A Cancer Journal for Clinicians, 53,* 356–371.

Gagliano, M. E. (1988). A literature review on the efficacy of video in patient education. *Journal of Medical Education, 63,* 785–792.

General Medical Council. (2003). *Tomorrows doctors.* GMC.

Goddard, M., & Hobden, C. (2003). *Patient choice: A review.* York: Centre for Health Economics, University of York.

Ha, J. F., & Longnecker, N. (2010). Doctor-patient communication: A review. *The Ochsner Journal, 10,* 38–43.

Heneghan, C., Alonso-Coello, P., Garcia-Alamino, J. M., Perera, R., Meats, E., & Glasziou, P. (2006). Self-monitoring of oral anticoagulation: A systematic review and meta-analysis. *Lancet, 36,* 404–411.

Ho, P. M., Magid, D. J., Masoudi, F. A., McClure, D. L., & Rumsfeld, J. S. (2006). Adherence to cardioprotective medications and mortality among patients with diabetes and ischemic heart disease. *BMC Cardiovascular disorders, 6,* 48.

Institute of Medicine. (2004). *Health literacy: A prescription to end confusion.* Washington, DC: The National Academic Press.

Kenny, T., Wilson, R. G., Purves, I. N., Clark, J., Newton, L. D., Newton, D. P., & Moseley, D. V. (1998). A PIL for every ill? Patient information leaflets (PILs): A review of past, present and future use. *Family Practice, 15,* 471–479.

Kirkcaldy, B., Siefen, R. G., Merbach, M., Rutow, N., Brahler, E., & Wittig, U. (2007). A comparison of general and illness-related locus of control in Russians, ethnic German migrants and Germans. *Psychology, Health and Medicine, 12,* 364–379.

Kitching, J. B. (1990). Patient information leaflets – the state of the art. *Journal of Royal Society of Medicine, 83,* 298–300.

Kraetschmer, N., Sharpe, N., Urowitz, S., & Deber, R. B. (2004). How does trust affect patient preferences for participation in decision-making? *Health Expectations, 7,* 317–326.

Krenzischek, D. A., Wilson, L., & Poole, E. L. (2001). Evaluation of ASPAN's preoperative patient teaching videos on general, regional, and minimum alveolar concentration/conscious sedation anaesthesia. *Journal of Perianaesthesia Nursing, 16,* 174–180.

Mansell, D., Poses, R. M., Kazis, L., & Duefield, C. A. (2000). Clinical factors that influence patients' desire for participation in decisions about illness. *Archives of Internal Medicine, 160,* 2991–2996.

McGuckin, M., Taylor, A., Martin, V., Porten, L., & Salcido, R. (2004). Evaluation of a patient education model for increasing hand hygiene compliance in an inpatient rehabilitation unit. *American Journal of Infection Control, 32,* 235–238.

McGuckin, M., Waterman, R., Porten, L., Bello, S., Caruso, M., Juzaitis, B., ... Ostrawski, S. (1999). Patient education model for increasing handwashing compliance. *American Journal of Infection Control, 27,* 309–314.

McGuckin, M., Waterman, R., Storr, J., Bowler, I., Ashby, M., Topley, K., & Porten, L. (2001). Evaluation of a patient empowering hand hygiene programme in the UK. *Journal of Hospital Infection, 48,* 222–227.

Mullen, P. (1997). Compliance becomes concordance. *British Medical Journal, 314*, 691.

Office for National Statistics. (2008). *Health Statistics Quarterly, 39.*

O'Cathain, A., Walters, S. J., Nicholl, J. P., Thomas, K. J., & Kirkham, M. (2002). Use of evidence based leaflets to promote informed choice in maternity care: Randomised controlled trial in everyday practice. *British Medical Journal, 324*, 643–646.

O'Connor, A., & Edwards, A. (2001). The role of decision aids in prompting evidence-based patient choice. In A. Edwards & E. Elwyn (Eds.), *Evidence-based patient choice: Inevitable or impossible?* Oxford, UK: OUP.

Odegaard, K. J. (2004). Self-management in anticoagulation – a meta-analysis. *Tidsskr Nor Laegeforen* [Journal of the Norwegian Medical Association]*, 124*, 2900–2903.

Pitkethly, M., MacGillivray, S., & Ryan, R. (2008). Recordings or summaries of consultations with people with cancer. *Cochrane Database of Systematic Reviews*, CD001539.

Roth-isigkeit, A., Ocklitz, E., Bruckner, A., Ros, L., Dibbelt, H., & Friedrich, H. (2002). Development and evaluation of a video program for presentation prior to elective cardiac surgery. *Acta Anaesthesiologica Scandinavica, 46*, 415–423.

Scott, T., Entwistle, V. A., Sowden, A. J., & Watt, I. (2001). Giving recordings or written summaries of consultations to people with cancer: A systematic review. *Health Expectations, 4*, 162–169.

Siebenhofer, A., Berghold, A., & Sawicki, P. T. (2004). Systematic review of studies of self-management of oral coagulation. *Thrombosis and Haemostasis, 91*, 225–232.

Sihota, S., & Lennard, L. (2004). *Health literacy: Being able to make the most of health.* London, UK: National Consumer Council.

Stewart, D. E., Wong, F., Cheung, M., Dancey, J., Meana, M., Cameron, J. I., . . . Rosen, B. (2000). Information needs and decisional preferences among women with ovarian cancer. *Gynaecology Oncology, 77*, 357–361.

Thorndike, E. L. (1901). Animal intelligence: An experimental study of the associative processes in animals. *Psychological Review Monograph Supplement, 2*, 1–109.

Unruh, K. T., & Pratt, W. (2007). Patients as actors: The patient's role in detecting, preventing, and recovering from medical errors. *International Journal of Medical Informatics, 76S*, S236–S244.

van den Bemt, P., Egberts, A., Lenderink, J., Verzijl, K., Simons, W., van der Pol, J., & Leufkens, H. G. (1999). Adverse drug events in hospitalised patients. A comparison of doctors, nurses. *European Journal of Clinical Pharmacology, 55*, 155–158.

Vincent, C., & Coulter, A. (2002). Patient safety: What about the patient? *Quality and Safety in Health Care, 11*, 76–80.

Volk, R., Cass, A., & Spann, S. (1999). A randomised controlled trial of shared decision making for prostate screening. *Archives of Family Medicine, 8*, 333–340.

Wagner, E. H., Barrett, P., Barry, M. J., Barlow, W., & Fowler, F. J., Jr. (1995). The effect of a shared decision making program on rates of surgery for benign prostatic hyperplasia: Pilot results. *Medical Care, 33*, 765–770.

Yang, B. Y., Thumula, V., Pace, P. F., Banahan, B. F., Wilkin, N. E., & Lobb, W. B. (2009). Medication nonadherence and the risk of hospitalization, emergency department visits and death among Medicare Part D Enrollees with diabetes. *Drug Benefit Trends, 21*, 12.

Migrant Health

Idioms of Distress and Health Services

Jutta Lindert

Protestant University of Applied Sciences, Ludwigsburg, Germany

This chapter reviews the current state of knowledge on migrants' health and their idioms of distress. Good health is crucial for the successful resettlement of migrants in a new country (Lassetter & Callister, 2009). However, reliable empirical information on the epidemiology of health and their idioms of distress among migrants remain scarce (Anikeeva et al., 2010; Friis et al., 1998; Peeters, 1985), posing an obstacle to tailoring health care services to this population group (Lindert et al., 2009).

Generally, even in the absence of comprehensive data on migrants' health and migrants' idioms of distress, societies are conscious that the health status, idioms of distress, and health care needs vary among population groups. Nevertheless, caution should be exercised in making generalizations on migrants as a homogeneous group. Migrants are diverse groups, including people with diverse migration histories (e.g., voluntary or forced migration) and coming from a variety of countries. In the context of recent migration, migrants live increasingly in "transcultural identities." In those transcultural identities the country where migrants come from is not the only, or even the most central, aspect for health and idioms of distress as migrants like nonmigrants negotiate multiple identities, including age, gender, education, and professional background (Nadeau & Measham, 2006).

Moreover, health and idioms of distress may be transformed during the process(es) of migration and over time. Where variations between migrants and nonmigrants have been reported, there has been much argument about the likely reasons. Explanations have been offered in terms of the genetic make-up of different ethnic groups, which might predispose migrants to experience more or less mental illness than others; in terms of the lifestyle imported from the country of origin; in terms of selective migration (those with illness being less likely to leave their country of origin); or in terms of the social and economic conditions in which migrants find themselves during migration, including loss of relatives and relationships, poverty, inadequate housing, and discrimination. The direction of variation in health and in idioms of distress is not known precisely, but health care providers need to be aware of migrants' potentially specific idioms of distress (Nichter, 1981; Parsons, 1984; Parsons & Wakeley, 1991).

Low awareness among health professionals of potential idioms of distress may affect the perceived need of health services and the quality of health and psychosocial services offered and received (Fassaert, de Wit et al., 2009a, 2009b). Health care providers and migrants may have different idioms of distress, and misperceptions and misunderstandings may seriously hamper health care delivery. There are certain areas of healthcare, such as the existing asynchrony of perspectives on health and illness between caregivers and the migrant community, that have not yet been sufficiently addressed by health care providers. Furthermore, the responsibility of health care providers to respond to the needs and priorities for migrants' health must include a sociocultural perspective to migrants' social and economic conditions and to the idioms which the groups use to express bodily sensations. Without this more integral perspective, there is a risk for a mismatch of needs and care and for the medicalization of problems derived from migrants' social situations.

This chapter begins by reviewing the history and the concept of "idioms of distress," then provides an overview of the pattern of migration and the history of society's response to the health aspects of migration. This is followed by an exploration of what is known about the idioms of distress of migrants, ranging from somatic complaints to mental disorders. It is also important to know how these idioms of distress change in the process of migration and of settlement in the host countries. Therefore, before concluding this chapter, the process of migration and potential changes in idioms of distress during the migration trajectory will be described. The chapter concludes by drawing lessons on how health care providers might better meet the health care needs of migrants by understanding the concept of "idiom of distress" and the social meaning of these idioms.

Idioms of Distress – History of the Concept

Characteristic modes of expressing suffering and bodily sensations are called "idioms of distress" (Choudhury & Kirmayer, 2009; Hinton, 2006; Hinton, Howes et al., 2008a, 2008b). An idiom of distress was first defined by Mark Nichter (Nichter, 1981) in the following way:

In any given culture, a variety of ways exist to express distress. Expressive modes are culturally constituted in the sense that they initiate particular types of interaction and are associated with culturally pervasive values, norms, generative themes, and health concerns (p. 379).

Idioms of distress reflect values and themes found in the societies in which they originate. They have become a rather new paradigm in medicine to characterize reactions that are used to describe health-related symptoms and distress of special groups, for example, migrant groups.

Idioms of distress are those particular ways in which members of groups express affliction. These descriptions of distress vary across groups, depending on traditions for experiencing distress (Ewing, 2005). This concept has been used in medical anthropology and transcultural psychiatry to describe the culturally specific experiences of psychosocial and physical suffering. While the distress experiences seen in diverse cultural groups

Models of health and disease

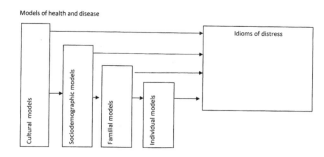

Figure 1. Models of health and disease.

sometimes signify the presence of physical or psychological disorders, they may also be culturally coded ways of expressing social discontent/discomfort and they may be functional in specific environments.

The construct of "idiom of distress" at least partly has replaced the earlier model of "culture bound" health-related syndromes and distress. Health-related syndromes and distress are not expressed in the same way across all cultures or subgroups of populations. The term "idioms of distress" can be used to describe specific health-related symptoms that occur in some societies or subgroups of societies and that are recognized by members of those societies or subgroups as health related. An example of an idiom of distress is somatization: People complain of physical symptoms which are mainly caused by emotional or mental worry, anxiety, or stress. Somatic complaints may be aches and pains, headaches, palpitations, and dizziness (Kirmayer & Sartorius, 2007).

The sources of the diversities of idioms of distress are individual models, familial models and varying cultural models, and the health services profile of the country (see Figure 1). Cultural models are models that influence together with individual models perceptions, beliefs, values, and behavioral practices.

Idioms of Distress

Cultural models direct attention and bodily sensations toward culturally relevant bodily expressions (Hinton, 2006). The individual learns in his or her environment which physical and emotional sensations, changes, and experiences should be acknowledged and articulated. In this way, cultural models shape how much attention one pays to one's constantly fluctuating bodily sensations. The health care services in the respective countries may contribute to the cultural models as bodily sensations may be accepted as cause for help-seeking behavior but not mental distress per se. While we know that complaints of physical symptoms can be seen in migrant patients, additional mental health symptoms might remain unrecognized (Cramer et al., 2007; Fassaert, de Wit et al., 2009a, 2009b; Regier, 2007).

Ethnographic and clinical studies of depression in diverse Asian groups have revealed that this group has a tendency to experience negative, depression-like emotions as symbolic and holistically interrelated with somatic sensations and interpersonal disharmony, suggesting an inclination to endorse a variety of somatic distress symptoms. Koreans are reported to have high prevalence rates of symptoms of depression in both Korea and in Korean immigrants in the US. Ethnographic studies of highly distressed Koreans have identified several idioms of distress that resemble symptoms of depression. These include *Han* (a form of regret or resentment syndrome), *Hwa-byung* (an anger syndrome), and *Shingyungshayak* (similar to the Chinese diagnosis of neurasthenia). *Han* has been described as a passive, chronic regret, and resentment syndrome, and includes the sensation of an obstruction by a lump in the epigastric and respiratory regions (Cho et al., 1998).

Herewith, idioms of distress constitute individually embodied sensations that are often based on local ideas associated with the functioning of the body and mind (Hinton, Howes et al., 2008a, 2008b). Physiologically, however, the conditions to which the idioms give rise to are no less real as a result. Biological mechanisms are recruited for their expression and may result in chronic disease over time, especially in vulnerable individuals. One of the main functions of idioms of distress is that they convey a wide range of personal and social concerns in a way recognizable by people from the same background, who are then alerted that the person relating the idioms of distress may need help.

One of the most common idioms of distress among migrants and among certain population groups of nonmigrants, for example, persons from lower socioeconomic strata is somatization, the expression of distress in terms of physical suffering (Aragona et al., 2010; Machleidt & Assion, 2007). Somatization occurs widely and is believed to be especially prevalent among persons from a number of ethnic minority backgrounds.

Box 1
Idioms of distress are those particular ways in which members of groups express affliction.
Idioms of distress vary across groups, depending on traditions for experiencing and communicating distress.
Idioms of distress are personal and group related ways of expression.

Pattern of Migration

People tend to migrate to improve their living conditions and the living conditions of their families. The last decade has been called the "decade of ethnicity," with theoretical interest revolving around the way in which "culture and psyche" interact (Shweder & Sullivan, 1993). Kirkcaldy, Furnham, and Siefen (2009) discuss the economic factor that exerts a role in the migration process, especially evident from "immigration patterns towards more industrialized, economic stable countries. There are push and pull factors. Migrants are pushed by poverty, famine, illness, and political oppression while being pulled by opportunities for a better life for themselves and their families." (p. 328). This might include more career opportunities in the country of destination, better quality of working conditions, and/or moving away from political instability and the experience or the threat of violence in the home country.

Conversely, motives to migrate are frequently complex, having economic, increasingly ecological, psychological, and cultural determinants. Migration is often stepwise as people tend to move from poorer regions to richer regions within a country and then to higher income countries. Globalization has helped to drive international migration and the number of people migrating is expected to increase even more in the context of the financial crisis. In the following the diverse groups of migrants will be described as "migrants" without differentiating between the various groups of migrants. We focus in this chapter on health care needs and idioms of distress of migrants.

Although in general, people migrate to improve life chances for themselves or their children and expect gains in well-being, a large body of literature suggests that migration can be a stressful process, with potentially negative impacts on health and on mental health (Bhugra, 2001).

In fact, the World Health Organization (WHO) claims that "[...] usually migration does not bring improved social well-being; rather [...] it often results in [...] exposing migrants to social stress and increased risk of mental disorders" (WHO, 2001, p. 13). The available evidence suggests that the impact of migration on health and on mental health may differ among different types of migrants (e.g., permanent and nonpermanent labor migrants, migrants forcibly uprooted by wars, conflicts, or political violence (e.g., refugees and asylum seekers) (Lindert, Brahler et al., 2008).

Four broad phases have been identified in the development of interest for the health problems of migrants. The first phase is characterized by an interest in unusual *infectious diseases* of migrants. The second phase was around biological differences, with a focus on *genetically inherited diseases*. The third phase was characterized by focusing on the *population patterns* of disease with a strong emphasis on migrants groups comparisons. Fourth, it was an issue to *adapt health care services and research* to meet the needs of migrants. Apparently, the impact of migration on idioms of distress, on the perception of physical and emotional states of migrants and on their help-seeking has been downsized in some available studies. The respective idiom of distress influences the evaluation and determines the action one takes in response to bodily sensitizations.

Migration patterns change over time. In 2009, the aging of migrants and migrants from violent events were of special concern for health care services. The five countries with the largest number of migrants are the US, Russia, Germany, Saudi Arabia, and Canada (United Nations, 2010). The five countries with the highest percentage of migrants in 2009 are Quatar, The United Arab Emirates, Kuwait, and Jordan. Asia has the largest number of young migrants and Europe has the largest number of older migrants. In

2010, Europe hosted the highest number of international migrants aged 20–64: 50.5 million or nearly a third of all international migrants of working age. They account for 11% of the working age population in the continent. Asia, the most populous world region, hosts the second largest number of international migrants of working age (42 million), which represent 27% of all international migrants aged 20–64 and just 1.7% of the working age population in Asia. In Northern America, the 39.3 million international migrants of working age present in 2010 accounted for nearly 19% of the working age population in the region. As long-established countries of immigration, Canada and the US remain major magnets for international migrants. Asia hosts 12.9 million international migrants under the age of 20 years, representing 39% of the total population. Europe hosts 11.9 million international migrants aged 65 or over, representing 44% of all older migrants (Fund, 2010).

A special group of migrants are refugees. Refugees are the result of disasters, such as war, conflict, and natural disasters, which cause population displacement. The 1951 United Nations Refugee Convention states that a refugee is an individual who "owing to a well-founded fear of being persecuted for reasons of race, religion, nationality, membership of a particular social group or political opinion, is outside the country of his nationality, and is unable to, or owing to such fear, is unwilling to avail himself of the protection of that country" (United Nations General Assembly, 1951). Some refugees, however, flee from conflict, violence or persecution on a small-scale or individual basis, making their way to countries of asylum. Persons of special concern are individuals who do not meet the formal criteria for obtaining refugee status according to the United Nations High Commissioner for Refugees (UNHCR) in some countries. This group included in 2006 asylum seekers (0.8 million), returned refugees (1.1 million), internally displaced persons (IDPs; 6.6 million), and stateless persons (3.8 million). According to UNHCR, in 2009 worldwide there are approximately 43 million forcibly displaced people.

Worldwide trends of refugee resettlement mean that they are contributing to more culturally diverse societies in developed countries. When people are forcibly displaced from one area to another, several factors might contribute to specific idioms of distress because of the experience of forced displacement (Hinton & Lewis-Fernandez, 2010; Hinton et al., 2010).

Idioms of distress can be a useful marker for the presence of traumatic events among refugees, independent of the presence or absence of psychiatric diagnoses. In a sample of highly traumatized migrants from Latin America the presence of cultural idioms of distress was found (e.g., "susto") but not of symptoms of psychiatric diseases (Hinton & Lewis-Fernandez, 2010; Lewis-Fernandez et al., 2010).

Box 2
Migration is dynamic and rapidly changing both pattern and population composition.
Immigrants and their families comprise population groups of special interest for health care provide.

Phases of Migration and Idioms of Distress of Migrants

Berry (1992) formulated a multiphase model of the integration process commencing with contract/observation and transition into a conflict phase with an associative increase in stress, which eventually decreases in a stage of adaptation or stabilization. This theory has been augmented by others, for example, by Ritsner & Ponizovsky (1999), but is under discussion now. This model related to the pattern of migration before the era of transcultural migration with several migrations following each other.

Idiom of distress is neither regarded as a closed nor as an entity, but rather as a multiple, relational being-in-the-world that is captured by his or her surroundings, engaging with past, present, and future situations. Crucially, this approach acknowledges that idioms of distress are not only shaped by the culture of origin directly, but also by memories and imagination. Certain events during the life course and especially during the phases of migration can have a long-lasting impact on one's perception of distress.

The "others" in the migration process are not only other human beings and cultures but animals, landscapes, material objects, images, or events. In this context, it is vital to realize that migrants' health and migrants' idioms of distress are not static but are associated with migration-related phases and the encounters during these phases. Movement related phases are the pre-migration phase, the displacement phase itself, the post-migration phase, and the resettlement phase. Each migration phase is associated with potential health risks and vulnerabilities and in each phase the idioms of distress may change according to the environment as idioms of distress may be looked upon as discourses and embodied experiences (see Figure 2).

Pre-Migration Phase

The pre-migration phase constitutes the first phase, it means the traditional environment in which the idiom of distress is formed by the environment and understood in the respective

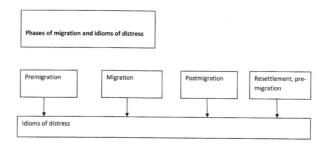

Figure 2. Migration phases and idioms of distress.

environment. Related to the idiom of distress of the migrant is the epidemiological profile of the country of origin, and the structure of the health system (e.g., accessibility and performance). The idiom of distress is formed in this special environment. The performance of the health system will, in part, determine the idiom of distress.

Migration Phase

The second phase of the migration encompasses the displacement period. In this phase, the idioms of distress may change because of the migration and due to the changing environment.

Kirkcaldy et al. (2005) monitored somatic complaints among Russian immigrants in Germany during the initial 18 months after migration. An increase in complaints was observed during the first phase (6 months) after arrival, consistent with the migration hypothesis. The authors were cautious in assuming physical complaints were necessarily related to actual physical health. Pain symptoms and signs of headache and fatigue suggested excessive strain resulting possibly from the extreme demands of communicating in an unfamiliar language as well as reorienting in a novel/host community. After 18 months, the degrees of complaints were below the level on arrival.

The Post-Migration Phase

The third phase of the migration comprises the post-migration phase. In this phase the idiom of distress may change again according to the new situation in the host country. Migrants may not be aware of available health care services, may not have legal or respected documentation in the host country of asylum, or may lack health insurance and other social safety nets. Cultural and linguistic barriers may exist that prevent populations from fully benefitting from available healthcare services. Financial barriers in the form of user fees, or lack of transportation, may render services inaccessible. Furthermore, the legal status of migrants – whether they are considered refugees with legal documentation, asylum seekers awaiting a decision, or failed asylum seekers – all have an impact on access to health care services. The access itself or the lack of access may be related to the idioms of distress as those may arise which are functional in the new environment. The post-migration phase can be a new pre-migration phase as migrations increasingly follow each other.

Migration involves coming into contact not only with new languages but with other forms of health care services and other idioms of distress. Idioms of distress are not static and the transformation of expressions of migrants' idioms of distress during the migration process needs further research.

The process of coming into contact is associated with subsequent changes in the original culture patterns of idioms of distress. Health care providers must remember that none of these processes are static and these acts keep occurring and the individual keeps responding to events by changing his or her concepts and his or her idioms of distress. In conclusion, when people migrate from one nation or culture to another they carry their knowledge and idioms of distress with them. Idioms of distress are both individual perceptions of bodily sensations and education and culturally shaped sensations and idioms to express feelings of distress. A number of studies suggest that cultural groups differ in the extent to which members perceive and monitor bodily states (Keyes & Ryff, 2003). Significant differences between migrant groups in the perception, interpretation, and in the response to bodily states are reported. In addition to objective disparities in health, the obvious differences in health of migrants and nonmigrants may be related to those idioms of distress of migrants that do not match the idioms of distress of nonmigrants (Kirmayer, 2008; Kirmayer et al., 2010).

For example, a study of Punjabi women who had been in the UK for a number of years found that they maintained the belief that depression was not a medical condition (Jacob et al., 1998). Their help-seeking was related to their idioms of distress, which led them to seek help from religious practitioners and by reading scriptures rather than seeking medical help from professional health care services. It has been suggested that differences in certain areas of health between groups may decrease if idioms of distress are taken into account, for example, disparities in mental health between countries disappeared as somatization increased (Keyes & Ryff, 2003).

As migrants encounter new opportunities or hardship during migration, or negotiate new relations, they are exposed to new emotional vocabularies and ways of "feeling." The longer they stay abroad, the more acquainted they become with new ways of expressing emotions and the more they have to reconcile these views with the emotional knowledge and the idioms they carry. These idioms of distress which change during the migration process are related to the utilization of health care services and to help-seeking behavior.

Utilization of Health Care Services and Idioms of Distress During Migration

Idioms of distress carry important consequences for willingness to offer and to seek health services. Among adults, the evidence is considerable that persons from migration backgrounds are less likely than nonmigrants to utilize health care services in the mental health sector (Lindert, Schouler-Ocak et al., 2008). Again, Kirkcaldy, Siefen, and Furnham (2009) use the label "cultural disparity" and suggest that migrants may report more or less distress of a specific kind than natives due to cultural norms in manifesting distress.

Health care services may offer a poorer service to ethnic minority groups for a variety of reasons (e.g., policies based on the needs of nonmigrant populations and institutional racism). There is evidence that policies based solely on the needs of nonmigrant populations and/or institutional racism are in action but less is known about the use of health care services associated with idioms of distress (Bhui & Bhugra, 2002, 2003). Findings suggest that there are differences among migrant groups in idioms of distress and perceived need for healthcare that may partially account for the low rates of health care among migrants.

The available evidence indicates that the utilization of health care services among migrants shows patterns of under- and overutilization, but studies with representative samples are still scarce (Baarnhielm & Ekblad, 2000). The literature attributes underutilization of health services by migrants to a nonexclusive group of barriers relating to migration background, ethnicity, culture, health systems, and societal responses to migrants. Barriers identified by researchers focusing on the health system include limited access to health professionals from the same culture, high cost of services, lengthy waiting times for specialist counseling services, and, for many refugees, difficulties in accessing mental health services because of legal restrictions. Other system-level barriers include service complexity, bureaucracy, and fragmentation. Overutilization of health services may be related to idioms of distress which perceive pain differently from the majority population.

Particularly salient to the issue of service utilization is the level of match between services offered and those accessing them (Ingleby, 2005). Matching of offer and needs is possible when the expectations and possibilities of the service providers and the expectations of the help-seeking individuals match. This might not be the case if service providers are not aware of idioms of distress and of the potential mismatch of their own idioms of distress and those of migrants.

Conclusion

We contend that academics and health care providers have not paid sufficient attention to idioms of distress and embodiment among migrants. We believe that clinicians and researchers must develop reliable ways to measure idioms of distress phenomena for migrants. New methods, for example, mixing qualitative and quantitative methods, would be needed. Research on the incidence of an illness for any cultural group requires assessment with an instrument or assessment tool, and the general practice worldwide in research has been to use translated versions of western instruments. The widespread use of these measures across migrants requires assumptions. Firstly, the assumption that there is phenomenological equivalence between the symptoms on self-assessment indicators for the members of all of these groups, that is, the symptoms are experienced in the same way, and mean the same thing. Secondly, there is a tacit assumption that the measure in question assesses all facets of the relevant symptoms and indicators necessary to accurately and adequately capture the phenomenon of interest. Unfortunately, few studies have tackled these questions of phenomenological equivalence using symptom inventories, for example, the cross-cultural equivalence of psychometric and medical instruments for assessment with large groups in order to expand the symptom list to capture symptoms relevant to migrants. Specifically, we need to learn more about the idioms of distress that migrants identify as most salient to their problems.

In conclusion, available evidence supports the value of assessing idioms of distress in health evaluations alongside illness (Hinton & Lewis-Fernandez, 2010). The idioms of distress may add useful clinical information, pointing to additional sources of morbidity and even potential psychological mechanisms that underlie and help shape the clinical presentation of illness.

Their broader inclusion in health research may help explain some of the missing variance in the relationship between symptomatology and levels of morbidity and distress among migrants (Lewis-Fernandez et al., 2010). There seems to be sufficient evidence to suggest that a focus on differences in health which fails to address idioms of distress will not fully meet the needs of migrants.

References

Anikeeva, O., Bi, P., & Han, G.-S. (2010). The health status of migrants in Australia: A review. *Asia-Pacific Journal of Public Health, 22*, 159–193.

Aragona, M., Catino, E., & Geraci, S. (2010). The relationship between somatization and posttraumatic symptoms among immigrants receiving primary care services. *Journal of Traumatic Stress, 23*, 615–622.

Baarnhielm, S., & Ekblad, S. (2000). Turkish migrant women encountering health care in Stockholm: A qualitative study of somatization and illness meaning. *Culture, Medicine and Psychiatry, 24*, 431–452.

Berry, J. W. (1992). Acculturation and adaptation in a new society. *International Migration, 30*, 69–85.

Bhugra, D., & Jones, P. (2001). Migration and mental illness. *Advances in Psychiatric Treatment, 7*, 216–233.

Bhui, K., & Bhugra, D. (2002). Explanatory models for mental distress: Implications for clinical practice and research. *British Journal of Psychiatry, 181*, 6–7.

Bhui, K., & Bhugra, D. (2003). Explanatory models in psychiatry. *British Journal of Psychiatry, 183*, 170.

Cho, M. J., Nam, J. J., & Suhc, G. H. (1998). Prevalence of symptoms of depression in a nationwide sample of Korean adults. *Psychiatry Research, 81*, 341–352.

Choudhury, S., & Kirmayer, L. J. (2009). Cultural neuroscience and psychopathology: Prospects for cultural psychiatry. *Progress in Brain Research, 178*, 263–283.

Cramer, V., Torgersen, S., & Kringlen, E. (2007). Socio-demographic conditions, subjective somatic health, Axis I disorders and personality disorders in the common population: The relationship to quality of life. *Journal of Personality Disorders, 21*, 552–567.

Ewing K. P. (Ed.), (2005). *Immigrant identities and emotion. Companion to psychological anthropology.* Oxford, UK: Blackwell.

Fassaert, T., de Wit, M. A., & Dekker, J. (2009a). Perceived need for mental health care among non-Western labour migrants. *Social Psychiatry and Psychiatric Epidemiology, 44*, 208–216.

Fassaert, T., de Wit, M. A., Verhoeff, A. P., Tuinebreijer, N. C., Gorissen, W. H. M., Beekman, A. J. F., & Dekker, J. (2009b). Uptake of health services for common mental disorders by first-generation Turkish and Moroccan migrants in the Netherlands. *BMC Public Health, 9*, 307.

Friis, R., Yngve, A., & Persson, V. (1998). Review of social epidemiologic research on migrants' health: Findings, methodological cautions, and theoretical perspectives. *Scandinavian Journal of Social Medicine, 26*, 173–180.

Hinton, D. E. (2006). Transcultural Psychiatry. *Journal of Analytical Psychology, 51*, 615–617.

Hinton, D. E., Howes, D., & Kirmayer, L. J. (2008a). The medical anthropology of sensations. *Transcultural Psychiatry, 45*, 139–141.

Hinton, D. E., Howes, D., & Kirmayer, L. J. (2008b). Toward a medical anthropology of sensations: Definitions and research agenda. *Transcultural Psychiatry, 45*, 142–162.

Hinton, D. E., & Lewis-Fernandez, R. (2010). Idioms of distress among trauma survivors: Subtypes and clinical utility. *Culture, Medicine and Psychiatry, 34*, 209–218.

Hinton, D. E., Pich, V., & Pollack, M. H. (2010). Khyal attacks: A key idiom of distress among traumatized cambodia refugees. *Culture, Medicine and Psychiatry, 34*, 244–278.

Ingleby D. (Ed.), (2005). *Forced migration and mental health: rethinking the care of refugees and displaced persons.* International and Cultural Psychology Series. New York, NY: Springer.

Jacob, K. S., Bhugra, D., & Mann, A. H. (1998). Common mental disorders, explanatory models and consultation behaviour among Indian women living in the UK. *Journal of the Royal Society of Medicine, 91*, 66–71.

Keyes, C. L., & Ryff, C. D. (2003). Somatization and mental health: A comparative study of the idiom of distress hypothesis. *Social Science & Medicine, 57*, 1833–1845.

Kirkcaldy, B. D., Furnham, A., & Siefen, G. (2009). Migration and health: Psychosocial determinants. In A. A. Antoniou, C. L. Cooper, G. P. Chrousos, C. D. Spielberger, & M. W. Eysenck (Eds.), *Handbook of managerial behaviour and occupational health.* Cheltenham, UK: E. Elgar.

Kirkcaldy, B. D., Siefen, R. G., Wittig, U., Schüller, A., Brähler, E., & Merbach, M. (2005). Health and emigration: Subjective evaluation of health status and physical symptoms in Russian-speaking migrants. *Stress and Health, 21*, 295–309.

Kirmayer, L. J. (2008). Culture and the metaphoric mediation of pain. *Transcultural Psychiatry, 45*, 318–338.

Kirmayer, L. J., Narasiah, L., Munoz, M., Rashid, M., Ryder, A., Guzder, J., . . . K. Pottie. (2010). Common mental health problems in immigrants and refugees: General approach in primary care. *Canadian Medical Associate Journal.* Advance online publication. doi: 10.1503/cmaj.090292.

Kirmayer, L. J., & Sartorius, N. (2007). Cultural models and somatic syndromes. *Psychosomatic Medicine, 69*, 832–840.

Lassetter, J. H., & Callister, L. C. (2009). The impact of migration on the health of voluntary migrants in western societies. *Journal of Transcultural Nursing, 20*, 93–104.

Lewis-Fernandez, R., Gorritz, M., & Guarnaccia, P. J. (2010). Association of trauma-related disorders and dissociation with four idioms of distress among Latino psychiatric outpatients. *Culture, Medicine and Psychiatry, 34*, 219–243.

Lindert, J., Brähler, E., & Priebe, S. (2008). Depression, anxiety and posttraumatic stress disorders in labor migrants, asylum seekers and refugees. A systematic overview. *Psychotherapie, Psychosomatik, Medizinische Psychologie, 58*(3–4), 109–122.

Lindert, J., Ehrenstein, O. S., & Brähler, E. (2009). Depression and anxiety in labor migrants and refugees – a systematic review and meta-analysis. *Social Science & Medicine, 69*, 246–257.

Lindert, J., Schouler-Ocak, M., Heinz, A., & Priebe, S. (2008). Mental health, health care utilisation of migrants in Europe. *European Psychiatry, 23*, (Suppl. 1) 14–20.

Machleidt, W., & Assion, H. J. (2007). Immigrants in the general medical practice. Good patient-doctor-patient relationship protects against somatization. *MMW Fortschritte der Medizin, 149*, 30–31.

Nadeau, L., & Measham, T. (2006). Caring for migrant and refugee children: Challenges associated with mental health care in pediatrics. *Journal of Developmental & Behavioral Pediatrics, 27*, 145–154.

Nichter, M. (1981). Idioms of distress: Alternatives in the expression of psychosocial distress: A case study from South India. *Culture, Medicine and Psychiatry, 5*, 379–408.

Nichter, M. (2010). Idioms of distress revisited. *Culture, Medicine and Psychiatry, 34*, 401–416.

Parsons, C. D. (1984). Idioms of distress: Kinship and sickness among the people of the Kingdom of Tonga. *Culture, Medicine and Psychiatry, 8*, 71–93.

Parsons, C. D., & Wakeley, P. (1991). Idioms of distress: Somatic responses to distress in everyday life. *Culture, Medicine and Psychiatry, 15*, 111–132.

Peeters, R. F. (1985). Migration and health: A literature review. II. Descriptive studies. An inventory of available studies concerning migrants' health with emphasis on Moroccans in Belgium and the Netherlands. *Archives of Belgica, 43,* 444–460.

Regier, D. A. (2007). Somatic presentations of mental disorders: Refining the research agenda for DSM-V. *Psychosomatic Medicine, 69,* 827–828.

Ritsner, M., & Ponizovsky, A. (1999). Psychological distzress through immigration. The two-phase temporal pattern. *International Journal of Social Psychiatry, 45,* 125–139.

Shweder, R. A., & Sullivan, M. A. (1993). Cultural Psychology: Who needs it? *Annual Review of Psychology, 44,* 497–527.

United Nations D. oeasa population division. (2010). *International migration 2009.* New York, NY: United Nations.

United Nations. (2010). *Population Facts.* Retrieved from http/www.un.org/esa/population/publications/popfacts/popfacts_2010-6.pdf.

World Health Organization. (2001). *World Health Report 2001. Mental health: New understanding, new hope.* Geneva: World Health Organization.

Drug Abuse Among Immigrants and the Role of Professionals in the Treatment Process

Alexander-Stamatios Antoniou[1] and Marina Dalla[2]

[1]University of Athens, Greece
[2]University of Athens and 18 ANO Dependence Unit, State Psychiatric Hospital of Athens, Greece

Chemical dependency and alcohol abuse represent one of the most threatening public health hazards in Europe (and elsewhere), and has been shown to be related to inferior educational performance, delinquency, and self-injurious behavior. Providing effective forms of treatment modalities for people with substance abuse problems is perceived as a "central pillar" to the European nations' response to drugs, with estimates of over one million persons in the EU receiving treatment every year. This chapter focuses on one country, Greece, and its problems with drug abuse, albeit this could be seen as typical of many nations, and hopefully the findings, recommendations, and suggestions for social health policy makers and health professionals will be helpful for other countries.

Greece as a Plural Society

This chapter concentrates on immigration and drug abuse together with models for professionals treating refugee and immigrant drug abusers in a European country (Greece). It is guided by four key questions: (1) How do immigrants deal with immigration and acculturation? (2) What are the risk factors related to drug abuse among immigrants and refugees? (3) What are the differences in drug abuse among immigrants and natives in Greece? (4) How can professionals become more culturally sensitive in servicing immigrant and refugee drug abusers and their families?

We report some of the main findings on the prevalence of illicit drug use among immigrants in Greece aged 19 years or older in comparison to native Greeks. Estimates for immigrants and native drug abusers are based on data collected during 2005–2009 from adults on the Drug Dependence Unit-State Psychiatry Hospital of Attica. Sample sizes were: $N = 67$ (54.5%) immigrants (Countries: Albania, former Soviet Union, Arabic countries) and $N = 56$ (45.5%) native Greeks. The data collection method used in this study involved face-to-face structured interviews that examined personal and demographic information (age, education in years, and country of birth), marital status, living conditions and housing, health status (HIV/AIDS), criminal and deviant behaviors, and information about the lifetime use of illicit substances. Immigrants are seen to differentiate their behavior in relation to drug abuse involvement and drug abuse treatment.

Starting in the mid 1980s, but especially during the 1990s, Greece turned from a country that was a source of immigrants into an immigration country. According to the Organization for Economic Cooperation and Development (OECD, 2000), the number of immigrants in the country was 1 million (10% of the Greek population). Major population inflows toward Greece include Albanian immigrants that constitute 56% of the total foreigners in the country. An estimated 13.3% of immigrants had come from the former Soviet Union and other countries of Eastern Europe, including Bulgaria and Romania (Baldwin-Edwards, 2004). Since 2003, the influx of Asian (Pakistani, Bangladeshi, and Indian) and Arab (Syrian and Egyptian) immigrants has sharply increased. It is estimated that the total number of Asian and Arab immigrants in Greece is no less than 130,000, representing roughly 10% of immigrants (Markoutsoglou, Kasou, Moshotos, & Ptohos, 2007). The same study also reported that immigrants from Sub-Sahara countries (Nigeria and Ethiopia) constituted approximately 2% of foreigners, although there were no entirely reliable data sources regarding their exact number. In addition, Germans, Britons, Italians, and other Europeans appeared as sizeable foreign communities, accounting for around 2% each of the total foreign population. A further group included ethnic Greek immigrants, including Pontics from the Black Sea region (152,204 Pontic Greeks) and Vorioepirotes (100,000), ethnic Greek-Albanian citizens (Gropas & Triandafyllidou, 2005) who had either been given Greek citizenship or awarded 5-year residency cards.

It is interesting to note that many of the immigrants entered the country irregularly, at least initially. Currently, about three quarters of the immigrant population have work and permit status (Gropas & Triandafyllidou, 2005). However, in 2008 there were between 200,000 and 250,000 undocumented immigrants in Greece (Lianos, Kanellopoulos, Gregou, Gemi, & Papakonstantinou, 2008). The pluralism of Greek society is reflected in the Greek National Health System. The percentage of hospitalized migrants in the General Hospital of Attica for the year 2003 was 6.2%, a percentage that approached the percentage of foreigners in comparison with the total population (Maratou-Alipranti & Gkazon, 2005).

Acculturation of Immigrants and Refugees

The process of migration can be understood as a transition life event (Suárez-Orozco, 2000) consisting of the pre-migration and departure phase and the transition and adaptation to a new country. The decision to migrate due to a perceived lack of prospects that a person has in his/her own country, related to economical or political conditions (Ward, Bochner, & Furnham, 2001), removes individuals from predictable contexts and creates a sense of loss (Suárez-Orozco & Suárez-Orozco, 2001). This sense of loss relates not only to one of belonging, but also the loss of family and social networks, customs, and language and even to the experience of homesickness (Stroebe, van Vliet, Hewstone,

& Willis, 2002). Following an initial period of hopes and expectations, many immigrants experience a sense of confusion in role, values, and identity, which can result in the experience of anxiety, disorientation, suspicion, and bewilderment (Oberg, 1960). Accordingly as the realities of the new situation are confronted, individuals may begin to experience a variety of psychological problems due to acculturation.

Acculturation implies cultural and psychological changes of persons in first-hand contact with persons representing another culture (Sam, 2006). Pressures on the individual to contend with the host society can lead to increased stress, or acculturative stress as a generalized physiological and psychological state brought about by the experience of stressors in the new environment (Berry, 2003). For example, stress is likely to be minimal and personal consequences are generally positive when the acculturation trajectory is bicultural as a result of a connection to both the country of origin and that of the mainstream culture. Alternatively, when an individual's adaptive resources are insufficient to support adjustment to a new cultural environment, or when individuals lack connection to both cultures, stress will be higher and its effects more negative (Berry, 2003). Acculturative stress is a common experience of first generation immigrants (Ward et al., 2001). Second generation and later generation immigrants may experience acculturative stress owing to the conflicts that arise out of their bicultural socialization (Roysircar-Sodowsky & Maestas, 2000). Longitudinal evidence suggests that acculturative stress has been frequently associated with the development of emotional and behavioral problems among immigrants (Organista, Organista, & Kurasaki, 2003), including substance abuse (Straussner, 2002).

Substance Abuse Among Immigrants

Drug dependence is characterized by a need for a markedly increased amount of abuse of legal drugs (e.g., alcohol and prescription drugs) as well as illegal drugs (e.g., cocaine, heroin, methamphetamines, and other substances), with the presence of physiological and behavioral symptoms associated with compulsive use, increased tolerance, and withdrawal symptoms (APA, 2000). Substance abuse and dependence is identified as a significant health problem for all European societies (Diamanduros, 2005). In addition, it is a serious social and public problem because it is widely associated with delinquent activities (Losoya et al., 2008), HIV, hepatitis B and C transmission through the sharing of needles, poverty, and social exclusion (WHO, 2008).

Research findings on substance use patterns among immigrant populations are mixed, with some studies indicating that substance use increased with increased time in the new country (Gfroerer & Tan, 2003). Acculturation processes with low educational aspirations for children of immigrants has been associated with high levels of substance abuse (Vega & Gil, 1999). Other studies have reported a decrease in substance use and mental health problems over time and with increased levels of acculturation (Caetano & Clark, 2003; National Institute on Drug Abuse [NIDA], 2001). Even within subgroups of immigrants, there is wide variability in substance use patterns. According to previous studies, immigrants from the former Soviet Union faced with the highly complex challenge of acculturation often develop emotional and behavioral problems that include mental illness, delinquency, and alcohol and drug abuse (Isralowitz, Straussner, Vogt, & Chtenguelov, 2002). Their experiences in their new countries, where drugs and alcohol are readily available at low prices, may lead to some immigrants experiencing a tendency to turn to substance abuse as a way of coping. Early research shows that substance abusers from the former Soviet Union, especially those using drugs, are mainly bilingual males in their early twenties. Unlike other young people in the New York City area, this population does not start with "gateway" drugs, such as marijuana or ecstasy, but goes straight to injecting heroin (Isralowitz et al., 2002).

The mixed findings from research with immigrant and minority populations point to the need for considering a coexistence of stressors that can increase vulnerability of immigrants to use or experiment with illicit drugs. Most studies have relied on acculturation and acculturative stress effects on licit and illicit drug use by immigrant adolescents (European Monitoring Centre for Drugs and Drug Addiction [EMCDDA], 2003). Additional research addresses the culture itself, including the role of cultural values on the initial or continued substance abuse by minority youth (Robbins & Mikow, 2000), and on reactions to different substances (Straussner, 2002).

Risk Factors Related to Drug Abuse Among Immigrants

Acculturative stress, or the challenge of assimilating into the dominant culture, has been implicated as a mechanism for increased substance use among immigrants (NIDA, 2001). The process of acculturation implies role strains, cognitive manipulations, and affective states that are potentially stressful and responsible for the nonadaptive attitudes and behaviors of immigrants (Berry, 1997). An important premise of the acculturative stress process is that stressors are harmful and coping resources are inadequate for solving problems; demands must exceed resources to produce a negative outcome. Drug use is one possible negative outcome (Alaniz, 2002; Castillo & Henderson, 2002). Mental health professionals have described the common symptoms that most immigrants present and have labeled it "chronic and multiple stress syndrome" (Carta, Bernal, Hardoy, & Haro-Abad, 2005). Immigrants affected by this syndrome present depressive symptomatology with atypical characteristics. The development of this condition occurs progressively as the immigrants encounter difficulties that take place during the migration and acculturation process. This can manifest in difficulties in finding a job and housing, problems in obtaining documents, or experiences of racism encountered in a new country. According to specialists, chronic and multiple stress syndrome should constitute a category situated in between adjustment disorders and posttraumatic stress disorder.

Another hypothesis is that exposure to a new culture brings with it increasing familiarity with the social contexts of drug use, as well as opportunities for drug use in peer group situations, in which youth often construct spaces of competence in the underground (Suárez-Orosco, 2000). These peer groups function on the periphery of multiple sociocultural worlds and include individuals who may feel confused, frustrated, and inferior. Consequently, the use of substances is adopted as a method of socialization into the new society. Thus, the addicts acquire friends or peers and are in this way grown-up, independent, and successful.

Despite the plausibility of both explanations, they are neither satisfactory nor comprehensive. Becoming a drug user is a complex, multipathed process that has no unitary explanation. While it is evident that immigrant youth who have greater exposure to a new culture may become more delinquent or use more illicit drugs, this fact alone cannot explain which youths are susceptible among all youths so exposed. Similarly, the argument that acculturative stress increases drug use among immigrants fails to identify the factors or conditions that differentiate users from nonusers. Added stressors from the process of immigration itself can lead to increased risk for emotional disturbance and drug abuse in newer immigrants. These may include previous traumatic experiences in their homelands (war and torture), many of which may have prompted the decision to emigrate in the first place. These are often compounded by the loss of extended family and kinship networks (and even separation from nuclear family members, such as children separated from their parents), in addition to a lack of social support and assimilation or marginalization (Caetano, Clark, & Tam, 1998). Such experiences create vulnerability in children and adolescents due to their incomplete biopsychosocial development, dependency, inability to understand certain life events, and underdevelopment of coping skills. These risk factors for drug use operate through increasing the probability of incorporation of deviant norms, generally by increasing the chances of involvement with deviant peers (Beauvais & Oetting, 1999).

Accumulating data indicate that unaccompanied children and adolescents and those separated from family members are consistently argued to be at greater risk for psychiatric and mental health problems than their accompanied peers (Sourander, 1998). By definition, an unaccompanied immigrant child is an individual under 18 years of age who has been separated from both parents and is not being cared for by an adult who has a responsibility to do so (Servan-Schreiber, Le Lin, & Birmaher, 1998; Sourander, 1998). Unaccompanied adolescents and youths are particularly vulnerable as their increasing autonomy often causes them to relive past separations, creating difficulties in adjustment. Separation of children from their parents (for whatever reason) can directly affect the parent-child relationship and may result in increased vulnerability and risk for children. On reunification, parents and children have to adjust to living together again. The parental viewpoint of separation-reunion is often very different from that of their children. Parents have expectations that their children will be happy, affectionate, and obedient. In the absence of such behaviors, parents may perceive the child as ungrateful and experience hurt and anger when faced with a hostile or unappreciative child (Suárez-Orozco, 2000). The symptom of addiction in these cases provides a form of "pseudo-individuation" at several levels, containing elements of the fear of being separated or abandoned, and presenting an attempt to punish the parents by engaging in acting-out behavior.

Moreover, a variety of problems exist when one parent, especially the man, migrates first, and, if married, leaves behind a wife and children, and the reunion occurs after he has become established in the new country (Suárez-Orozco & Suárez-Orozco, 2001).

The temporary loss of relationships and contact with the family, and the disruption of family support are related to the sense of loneliness and the lack of an accessible attachment figure (Peplau & Perlman, 1982). Drug addiction in this case, especially to heroin, does indeed appear to have many adaptive, functional qualities in terms of reducing negative emotional states of isolation, loneliness, and lack of family.

Contact with the new culture and conflicts that that are rooted in different rates of acculturation in the family (e.g., highly assimilated children and adherence of parents in the traditional values) lead to the disruption of the core family processes (perceived roles, hierarchy, exercise of power, and models of interaction), even in the case where the entire family immigrate. Weakness on the side of the parents in terms of supporting their children (perhaps because their economic needs force them to leave their children alone without observation for extended hours) can be highly problematic. Similarly, other problems, such as mental disturbance or divorce (Hjern, Angel, & Jeppson, 1998; Suárez-Orozco & Suárez-Orozco, 2001) can have a serious and negative impact. At the same time, the speedier acculturation of children due to their young age, together with their integration into the educational system, may result in parent-child conflicts concerning issues such as dress code, dating, and school performance, together with rights and obligations within the family (Booth, Crouter, & Landale, 1997). When the intensity of conflicts becomes unbearable and the youngster is unable to trust other people outside of the familial environment, drug abuse may present a means of making the negative emotions more tolerable. Using drugs may be considered to be a way of expressing frustration and anger, especially when young people are unable to deal with their parents directly. Young drug abusers may be bound up with a simultaneous need to defy their parents and to punish themselves for their own rebellion.

Acculturation strategies regarding the way in which immigrants regulate the proximity and the distance in the transformation of identity and in the relations with the country of origin and country of reception (Akhtar, 1999) are considered to have different effects on mental health (Sam, 2006). Moreover these strategies differentially impact in terms of substance abuse problems. If young people feel isolated, because they are unable to accomplish integration or feel rejected by the mainstream culture, or if their ethnic group is viewed by the majority culture as devalued and denigrated, they may identify and internalize these negative perceptions. This, in turn, may lead to negative emotions about the self, which, in turn, may lead to substance abuse. At the other end of the continuum, they may develop an adversarial identity, standing in defiance of the majority culture, which is seen as depriving them of social and financial aspirations and marginalizing them. In these situations, some young people who are not able to embrace their own culture and who develop an adversarial identity against the mainstream culture, construct spaces of competence in the underground and may join gangs. For these youth, gangs offer a sense of belonging, solidarity, protection, discipline, and warmth. These groups structure the anger many feel towards the society that violently rejected their parents and themselves (Suárez-Orozco, 2000).

The path to acculturation is additionally problematic for undocumented immigrants who are illegal working citizens, persons with forged papers or who have assumed false identities with real papers, or persons with pending immigration status (Karl-Trummer, Metzler, & Novak-Zezula, 2009). Undocumented alien status is a persistent psychoenvironmental stressor that increases vulnerability to the development of socioemotional problems that arise from exposure to stresses (Cavazos-Rehg, Zayas, & Spitznagel, 2007). Having no legal status, undocumented children grow up without the same opportunities as other children. Although these children are schooled, their transition to adulthood marks their entry into an undocumented life with legal limitations that is associated with fear of deportation and restriction to access employment and housing (Rumbaut & Komaie, 2010). In these situations, youth often develop their identity in alternative economies where drug-dealing and drug-taking is an important feature (Suárez-Orozco, 2001).

Drug addiction is often associated with homelessness among immigrants. People sleeping rough or relying upon overnight shelters constitute a population vulnerable to drug dependence (Anderson et al., 2006). For immigrants, and especially refugees, being homeless involves not only a loss of shelter, but moreover a loss of the social aspects of a home, which may translate into a state of emotional isolation and feelings of hopelessness (Hiebert, D'Addario, & Sherrell, 2005). To experience a good time, to forget problems, and the influence of street life culture are some of the reasons why people turn to drugs when they experience homelessness (Logothetis, 2003).

Additional factors that are connected with the pathology of usage are the loss of social resources, such as low economic and social level of the parents (Howard & Hodes, 2000), unemployment and economic poverty, low social status, the failure of the school as a basic institution of children's socialization (Hyman, Vu, & Beiser, 2000), and a lack of future opportunities (Caetano et al., 1998). The lack of economic resources may lead some individuals into selling and then using illegal substances to attain economic independence (Straussner, 2002).

Drug Dependence Among Immigrants and Refugees in Greece: The Experience of 18 ANO

Drug dependence may be an emerging problem among immigrants living in Greece (or elsewhere). The percentage of immigrant users in drug-specialized services in the years 1995 and 2003 was 2.1% (Kontogeorgiou, Pouloudi, Spyropoulou, & Terzidou, 2006). However, according to the Research Centre of 18 ANO Dependent Unit of Psychiatric Hospital of Attica there was a significant increase in the number of immigrant users admitted for treatment from 2005 to 2010. In 2009 alone, there were about 100 new immigrant users seeking treatment in the 18 ANO Dependent Unit Centre. In recent years, the 18 ANO Dependence Unit, which operates under the Ministry of Health and implements programs of internal residence and external supervision for general population, has been working to respond to the needs of addicted immigrants and refugees by developing and integrating a cultural, psychosocial model of substance abuse intervention. According to this model, the multi-stage therapeutic process consisting of sensitization (0–3 months), psychological recovery (main treatment about 6–8 months), and social reintegration (8–12 months) is sensitive to cultural values and experiences of immigrant groups, while addressing the common etiological factors of substance abuse. The therapeutic team consists of specialized personnel such as psychologists, psychiatrists, social workers, nurses, etc., who through psychoanalytic and behavioral approaches, psychodrama, and educational activities support the rehabilitation and recovery process of people seeking admission to the 18 ANO Dependence Unit. An important aspect of the later phase of the treatment process is to provide bridges to social resources in the community and to provide information about supportive networks that facilitate the integration of individuals who have completed the program in the community.

We present information from a study on the prevalence of illicit drug use among male immigrants aged 19 years or older ($M = 30.96$, $SD = 7.26$) in Greece in comparison to native Greeks ($M = 31.30$, $SD = 7.06$). Estimates for immigrants and native drug abusers are based on data collected during 2005–2009 from adults on the Drug Dependence Unit at the State Psychiatry Hospital of Attica. Sample sizes were: $N = 67$ (54.5%) immigrants and $N = 56$ (45.5%) native Greeks. Of immigrants, 34.1% ($N = 42$) were from the former Soviet Union (Armenia, Georgia, Ukraine, and Moldova), 11.4% ($N = 14$) from Asiatic countries (India, Iraq, Iran, Afghanistan, and Bangladesh), and 8.9% ($N = 11$) from countries of Eastern Europe (Albania, Poland, and Bulgaria). In the above sample, 18 people (17.5%) were married, 72 (69.9%) single, and 12 (11.9%) divorced. Although some immigrants were married, their children and wife lived in their country of origin.

Materials

The data collection method used in this study involved structured interviews with the subjects, incorporating procedures that would be likely to increase respondents' cooperation and willingness to report honestly about their illicit drug use behavior. The interviews considered personal and demographic information (age, education in years, and country of birth), marital status (single, married, cohabiting, divorced, and widowed), living status (stable or unstable accommodation), employment status, health status (HIV/AIDS), criminal and deviant behaviors, as well as information relating to lifetime use of illicit substances. The interviews were conducted following the subject's decision to participate in the program of drug rehabilitation.

Results

Education level. Immigrant abusers displayed the same education level compared with Greek abusers. Most people were lyceum graduates (38.8%), followed by lower second education graduates (25.6%), university and college graduates accounted for 14%, and 19% of the sample had completed primary school.

Marital status. Out of the total of immigrants, 55.4% were single, 26.2% married, 12.3% divorced, 4.6% cohabiting, and 1.2% widowed. Over 78.2% of Greek people were single, 14.5% married, 5.5% divorced, and 1.8% widowed, $\chi^2(4, n = 120) = 9.62, p < .05$.

Living status. Unstable accommodation was reported by 29.7% of immigrants and 22.2% of native Greeks.

Employment status. With regard to employment status, immigrants displayed a considerably higher unemployment rate compared with Greek natives: 66.7% compared to approximately 48.2%, respectively; $\chi^2(1, n = 122) = 6.70, p = .01$.

Social security. The rate of immigrants without social security (50%) is remarkably higher than the rate of natives (21.4%); $\chi^2(1, n = 122) = 9.23, p < .01$.

Health status. The rate of immigrants that were not users of the health care system (44.4%) was significantly higher than the rate of native Greeks (28.6%), $\chi^2(1, n = 120) = 9.0, p = 0.05$. Furthermore, more immigrants (65.6%) than natives (28.6%) had no information about AIDS, $\chi^2(1, n = 120) = 16.79, p < .001$, and hepatitis infection (56.3% versus 25%), $\chi^2(1, n = 120) = 3.68, p < .05$.

Legal status. Prior arrest and imprisonment were reported by 32.5% of the sample. There were no significant differences between groups.

Total negative life experiences. We calculated the level of adversity of drug abusers including their marital status (divorced and widowed), living status (unstable accommodation), employment status (unemployment), social security (no social security), health status (hepatitis), and legal status (prior arrest and imprisonment) as a total adversity score. A score can then be calculated on a scale of 0–6 for negative life experiences. According to the results, 12.2% of the sample reported no sociodemographic adversity; one risk factor was reported by 30.9% of people, 33.3% reported two risk factors and 23.5% indicated three or more negative experiences. Most immigrants from Asiatic countries (57.1%) followed by immigrants from countries of Eastern Europe (36.4%) and the former Soviet Union (21.4%) reported three or more negative life experiences. Only 14.3% of Greek people reported three or more negative life experiences, $\chi^2(9, n = 123) = 21.96, p < .01$ (see Table 1).

Table 1. Distribution of participants according to origin and number of risk factors

Risk factors	Former Soviet Union		Eastern Europe		Asiatic countries		Greece		Total	
	f	%	*f*	%	*f*	%	*f*	%	*f*	%
0	4	9.5	–	–	–	–	11	19.6	15	12.2
1	11	26.2	2	18.2	3	21.4	22	39.3	38	30.9
2	18	42.9	5	45.5	3	21.4	15	26.8	41	33.3
3–6	9	21.4	4	36.4	8	57.1	8	14.3	29	23.6
Total	42	34.1	11	8.9	14	11.4	56	45.5	123	100

Substance abuse. With respect to primary drugs, heroin was the main illicit substance used by 82.6% of the sample. This compared to 9.1% who reported cocaine as their main substance, and the other 8.3% reported others drugs such as amphetamines, benzodiaze-pines, marijuana, and hashish. The vast majority of the sample immigrants from the Former Soviet Union reported heroin as their main substance of abuse, $\chi^2(1, n = 121) = 7.81,$ $p < .01$. Furthermore, in comparison to other groups, the method of substance use among the most immigrants from Soviet Union occurs intramuscularly (65%) and through multi-person use of the needles and syringes (42.1%), $\chi^2(1, n = 115) = 13.68, p < .05$.

The path to drug addiction begins with the act of taking hashish or marijuana for about 75% of the Greek people, Asian immigrants, and immigrants Eastern Europe. Most people from Former Soviet Union (31.3%) began by using heroin, $\chi^2(1, n = 108) = 4.53, p < .05$. In regard to co-occurrence of different types of substance use, differences between groups were observed: Cocaine was associated with marijuana use in immigrants, whereas between natives multiple substance use was observed, $\chi^2(1, n = 108) = 26.58, p < .001$.

Age at first involvement with illicit substance use. The age at first involvement with elicit substances is older for Asian immigrants ($M = 23.14$ years) and younger for immigrants from Eastern Europe, $M = 15.55; F(3, 113) = 7.82, p < .01$. The mean age of first illicit substance use for immigrants from former Soviet Union is 21.5 years, whereas for Greek people it is 16.8. The age range for immigrants was between 10 and 48 years, whereas for natives it was between 12 and 30.

The mean length of use reported by natives was 8.3 years and by immigrants 5 years, $F(1, 116) = 11.04, p < .01$. There were no differences between immigrant groups.

Counseling and substance abuse treatment. The length of involvement of immigrants and natives in the treatment program was the same. However, immigrants, regardless of their origin, were two times less consistent than natives in attending their appointments, $F(1, 113) = 3.99, p < .05$ (see Table 2).

In addition, it emerged that many immigrant drug abusers tended to use treatment to reduce their level of drug abuse and not to eliminate the problem, $\chi^2(1, n = 116) = 4.96,$ $p < .05$.

Conclusions

Immigrant status (i.e., being an immigrant) appears to be associated with accumulative negative life experiences across the family, the community, and the individual. About 40% of immigrants, mostly from Asian countries (about 60%), reported three or more neg-ative experiences, such as unstable accommodation, unemployment, lack of social secu-rity, prior arrest or imprisonment, and health problems. Previous research confirms the association between sociodemographic characteristics of immigrants and refugees and mental health (Organista et al., 2003). Being of lower economic status was correlated with more isolation and limited opportunities, which, in turn, lead to lower acculturation and difficulties in seeking employment and social support. Homelessness or unstable accom-modation is a common problem among many immigrants seeking services. This factor

Table 2. Means and standard deviation of involvement of immigrants and natives in treatment program

Involvement in therapy	Greeks		Immigrants		F value
	M	SD	M	SD	
Length of involvement – months	3.12	4.34	2.46	5.15	0.53
Appointments	9.41	11.3	5.5	9.58	3.99*

Note. $*p < .05$

comprises a significant barrier to engagement in the treatment program and becoming drug free. All of the above factors become exacerbated by the experience of being undocumented.

Many problems associated with drug abuse among immigrants and refugees are exacerbated by underutilization of mental health services. Immigrants accounted for 44.4% of the cases that do not use the health care system, compared with 28.8% of native Greeks. Of concern is the fact that many immigrants have no information concerning whether they are infected by AIDS or hepatitis. According to the above results, immigrants face a social and economic environment of inequality that includes unstable accommodation, unemployment, and a lack of social security. Other barriers that affect underutilization of mental health services may be differences in language and culture, stigmatization, and the failure of services to target immigrant groups (EMCDDA, 2003; Makimoto, 1998).

Drug abusers, natives, and immigrants, are more inclined to use heroin as a main illicit substance, and their use is mostly a combination of heroin with other substances. However, numerous factors tend to differentiate immigrants and native drug abusers including patterns of injection heroin use; intramuscular in combination with multi-person use of needles and syringes was present among most immigrants. Multi-person sharing of syringes is associated with rapid transition of HIV among illicit drug users, with HIV incidence rates as high as 20–50 per 100 persons. Moreover, most illicit drug users who continue to inject may be unable to obtain a sufficient number of syringes to effectively reduce their risk of acquiring and transmitting blood-borne viral infections (Batki & Nathan, 2004).

An extremely important outcome from this study concerned the speed at which immigrant substance users' progress from mild to severe involvement. The faster progression of immigrants compared to natives was in contrast to the later initiators of substance use among immigrants. The results also suggest that it is important to investigate whether immigration and acculturation may play a role in addictive liability, above and beyond what is accounted for by other factors. Although, heroin is the most common substance among immigrants and natives, the path to addiction is different between groups. For example, Russian immigrants had higher rates of excessive drinking relative to other groups; their path to substance abuse begins with using heroin. Rates of heavy drinking among Russians have been identified in previous studies (Bobak et al., 2004; Rahav,

Hasin, & Paykin, 1999). According to Tapilina (2007) Russians do not drink more frequently than others, but they consume very large quantities of alcohol. This is in part explained by cultural tradition that encourages excessive drinking among men.

In a similar fashion, immigrants are seen to differentiate their behavior in relation to drug abuse treatment. They are seen as having increased probability for missing appointments and in addition are seen to seek a medical fix for their addiction. Substance abuse staff found that many immigrants enter the program with misconceptions about addiction and unfamiliarity with the process of recovery. Their tendency to perceive more organic or somatic involvement in drug abuse has to do with the cultural meaning of somatic complaints (Tanaka-Matsumi & Draguns, 1997). Somatic complaints are less stigmatized among some cultures and somatization justifies an acceptable medical intervention. On the other hand, specialists must be cognizant of the immigration experience itself, on account of the stress and the lack of social and economic resources for coping that may deter immigrant people from using services and receiving appropriate care.

Multicultural Competent Treatment of Drug Abuse Among Immigrants and Refugees

It is important to begin substance abuse treatment among immigrants and refugees with a comprehensive assessment of drug abuse and its effect on the life of the people (Straussner, 2002). However, the pathway to recovery should take into account cultural and migration circumstances that serve as an agent in the rise of addiction problems. The therapist of an immigrant drug abuser must take into account cultural factors that include belief systems about drug abuse and concepts of health and disease (Lindert, Schouler-Ocak, Heinz, & Priebe, 2008). For example, seeking medical treatment for their addiction, immigrants express their problem in a psychosomatic form, which is consistent with low shame and stigma and the perceived legitimacy to seek help for bodily complaints (Kleinman, 1980). Recovery from drugs is a long process characterized not only by abstinence from illicit drugs (and alcohol). Recovery is about reclaiming physical and psychological health and having a vision of good quality of life (The Betty Ford Institute Consensus Panel, 2007). This perspective is quite different from the deficit approach or medical model that lead to partial recovery that includes two main features: (a) a reduced frequency, duration, and intensity of drug abuse and the reduction of problems related to drug dependence, (b) the sustained abstinence from illicit drugs, but the failure to achieve sociopsychological and occupational health (White, 2007). Thus, the focus of the mental health professionals is to support immigrants' motives for engaging in drug treatment programs by developing therapeutic alliance as a useful way for understanding issues when working with immigrants and refugees.

Many immigrants are vulnerable to barriers against following intervention programs, based on cultural beliefs combined with a low conception of drug abuse risk. Other drug abusers trying to maintain their recovery from heroin dependence may find it difficult to deal with alcohol. Pre-immigration stressors may be important for drug addiction of immigrants and refugees. Refugees have several factors in common including exposure to violence, war, and torture, long separation from family and loved ones (van der Veer, 1998), and, in many cases, loved ones have been killed and possessions and homes are destroyed (Fazel & Stein, 2003). Some immigrants in our study report to us negative life events, which are culture general, such as divorce or losing one's parent, etc.

The process of migration in a globalized context includes new definitions of family life and different forms of family stress that begin in the pre-immigration stage (Falicov, 2007). Families with parents abroad and children with parents abroad as a result of segmented migration are characterized as distinct social groups. Research has noted that immigrant children experience separation from family members in which certain members of the family migrate first, and later, after their establishment, send for other family members (Suárez-Orozco, Todorova, & Louie, 2002). A long period of separation is particularly disruptive to adolescents who have to adapt to a new culture and to two sets of traumatic separations: First from their parents and later from the people who became their primary caretakers during the time that they were geographically separated from their parents. For example, S. from Bulgaria was 16 years old, when his mother moved to Greece. He lived with his grandmother, because his father had died. He was reunited with his mother after 6 years, when he became involved with drugs. Another respondent, from the former Soviet Union expressed extreme sadness at the loss of ties with his mother living in Greece and his alcoholic father in his country when he was about 10 years old. Although he referred to the economic benefits from his mother's migration and understood the reasons behind his mother's decision, he felt abandoned by her for a long time.

Sometimes we can talk about transnational families and virtual long-distance communication among parents and their children through new technologies (Falicov, 2007). Long distance parenthood using phone and internet has been referred to by many immigrants in our study, especially those coming from the former Soviet Union countries. The reunion after many years is seen more as a disorienting meeting of strangers than a true reunion. Young people have difficulty affirming parental authority after they have been independent or attached to another caregiver. In our clinical work, spousal separation, in particular, is another stressful situation for migrants.

The generational stress due to differing rates of acculturation between parents and teenagers makes family interactions stressful, leads to weakened quality of parent-child communication, and creates overreaction by parents to perceived loss of control over adolescent children (Szapocznik & Williams, 2000). According to clinical studies, immigrant teenagers must cope with different crises at the same time: The usual crisis of crossing from childhood to adulthood, the passing from one culture to another (Saucier et al., 2002), and generational stress due to acculturation that plays an important role in the disruptions of parent-child relationships. Immigrant parents often have to make dramatic sacrifices for a better future for their children. Within the new country, they set limits that are significantly more stringent than they would have if they had stayed in their country of origin. At the same time, they are often dependent upon their children. The children often learn the new language more quickly than their parents and consequently they often take on new roles as translators and advocates for their families. Alternating between parentifying the children and at the same time severely constricting their activities may create significant tensions within the family, adolescent defiance, and loss of family cohesiveness (Brook et al., 2001).

Risk factors for mental health in the post-emigration stage are associated with living conditions and legal status in the country of settlement. In an attempt to deal with their conditions, it is important to build connections either with the co-ethnic community or with the community of a larger society. The creation of networks provides immigrants with social support (Ward et al., 2001) in terms of emotional support, social companionship, tangible assistance, and informational support (Ong & Ward, 2005). Emotional support is expressed by display of love, care, concern, and sympathy; social companionship is viewed as the sense of belonging to a social group that provides company for a variety of activities; tangible assistance is demonstrated in concrete material or financial forms of help. Finally, informational support comprises of communicating and advising with regard to current personal difficulties concerning new surroundings. Increased levels of social support reduces exhibited levels of psychological problems among immigrants. Specifically, immigrants are helped in dealing with various stressors in the environment and facilitated in a positive adjustment process by getting advice and encouragement from sources of support.

To meet the needs of addicted persons from culturally diverse groups, health care providers must engage in the process of becoming culturally competent. Multicultural competence refers to the process in which the therapist continuously strives to achieve the ability and availability to effectively work within the cultural context of an individual, family, or community. This concept includes generic and specific awareness, knowledge, skills, and emotions (Draguns, 2002; Lindert et al., 2008; Pedersen, 2002). In general, intervention by drug rehabilitation of immigrants needs to be more culturally sensitive by combining specific culture patterns, experience of immigration and acculturation with universal aspects of treatment approaches. Work teams that are helpful and open to cultural diversity will improve parameters for immigrants with addiction.

Summary

By way of summary, Figure 1 describes the main issues suggested for work with immigrant and refuges addicted to illicit drugs. In this article, we argue that a myriad of stresses often accompany drug treatment of immigrants and refugees. Pre-migration stress, negative life events, separation from family and friends, and loss of social resources have been identified as risk factors for substance abuse among immigrants. Cultural diversity plays an important role in addressing differences in symptom expression (see the chapter by Lindert in this book) and in understanding factors that affect the accessibility and acceptability of services by immigrants and refugees. The dual emphasis on the universal and

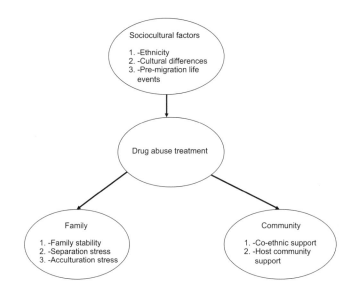

Figure 1. Context for drug abuse treatment among immigrants and refugees.

particular behavior of immigrants and refugees becomes a central professional issue in the development of multicultural competence for increasing success in counseling and treatment of different cultural groups.

References

Akhtar, S. (1999). *Immigration and identity. Turmoil, treatment and transformation.* London, UK: Jason Aronson.

Alaniz, M. L. (2002). Migration, acculturation, displacement: Migratory workers and "substance abuse". *Substance Use & Misuse, 37,* 1253–1257.

American Psychiatric Association. (2000). *Diagnostic and statistical manual of mental disorders-IV.* Washington, DC: American Psychiatric Association.

Anderson, I., Baptista, I., Wolf, J., Edgar, B., Benjaminsen, L., Sapounakis, A., & Schoibl, H. (2006). *Addressing homelessness in Europe. The changing role of service provision: Barriers of access to health services for homeless people.* European Federation of National Organisations Working with the Homeless (FEANTSA). Belgium: European Observatory on Homelessness.

Baldwin-Edwards, M. (2004). *Statistical data about immigrants in Greece Analytical study for managing migration according to standard of European Union.* Athens: Hellenic Migration Policy Institute.

Batki, S. L., & Nathan, K. I. (2004). HIV/AIDS and substance use disorders. In M. Galanter & H. D. Kleber (Eds.), *Textbook of substance abuse treatment* (pp. 555–563). Washington, DC: American Psychological Association.

Beauvais, F., & Oetting, E. O. (1999). Drug use, resilience and the myth of the golden child. In M. D. Glantz & J. L. Johnson (Eds.), *Resilience and development. Positive life adaptations* (pp. 101–106). New York: Kluwer Academic/Plenum Publishers.

Berry, J. W. (1997). Immigration, acculturation and adaptation. *Applied Psychology: An International Review, 46*, 5–68.

Berry, J. W. (2003). Conceptual approaches to acculturation. In K. Chun, P. Balls-Organista, & G. Marin (Eds.), *Acculturation: Advances in theory, measurement, and applied research* (pp. 17–37). Washington, DC: American Psychological Association.

Bobak, M., Room, R., Pikhart, H., Kubinova, R., Malyutina, S., Pajak, A., ... Marmot, M. (2004). Contribution of drinking patterns to differences in rates of alcohol related problems between three urban populations. *Journal of Epidemiological Community Health, 58*, 238–242.

Booth, A., Crouter, A. C., & Landale, N. S. (1997). *Immigration and the family: Research and policy on U.S. immigrants*. Hillsdale, NJ, UK: Erlbaum.

Brook, J. S., Brook, D. W., de la Rosa, M., Whiteman, M., Johnson, E., & Montoya, I. (2001). Adolescent illegal drug use: The impact of personality, family, and environmental factors. *Journal of Behavioral Medicine, 24*, 183–203.

Caetano, R., & Clark, L. C. (2003). Acculturation, alcohol consumption, smoking, and drug use among Hispanics. In K. M. Chun, P. B. Organista, & G. Marin (Eds.), *Acculturation. Advances in theory, measurement, and applied research* (pp. 207–223). Washington, DC: American Psychological Association.

Caetano, R., Clark, C. L., & Tam, T. (1998). Alcohol consumption among racial/ethnic minorities: Theory and research. *Alcohol Health & Research World, 22*, 233–238.

Castillo, M., & Henderson, G. (2002). Hispanic substance abusers in the United States. In G. X. Ma & G. Henderson (Eds.), *Ethnicity and substance abuse: Prevention and intervention* (pp. 191–206). Springfield, IL: Charles C. Thomas.

Carta, M. G., Bernal, M., Hardoy, M. C., & Haro-Abad, J. M. (2005). Migration and mental health in Europe (the state of the mental health in Europe working group: Appendix I). *Clinical Practice and Epidemiology in Mental Health, 9*, 1–13.

Cavazos-Rehg, P. A., Zayas, L. H., & Spitznagel, E. L. (2007). Legal status, emotional well-being and subjective health status of Latino immigrants. *Journal of the National Medical Association, 99*, 1126–1131.

Diamanduros, N. (2005). The European Ombudsman and EU Drugs Policy. In *"10th European Conference on Rehabilitation and Drug Policy – Drug addiction treatment and prevention in a United Europe: Diversity and Equality"* (pp. 13–23). Athens: Kethea & EFTC.

Draguns, P. J. (2002). Universal and cultural aspects of counseling and psychotherapy. In P. B. Pedersen, J. G. Draguns, W. J. Lonner, & J. E. Trimble (Eds.), *Counseling across cultures* (pp. 25–50, 5th ed.). London, UK: Sage.

European Monitoring Centre for Drugs, Drug Addiction (EMCDDA). (2003). *Annual Report 2003: The state of the drugs problem in the European Union and Norway: Drug and alcohol use among young people: Social exclusion and reintegration*. Lisbon: EMCDDA.

Falicov, C. J. (2007). Working with transnational immigrants: Expanding meanings of family, community, and culture. *Family Process, 46*, 157–171.

Fazel, M., & Stein, A. (2003). *Mental health of refugee children: Comparative study. British Medical Journal, 327*, 134.

Gfroerer, J. C., & Tan, L. L. (2003). Substance use among foreign-born youths in the United States: Does the length of residence matter? *American Journal of Public Health, 93*, 1892–1895.

Gropas, R., & Triandafyllidou, A. (2005). *Active civic participation of immigrants in Greece* Country report prepared for the European research project POLITIS, Oldenburg, Retrieved from www.uni-oldenburg.de/politis-europe.

Hiebert, D., D'Addario, S., & Sherrell, K. (2005). *The Profile of Absolute and Relative Homelessness Among Immigrants, Refugees, and Refugee Claimants in the GVRD: Final Report Prepared for the National Secretariat on Homelessness.* MOSAIC, Retrieved from http://www.urbancentre.utoronto.ca/pdfs/elibrary/HLN-among- Immigrants-Vancou.pdf.

Hjern, A., Angel, B., & Jeppson, O. (1998). Political violence, family stress and mental health of refugee children in exile. *Scandinavian Journal of Social Medicine, 26*, 18–25.

Isralowitz, R., Straussner, L., Vogt, I., & Chtenguelov, V. (2002). Toward an understanding of Russian speaking drug addicts in Israel, Germany and the United States. *Journal of Social Work Practice in the Addictions, 2*, 119–136.

Hyman, I., Vu, N., & Beiser, M. (2000). Post-migration stresses among Southeast Asian refugees youth in Canada: A research note. *Journal of Comparative Family Studies, 31*, 281–293.

Karl-Trummer, U., Metzler, B., & Novak-Zezula, S. (2009). *Health care for undocumented migration in the EU: Concepts and cases.* International Organization for Migration (IOM), Retrieved from http://europe.org/files/Health.pdf.

Kleinman, A. (1980). Major conceptual and research issues for cultural (anthropological) psychiatry. *Cultural Medical Psychiatry, 4*, 3–23.

Kontogeorgiou, K., Pouloudi, M., Spyropoulou, M., & Terzidou, M. (2006). Quantitative data on trends in the characteristics of drug users in treatment in Greece. In *Book of Proceedings: 10th European Conference on Rehabilitation and Drug Policy* (pp. 195–210). Athens: KETHEA & EFTC.

Lianos, Th., Kanellopoulos, K., Gregou, M., Gemi, E., & Papakonstantinou, P. (2008). *Estimate of the illegal immigrants population in Greece.* Athens: Hellenic Policy Institute.

Lindert, J., Schouler-Ocak, M., Heinz, A., & Priebe, S. (2008). Mental health, health care utilization of migrants in Europe. *European Psychiatry, 23*, 14–20.

Logothetis, T. (2003). *Inclusion for change: A review of the homeless and drug dependency trial's community reintegration program (March 2002–June 2003), Report 6.* South Melbourne: Hanover Welfare Services, Retrieved from http://www.health.vic.gov.au/drugservices/downloads/hddt_inclusion_for_change.pdf.

Losoya, H. S., Knight, P. G., Chassin, L., Little, M., Vargas-Chanes, D., Mauricio, A., & Piquero, A. (2008). Trajectories of acculturation and enculturation in relation to heavy episodic drinking and marijuana use in a sample of Mexican American serious juvenile offenders. *Journal of Drug Issues, 8*, 171–198.

Maratou-Alipranti, L., & Gkazon, E. (2005). *Immigration and health. The review of situation-challenges and perspectives of improvement* (in Greek). Athens: IMEPO-EKKE.

Makimoto, K. (1998). Drinking patterns and drinking problems among Asian- Americans and Pacific Islanders. *Alcohol Health & Research World, 22*, 270–275.

Markoutsoglou, M., Kasou, M., Moshotos, A., & Ptohos, Y. (2007). *Asian migrants in Greece origins, status and prospects.* Retrieved from http://www.idec.gr: Institute of International Economic Relations.

National Institute on Drug Abuse. (2001). *Monitoring the future: National survey results on drug use, 1975–2000. Volume II: College Students & Adults, Ages 19–40.* Bethesda, MD: U.S. Department of Health and Human Services NIH Publication No. 01–4925.

Oberg, K. (1960). Cultural shock: Adjustment to new cultural environment. *Practical Anthropology, 7*, 177–182.

OECD. (2010). *Combating the illegal employment of foreign workers.* Paris: OECD.

Ong, A., & Ward, C. (2005). The construction and validation of a social support measure for sojourners: The index of sojourner social support (ISSS) scale. *Journal of Cross-Cultural Psychology, 36*, 637–661.

Organista, P. B., Organista, K. S., & Kurasaki, K. (2003). The relationship between acculturation and ethnic minority mental health. In K. M. Chun, P. B. Organista, & G. Marin (Eds.), *Acculturation. Advances in theory, measurement and applied research* (pp. 95–119). Washington, DC: American Psychological Association.

Pedersen, P. (2002). Ethics, competence and other professional issues in culture-centered counseling. In P. B. Pedersen, J. G. Draguns, W. J. Lonner, & J. E. Trimble (Eds.), *Counseling across cultures* (pp. 3–24, 5th ed.). London, UK: Sage.

Peplau, L. A., & Perlman, D. (1982). *Loneliness: A sourcebook of current theory, research and therapy.* New York, NY: Wiley.

Rahav, G., Hasin, D., & Paykin, A. (1999). Drinking patterns of recent Russian immigrants and other Israelis: 1995 National Survey Results. *American Journal of Public Health, 89,* 1212–1216.

Robbins, S. P., & Mikow, J. (2000). *Tobacco, alcohol and other drug use among minority youth: Implications for the design and implementation of prevention programmes.* Philadelphia, PA: University of Pennsylvania, Center for the Study of Youth Policy.

Roysircar-Sodowsky, G., & Maestas, M. V. (2000). Acculturation, ethnic identity and acculturative stress: Evidence and measurement. In R. H. Dana (Ed.), *Handbook of cross-cultural and multicultural personality assessment* (pp. 113–131). Hillsdale, NJ: Erlbaum.

Rumbaut, R. G., & Komaie, G. (2010). Immigration and adult transitions. *Spring, 20,* 43–65.

Sam, D. L. (2006). Acculturation and health. In D. L. Sam & J. W. Berry (Eds.), *The Cambridge Handbook of acculturation psychology.* Cambridge, MA: Cambridge University Press (pp. 452–468).

Saucier, J. F., Sylvestre, R., Doucet, H., Lambert, J., Frappier, J. Y., Charbonneau, L., & Malus, M. (2002). Cultural identity and adaptation to adolescence in Montreal. In F. J. C. Azima & N. Grizenko (Eds.), *Immigrant and refugee children and their families: Clinical, research, and training issues* (pp. 133–154). Madison, WI: International Universities Press.

Servan-Schreiber, D., Le Lin, B., & Birmaher, B. (1998). Prevalence of posttraumatic stress disorder and major depressive disorder in Tibetan refugee children. *Journal of the American Academy of Child & Adolescent Psychiatry, 37,* 874–879.

Sourander, A. (1998). Behavior problems and traumatic events of unaccompanied refugee minors. *Child Abuse and Neglect, 22,* 719–727.

Straussner, S. L. A. (2002). Ethnocultural issues in substance about treatment. In S. L. A. Straussner (Ed.), *Ethnocultural factors in substance abuse treatment* (pp. 13–28). New York, NY: The Guilford Press.

Stroebe, M., van Vliet, T., Hewstone, M., & Willis, H. (2002). Homesickness among students in two cultures: Antecedents and consequences. *British Journal of Psychology, 93,* 147–168.

Suárez-Orozco, C. (2000). Identities under siege: Immigration stress and social mirroring among the children of immigrants. In C. G. M. Tobben & Suárez-Orozco (Eds.), *Cultures under siege. Collective violence and trauma* (pp. 195–226). Cambridge, MA: Cambridge University Press.

Suárez-Orozco, C., & Suárez-Orozco, M. (2001). *Children of immigration.* Cambridge, MA: Harvard University Press.

Suárez-Orozco, C., Todorova, I. L. G., & Louie, J. (2002). Making up for lost time: The experience of separation and reunification among immigrant families. *Family Process, 41,* 625–643.

Szapocznik, J., & Williams, R. A. (2000). Brief strategic family therapy: Twenty five years of interplay among theory, research, and practice in adolescent behavior problems and drug abuse. *Clinical Child and Family Psychology Review, 3,* 117–135.

Tanaka-Matsumi, J., & Draguns, J. G. (1997). Culture and psychopathology. In J. W. Berry, M. H. Segall, & C. Kagitcibasi (Eds.), *Handbook of cross-cultural psychology: Volume 3. Social behaviour and application* (pp. 449–491). Boston: Allyn & Bacon.

Tapilina, V. S. (2007). How much does Russia drink? *Sociological Research, 46,* 31–46.

The Betty Ford Institute Consensus Panel. (2007). What is recovery? A working definition from the Betty Ford Institute. *Journal of Substance Abuse Treatment, 33*, 221–228.

van der Veer, G. (1998). *Counselling and therapy with refugees and victims of trauma*. Chichester, UK: Wiley.

Vega, W. A., & Gil, A. G. (1999). A model for explaining drug use behavior among Hispanic adolescents. *Drugs & Society, 14*, 57–74.

Ward, C., Bochner, S., & Furnham, A. (2001). *The psychology of culture shock* (2nd ed.). New York, NY: Routledge.

White, W. (2007). Addiction recovery: Its definition and conceptual boundaries. *Journal of Substance Abuse Treatment, 33*, 229–241.

World Health Organization. (2000). *Discussion paper-principles of drug dependence treatment*. United Nations: Office on Drugs and Crime.

Difficult Patients, Difficult Situations

Psychological Overview

Lorraine Sherr and Natasha Croome

University College London, UK

Difficult patients are often discussed anecdotally – their problems can be complex, their issues time consuming, and they challenge coping and emotions. They may disrupt the smooth running systems or expectations within healthcare provision. There are those who maintain that there is no such thing as a difficult patient, it is a matter of perception and of picking up cues in order to handle these appropriately. Difficult situations on the other hand also create problems in terms of reactions and the quality of care provided. They are often emotive and may have severe consequences. This may be because these topics are avoided, understudied or not well understood.

Psychology is the science of human behavior and as such may provide some insight into such challenges in health care. This chapter will address such difficulties by way of some selected examples. These will be outlined from a psychological perspective to give the reader an overview of current knowledge and a methodology of incorporating psychological perspective to broaden understanding. Difficult situations covered include examples of both common and less common experiences. Common difficulties summarized relate to the topics of dissatisfaction with communication, breaking bad news, problems adhering to treatment regimens, and mental health issues in nonmental health consultations. Less common situations include abandoned babies and abuse in pregnancy. The review will allow for an understanding of psychological approaches, prevention, identification, and interventions.

Dissatisfaction With Communication in Medical Care

For several decades it has been well established that many patients are dissatisfied with communication aspects of care – despite high satisfaction with medical care. This has revolutionized medical school education and communication skills have been incorporated into many curricula. However, there is no sound evidence that this has addressed the problem. Patients continue to express dissatisfaction with communication aspects of their care.

It is not surprising that extensive shortcomings in the abilities and proficiency of professional communication have been cataloged. Communication training is a relatively new innovation, time pressures devalue communication demands, skills may be lacking, and motivation may be low. Few studies examine the general situational factors which may confound communication expertise. Any medic working in an overcrowded situation for unreasonable lengths of time, carrying out repetitive work, in poor environmental conditions and with limited rewards will experience a drop in communication proficiency and motivation.

Numerous theories have been postulated to account for dissatisfaction with communication. Personality theories propose a patient typology where dissatisfaction may be common. However, the evidence suggests that those who are dissatisfied with communication are not generally dissatisfied – which argues against such personality theories. Other theories look at situational factors from the patient perspective, which contribute to dissatisfaction such as stress, unfamiliarity, or pain. Cognitive theories examine cognitive aspects of doctor patient interactions to point out how important it is to understand these factors in order to enhance satisfaction. Dissatisfaction with communications seems to matter – not only from a satisfaction point of view, but from good evidence that those who are dissatisfied are also more likely to take up more time, to require more medication, to stay longer in hospital, and to show lowered adherence to medical regimens.

An alternative approach is to provide training for patients who receive brief training prior to their consultation in an effort to enhance questioning, improve disclosure, raise satisfaction, and maximize the doctor patient interview (Kinnersley et al., 2008). Such training has been shown to improve question asking, reduce pre-consultation anxiety but the effects were small and entrenched behaviors may be difficult to change. When doctor training accompanied such patient training little add-on benefit was found. Other interventions that have been tried include decision aids (a systematic review identified 87 such aids, O'Connor et al., 2009) and these have been found to increase involvement and also lead to more informed decision making.

This opens the door to the importance of communication studies and the possibility that communication skills can be taught and integrated into consultations from both the doctor and patient perspective. The evidence seems to suggest that such interventions may enhance both the quality of the communication as well as an array of medical outcomes.

Breaking Bad News

Although bad news is common, many doctors find it difficult to master the skills of breaking bad news and many patients find the moment of bad news revelation a difficult experience. There is good evidence that the way in which any news is provided to a patient may affect their subsequent adaptation and coping. Any piece of information which causes an individual to change their expectation for their future negatively has been classified as bad news (Buckman, 1984). Many physicians find breaking bad news to patients stressful and often deliver the news in ineffective ways (Fallowfield & Jenkins, 2004). Almost half of the junior and two thirds of the senior doctors in one study, were shown to feel insufficiently knowledgeable to deliver bad news (Orgel, McCarter, & Jacobs, 2010). Factors such as inappropriate language, lack of empathy, and preparedness were the main reasons for poor previously experienced incidents (Orgel et al., 2010).

Due to doctors' uncertainty in this situation, protocols such as "SPIKES" (Baile et al., 2000) and "SCOPE" (SCOPE, 2003) were created for disclosing bad news to patients (Fallowfield & Jenkins, 2004). There are common factors between the different guidelines in particular: preparation before the interview, assessing the patients' reaction, and effectively communicating with the patient by giving them sufficient knowledge and information (Baile et al., 2000; SCOPE, 2003). Psychological insight can examine doctor and patient behavior at the time of news transfer, can provide insight into the impact and emotional reactions that patients may have so that doctors are better equipped and can anticipate and therefore prepare for reactions. Training can help doctors plan and refine skills of delivering such news.

Patients have highlighted the importance of trust as well as the use of adequate time and information in buffering the impact of the news (Gallagher, Arber, Chaplin, & Quirk, 2010). Patients desire their doctor to be honest and upfront about their diagnosis (Ishaque, Saleem, Khawaja, & Qidwai, 2010) but also empathetic (Quirk et al., 2008). When examining what creates a caring doctor's attitude the results showed the most important aspect may not be a set of behaviors or an attitude to adopt but an ability to take the patient's perspective and reflect on their responses (Quirk et al., 2008). Early studies showed that withholding news and negative diagnoses was often seen, but did not accord with patient's wishes. Maguire (1985) showed that doctors focus on information provision rather than addressing worries and concerns. The way the news is handled has a significant effect on both patient appraisal and subsequent psychological adjustment.

Delivering a terminal diagnosis is in particular a stressful situation for a physician (Friedrichsen & Milberg, 2006) as well as the patient. Doctors may have worries such as losing control by revealing their emotions and thus losing their professionalism (Friedrichsen & Milberg, 2006). Qualitative research on terminal patients and their families revealed areas which were particularly important for them in communication with their physician (Wenrich et al., 2001). They wanted their doctor to be willing to talk about dying, to encourage questions, to listen, and to be sensitive to when their patient is ready to talk about death. An important issue also raised was for the physician to achieve a balance between being honest with the prognosis and rejecting hope.

Delivering bad news to parents is also stressful. Research shows when delivering the news to parents of children with a chronic illness or disability it is important for physicians to inform the parents early on with straightforward and direct language and to exclude medical jargon (Ahmann, 1998). The communication should occur in private and the physician should support the parents' emotional expression to the news. An important point raised was to individualize the communication style and the information expressed (Ahmann, 1998).

If a diagnosis is communicated ineffectively it can lead to resentment, confusion, and distress (Fallowfield & Jenkins, 2004), thus it is important for physicians to feel confident and to follow medical guidelines when delivering bad news (Dosanjh, Barnes, & Bhandari, 2001). Parents of patients who were dissatisfied with their physician's communication showed self-reported depression to a greater degree than parents who were satisfied (Baird, McConachie, & Scrutton, 2000). When there is good communication between doctor and patient it can facilitate adjustment, acceptance, and understanding (Fallowfield & Jenkins, 2004).

Problems Adhering to Medicine Regimens or Medical Advice

Lack of adherence to medical treatment has quite severe ramifications. On the one hand it creates ongoing frustration in physicians (Melnikow & Kiefe, 1994) since adherence has shown to be positively associated with improved outcomes (Urquhart, 1996). On the other hand there are major public health implications of poor adherence such as failed treatment, emerging resistance and increased expenditure. Poor adherence is expected in 30–50% of patients, irrespective of disease, prognosis or setting (Donovan, 1995; Gold & McClung, 2006). Two hundred different variables have been analyzed to try and explain lack of adherence; however, none are consistent predictors (Donovan, 1995; Vermeire, Hearnshaw, Van Royen, & Denekens, 2001). Adherence to strict medical regimes, such as antiretroviral treatment in HIV infection or completing a course of antibiotics, have been studied and been shown to be complex challenges (Chesney, Morin, & Sherr 2000). Adherence interventions have been shown to be effective, so clearly good preparation and sensitive systems can enhance adherence and minimize the damage generated by adherence shortfalls (Smith et al., 2009).

Theories to explain nonadherence focus on the patient, the provider or the potion. At times it may be a complex harmony of all three factors. Interventions to promote adherence differ from strategies to reduce nonadherence. Planning, lifestyle appreciation, motivation, and patient support have been shown to be effective. The duration of treatment (short term, medium term, or lifelong) may affect adherence over time. Cognitive models which examine forgetting, recall, and understanding may contribute to improved adherence. Social models which provide an understanding of social circumstance, barriers such as stigma and the meaning of illness, may provide routes to enhance preparation and deal with potential obstacles in advance of treatment commencement. Practical interventions such as prompts and reminders, planning prior to treatment commencement, support of various kinds, and side effect management have all been effective in promoting adherence (Sandelowski, Voils, Chang, & Lee, 2009).

Guidelines, for example, ICEDD (Identify, Clarify, Educate, Decide, Document) from OMIC (Ophthalmic Mutual Insurance Company) have been created to help physicians with this difficult situation (Tsui & Alward, 2010). They help involve the patient in their care by clarifying the reason behind nonadherence and by the patient and doctor communicating to decide how the treatment plan should proceed (Tsui & Alward, 2010). Lack of adherence has been linked to patients not feeling the treatment is necessary (Lombas, Hakim, & Zanchetta, 2001); however, educating the patient about their illness and the risks associated with it has shown to increase rates of adherence (Cuddihy et al., 2004; Gold & McClung, 2006). Education alone is not sufficient in some areas to change behavior; therefore, research needs to examine other implementation plans which can be effective (Bui, Cavanagh, & Robertson, 2010).

Some difficulties in consultations may emerge simply because of language barriers. At times these may signal both language and cultural barriers which act in a complex way disrupting communications and may affect history taking, diagnosis, and treatment. Language discordance between physician and patient may hinder delivery of an effective treatment (Hornberge et al., 1996). Patients, who are able to communicate with their physicians in their primary language and have similar cultures, understand the information from their physician better and engage in the conversation more.

Mental Health Problems in Nonmental Health Consultations

Some difficult situations are related to the complexity of problems presented by patients. For example, many consultations include an element of mental health which is difficult to identify, accommodate, and incorporate. Studies claim that one third of General Practice consultations are related to mental health problems (Goldberg & Huxley, 1992). The majority of these problems are solely managed with primary care since only 10% of patients are referred (Verhaak, 1993). Studies show GPs fail to recognize up to half of all mental health problems in their consulting patients (Vasquez-Barquero, 1990) and fail to diagnose 50% of cases of major depression and anxiety disorders (Farvolden, McBride, Bagby, & Ravitz, 2003).

How patients present their symptoms may be the main cause (Sigel & Leiper, 2004). More than 50% of patients present with only somatic symptoms thus attributing mental health experiences to a physical illness (Bridges & Goldberg, 1985). Patients who know they have psychological symptoms may still not disclose them due to several worries such as stigma and feeling the problem is trivial (Cape & McCulloch, 1999). In primary care, patients are presenting earlier with symptoms that are less developed (Booton & Collerton, 1998); however, it is important for physicians to realize and recognize the link between physical and mental illness (Copsey Spring, Yanni, & Levenson, 2007). Somatic symptoms with a psychological background induce the highest perceived burden on GPs who feel that the lack of time in consultation hinders their ability to explore mental health components of physical presentations (Zantinge, Verhaak, Kerssens, & Bensings, 2005). Many physical illnesses carry with them a psychological burden and treatment often overlooks this while the focus is on the primary condition.

To help identifying patients, screening questionnaires are now available (Means-Christensen, Sherbourne, Roy-Byrne, Craske, & Stein, 2006) for example, a self-report version of PRIME-MD (Spitzer, Kroenke, & Williams, 1999). Screening on its own does not improve patients' outcomes (Palmer & Coyne, 2003) but when screening is combined with treatment and follow up the effects are much more beneficial (Sherman, 2002). GPs which have an interest in mental health or have had mental health training are more likely to recognize mental health symptoms (Hickie et al., 2001). During consultations, patient-directed gaze has been shown to be related to a patients' share of talking and number of health problems revealed especially psychological (Bensing, Kerssens, & van-der-Pasch, 1995). Patient-directed gaze was also related to an improved diagnosis of psychological symptoms thus it is important for physicians to implement this in their consultations (Bensing et al., 1995).

Patient outcomes often rely on good communication with their physician (Gask, Rogers, Oliver, May, & Roland, 2003). Research has shown patients want their GP to listen to them and remain optimistic before taking specific actions towards relieving their symptoms (Backenstrass, Joest, Rosemann, & Szecsenyi, 2007; Lester, Tritter, & Sorohan, 2005a, 2005b). An important concern that physicians should discuss with their patients is the fear of stigma which the majority of patients worry about (McNair, Highet, Hickie, & Davenport, 2002).

Patients often are not active in seeking care, for example, not making follow up appointments thus physicians need to be active in providing care that is beneficial for the patient (Gask et al., 2003). There are a range of well established effective interventions for mental health problems. However these can only be accessed if the mental health conditions are identified in the first place – be they the sole problem or an adjunct to other conditions. Recent NICE guidelines and systematic review evidence has shown the efficacy of interventions such as cognitive behavioral treatment (Butler, Chapman, Forman, & Beck, 2006).

Abandoned Babies

At times difficult situations can be a complex mixture of emotionally fraught circumstances coupled with a rare occurrence. Baby abandonment may be a good example of such a difficult phenomenon – it is relatively rare, yet has been tracked from ancient times. Clearly prevention of such circumstances is the ideal solution. The advent of contraception and termination of pregnancy has changed the frequency and nature of the phenomenon. Yet still this difficult situation is not prevented or avoided. There is a distinct lack of policy for handling abandoned babies (Mueller & Sherr, 2009) within healthcare settings. What is seen as a convergence of a medical, social, and legal phenomenon also has distinct psychological ramifications for the mother (and father) of the baby, those who find the baby, and the adult survivors of abandonment. Rare situations create problems as learning from experience is prevented and the crisis nature of the situation at the time of finding may result in omissions in care or attention to detail. This is true of a number of difficult and rare situations. Good health care should equip doctors and healthcare workers with guidance and protocols which are thought out in advance, which pool the body of learning and which are informed by longer term sequelae.

There are those that see baby abandonment along the continuum of infanticide. This is a relatively rare phenomenon. West, Friedman, and Resnick (2009) summarized 16 studies and found that perpetrators were frequently young, single, and often living with parents. Fathers who kill their babies, on the other hand were found to be affected by mental health triggers, revenge, and were often linked with subsequent suicide (West et al., 2009). It is unclear what the link between infanticide and abandonment is and whether parental characteristics from infanticide can be generalized to parents of abandoned babies.

Abandonment experience and frequency ranges in different international contexts. It may be fuelled by multiple factors such as alcohol and drug use which has been described in studies from Russia (Zabina et al., 2009). Over the course of the HIV epidemic infant abandonment has been monitored. In the early days of the epidemic the phenomenon of "boarder babies" was described where HIV positive parents abandoned babies at the hospital. After the advent of treatment and the finding that vertical transmission can be dramatically reduced, this practice has changed. Abandonment in the presence of HIV seems to be more highly associated with parental risk behavior categories in the first place, such as intravenous drug use (Bailey, Semenenko, Pilipenko, Malyuta, & Thorne, 2010). Abandonment has been associated with the unavailability of contraception services in the first place or access to termination of unwanted pregnancies. The social stigma of a baby born out of wedlock was seen as a trigger, which can be affected by changing social norms (Cohen, 2010). In China the one child policy may have affected abandonment rates, as do gender factors. The literature also shows that war or conflict and babies conceived under traumatic circumstances such as rape has resulted in infant abandonment (Chhabra, Palaparthy, & Mishra, 2009). Finally factors associated with coercion or unwanted pregnancies and possibly mental health considerations alone or in conjunction with the previous factors may contribute to a baby being abandoned.

If evidence based policies are to be created, then good data gathering and study must precede this. In many countries there is poor record keeping and the size and circumstance of the phenomenon is poorly understood (Sherr, Mueller, & Fox, 2009). Despite this, there have been a number of innovations. Safe Haven provision and baby hatches have been described in the last decade. For example, in the US 47 states have Safe Haven provision or laws (Kunkel, 2007). It is unclear whether infants abandoned under these policies differ from those abandoned in nonSafe Haven environments, thus it is unknown whether such provision affects the behavior, enhances the problem or creates different problems, let alone solves the abandoning problem. Monitoring and evaluation of the Safe Haven provision is inadequate. Policy availability generally for abandoned babies is poor and simple guidance could be made available.

Little is known about the reasons for abandoning as most mothers do not come forward. Mental health is often a key factor in later abandonments, but may differ from early neonatal abandonments. Those who abandon older children are usually reunited. In a study Sherr et al. (2009) found the biggest predictor of survival was "findability." Few consider the emotional needs of the adult survivor and the fact that records need to be kept for a long time if the child wants recourse to information in later life.

Abuse in Pregnancy

Abuse in pregnancy is an all too common experience. Abuse refers to any physical, psychological, or sexual assault on a woman that can cause pain, trauma, damage, and which can have an impact for considerable time beyond the incident. Such effects relate to both the mother and the infant. Often studies have shown a combination of physical and sexual abuse in pregnancy (Lau, Keung, Wong, & Chan, 2008). True prevalence and description has not been fully established. Some studies in the US put the prevalence as high as 7–11% of the pregnant population (Helton, McFarlane, & Anderson, 1987; Hilliard, 1985). In Norway, similar findings were reported (Schei & Bakketeig, 1989). Such levels of abuse cannot be simply seen as a function of overall abuse, as an American study found an increased incidence of abusive violence of 60.6% when comparisons were made between pregnant and nonpregnant women (Gelles, 1988). Some age factors may also be prevalent where younger women are more likely to be abused and more likely to be pregnant.

Women are often reluctant to report abuse, but are more willing to divulge it if questioned in a sensitive way by their carers. Durant, Colley, Gilbert, Saltzman, and Johnson (2000) showed that only a minority of women (22–39%) reported that abuse had been mentioned during their pregnancy care. This represents a missed opportunity, and systematic interviewing in a safe nonjudgmental environment may facilitate reporting of abuse and the subsequent provision of support. McFarlane, Parker, Soeken, and Bullock (1992) found that 8% of their sample voluntarily reported abuse with no prompting; the figure rose to 29% when questions from their medical staff addressed the issue. Plichta, Duncan, and Plichta (1996) showed that in a sample where 7.3% reported abuse, satisfaction with physician communication was low and satisfaction with care was low. Only 9.7% of abused women discussed abuse with a physician.

The research studies currently available on abuse pose numerous methodological problems rendering them difficult to generalize. There is a growing evidence base on abuse in pregnancy, implications for mother and infant, correlates and predictors as well as the efficacy of interventions. Saltzman, Johnson, Gilbert, and Goodwim (2003) used modeling to estimate abuse in pregnancy in 16 US states and concluded a rate of 7.2%. They note that abuse commenced prior to pregnancy for three quarters of women. Muhajarine and D'Arcy (1999) reported a prevalence of 5.7% abuse in a large Canadian sample. Stewart and Cecutti (1993) reported a prevalence of 6.6% during pregnancy and 10% before pregnancy. Fisher, Yassour, Borochowitz, and Neter (2003) described different forms of abuse, severe physical attack (8%), minor physical attack (17%), psychological abuse (24%), and sexual coercion (5.6%). Bullock and McFarlane (1989) found a higher prevalence of low birth weight where mothers had suffered abuse during pregnancy. McFarlane et al. (1992), in a study of 691 American subjects, found that one in six women in this prospective study had been abused, with 60% of this group reporting at least two occasions of abuse. Abuse was most common around the head. The perpetrator was almost always someone known to the pregnant woman – 78% had been abused by their husband or boyfriend. Particular risks were apparent in the cases of teenagers who reported multiple abuses (often by both their boyfriend and their parents). The authors noted that abused women were highly likely to be late attenders for antenatal care. Ludermir, Lewis, Valongueiro, de Araújo, and Araya (2010) notes the specific association between abuse and postnatal depression.

Stewart (1992) and Stewart and Cecutti (1993) studied a sample of 548 women in Canada. In addition to the physical abuse, the women recorded mental abuse, threats, forced sex, and fear of their partner. Yet the majority was still in the relationship, despite requiring medical treatment for the abuse. For 62%, the abuse increased during pregnancy, for 30% the level remained constant; only in 7% did pregnancy mark a decrease in abuse. Only 2.5% told the antenatal staff of the abuse.

Abuse of the pregnant woman can lead to direct and indirect effects on both mother and baby. There is a direct risk of trauma and physical damage to the mother. There is a similar risk to the baby, in the case of severe violence to the abdomen, which may cause conditions such as abruptio placentae, fetal fractures, ruptures, and hemorrhage (Boy & Salihu, 2004; Sammons, 1981). Boy and Salihu (2004) reviewed 296 publications and noted elevated maternal and infant mortality, operative delivery, low birth weight, and a number of other negative outcomes associated with abuse in pregnancy. Indirectly, the abuse may lead to emotional reactions, increased anxiety, depression, or the exacerbation of any illnesses. Tiwari et al. (2008) showed a link between abuse and elevated self-harming thoughts, lowered quality of life and higher mental health problems. Ludermir et al. (2010) in Brazil showed an association between abuse in pregnancy and postpartum depression. If a woman turns to over use of items such as alcohol, tobacco, medication, or illicit drugs to help her cope with the trauma, these will have documented deleterious effects on any developing fetus (Harlap & Shiono, 1980; Kline, Shrout, Stein, Susser, & Warburton, 1980; Zuckerman, Frank, & Hingson, 1989) as well as on the health of the mother. Altarac and Strobino (2002) noted a relationship between abuse in pregnancy and low birthweight of the infant, either directly from the abuse, indirectly from the stress or clustering with a series of sociodemographic factors that are risks for low birthweight as well as abuse.

Women who are the subject of abuse often display a range of common reactions, often referred to as the "battered women syndrome" (Walker, 1984). Some studies have typified such women as those who suffer from "learned helplessness," yet other studies (Gondolf & Fisher, 1988) have shown a high degree of behavioral adaptation and resourcefulness in the victims of abuse. However, all abused women run the risk of social isolation, of detachment from social support, of shame and guilt and they may simultaneously suffer from lowered self-esteem. Goodwin, Gazmararian, Johnson, Gilbert, and Saltzman (2000) carried out a comprehensive study on 39,348 women to examine the relationship between pregnancy intendedness and physical abuse. For this large sample abuse for those with unintended pregnancy during preconception year was reported at 12.6% and abuse during pregnancy was elevated to 15.3%. The rates were 5.3% for women who did not report an unintended pregnancy. Martin, Macie, Kupper, Buescher, and Moracco (2001) underlined the importance of not confining enquiry to the pregnancy and measured abuse before, during and after pregnancy in a sample of 2,648 women. They found fluctuations in prevalence from 6.9% before, 6.1% during, and 3.2% after pregnancy. They also noted that of the 77% who were injured, only 23% received medical attention, thus highlighting the fact that such incidents are associated with a reluctance to seek help. Similarly Stewart and Cecutti (1993) and McFarlane, Campbell, Sharps, and Watson (2002) emphasize the continuity of abuse before, during, and after pregnancy. The authors noted a significant increase in abuse incidents postpartum. This was confirmed by Hedin (2000) in Sweden who noted a group who were abused post partum who had not reported abuse previously.

Table 1. Studies on abuse during pregnancy

Author	Place	N	% Abuse
Bacchus, Mezey, & Bewley, (2004)	London	200	3
Bacchus et al. (2004)	London	892	6.4
Bohn et al. (2004)	US	1,004	15.9
Bowen et al. (2005)	Britain	7,591	Physical 1
			Emotional 4.8
			Victimisation 5.1
Cuevas et al. (2006)	Mexico	1,949	13
Curry (1998)	US	559	37
Dye et al. (1995)	US	364	15.9
Ezechi et al. (2004)	Nigeria	418	47.1
Fisher et al. (2003)	Israel	270	5.4
Goodwin (2000)	US	39,348	15.3
Greenberg et al. (1997)	US	261	33.3
Hedin (2000)	Norway	207	14.5
Hilliard (1985)	US	742	10.9
Johnson et al. (2003)	UK	475	17
Kaye et al. (2006)	Uganda	612	27.7
Keeling and Birch (2004)	UK	312	35.1
Lau (2005)	Hong Kong	1,200	11.2
Leung et al. (1999)	China	631	17.9
Ludermir et al. (2010)	Brazil	1,045	Psychological 28.1
			Physical 11.8
			Sexual 5.7
MacFarlane (1992)	US	691	17
MacFarlane (2002)	US	437	7.8
Martin et al. (2001)	US	2,648	6.1
Muhajarine and D'Arcy (1999)	Canada	543	5.7
O'Campo et al. (1994)	US	358	65
Parker et al. (1993)	US	691	26

(continued)

Table 1. Continued.

Author	Place	N	% Abuse
Purwar et al. (1999)	India	600	8.33
Sahin and Sahin (2003)	Turkey	475	33.3
Stenson et al. (2001)	Sweden	1,038	1.3
Stewart and Cecutti (1993)	Canada	548	6.6
Tiwari et al. (2008)	Hong Kong	3,245	9.1
Valladares et al. (2005)	Nicaragua	478	32.4
van der Hulst et al. (2006)	Netherlands	625	11.2
Varma (2007)	India	203	Physical 14
			Psychological 15
			Sexual 9
Webster (1994)	Australia	1,014	27.9
Yang (2006)	Taiwan	1,143	6.9
Yost (2005)	US	16,041	6

The phenomenon seems to be international, but with prevalence variations. Stenson et al. (2001) in Sweden ($n = 1038$) reported a rate of 1.3% during pregnancy and 2.8% in the year preceding pregnancy. They found an association with past abortion. Jewkes, PennKekana, Levin, Ratsaka, and Schrieber (2001) explored the phenomenon among respondents to a household survey ($n = 2,232$) which generated a sample of 1,306 women who reported physical abuse during a pregnancy at 9.1%, 6.7%, and 4.7% (depending on geographic location). Purwar, Jeyaseelan, Varhadpande, Motghare, and Pimplakute (1999) in India selected 600 pregnant women and noted that 25.33% reported abuse before pregnancy and 22% reported abuse during pregnancy – 8.3% reported increases in abuse during the pregnancy. Abuse was recurrent for the majority (92%). In Brazil, Moraes and Reichenheim (2002) studied 526 women and noted 33.8% reporting some form of physical violence, and 16.5% reporting severe violence. These rates are much higher than other centers. Savona Ventura, Savona Ventura, Drengsted, Nieldsen, and Johansen (2001) reported a rate of 11.7% in Malta. Gazmararian et al. (1996) attempted to synthesize studies on abuse and selected 13 studies with sound methodology. This composite account indicated a prevalence ranging from 0.9% to 20.1%. Gazmararian et al. noted that higher prevalence was noted where women were questioned later in pregnancy. Table 1 above summarizes international studies exploring the rate of abuse in pregnancy, providing details, geographical place of the study and prevalence. It shows that the range of abuse during pregnancy is from 1.3% (Sweden) through to 35.1% (UK) for the European nations and a range of prevalence from 6.0% to 65.0% in North America.

There is no literature which directly links child abuse with the abuse of pregnant women. There is a literature which relates femicide to abuse (McFarlane et al., 2002). These researchers used a complex methodology of exploring attempted and completed femicide cases identified from police and medical examiner records and comparing these to abuse in pregnancy controls. They found that the risk of becoming an attempted or completed femicide victim was three times higher for women who had been abused during pregnancy.

Finally the key question relates to prevention. Are there any interventions which can prevent or reduce abuse? The literature shows some advances in this respect. Empowerment interventions (Tiwari et al., 2005) were effective in reducing violence and improving self-esteem. Intensive advocacy has also been shown to have a positive effect in a recent Cochrane review (Ramsay et al., 2009). Cognitive behavioral therapy has been used for male partners to reduce abuse (Smedslund, Dalsbø, Steiro, Winsvold, & Clench-Aas, 2007), with occasional beneficial effects, but too few studies for definitive insight.

In general, when working with pregnant women, one can assume:

- Abuse may be present and should be explored, cataloged and support provided. Simply enquiry about abuse increases reporting rate.
- There is an increase in teenage abuse from parents and partners (sometimes both).
- Following abuse, there is a subsequent increase in negative outcomes for mother and infant, including miscarriages, low birth weight, still birth and depression.
- Abuse is largely not recognized or identified by health care staff.
- There is a possible association between abuse, suicidal behaviors and femicide.
- The prevalence of abuse to pregnant women is increasing.
- Pregnancy is no protection from abuse – a woman who was abused prior to pregnancy may well suffer abuse during the pregnancy.
- Indicators of risk include unintended pregnancy, abuse in the pre-conception phase (Martin et al., 2001) and those with challenging social conditions (living alone, entering care late, and smoking (Godwin et al., 2000, Savona Ventura et al., 2001) and a history of abortion (Stenson et al., 2001).
- Partner alcohol problem and number of negative life events in the preceding year may be a predictor (Muhajarine & D'Arcy, 1999).
- Interventions for both the pregnant woman and her partner may be beneficial.

Concluding Comments

This review has summarized some difficult situations encountered in health care. Traditional medical school training may not provide an insight into issues such as human behavior during doctor patient communications, mental health components of essentially physical health interviews and the human factor difficulties with processes such as breaking bad news. Some difficult situations occur every day while others are difficult by virtue of the fact that they are so rare. Abandoned babies and abuse in pregnancy are such examples.

What all these difficult topics have in common is a need to understand the psychological and human factors underpinning them and a need to explore how these can assist in preventing, reacting or adjusting to these difficult groups or situations. The examples in this chapter provide detailed insight into how social science understanding and rigor can be invoked to explore health related issues and provide an evidence base to inform doctors when faced with difficult situations, patients or problems.

There is considerable knowledge of human behavior that can be applied and a working knowledge of psychological approaches will help integrate this evidence base into challenging practice and ease the pathway for doctors. In so doing it can also assist in ensuring the best possible outcome for patients.

Dedication

This chapter is dedicated to my children, Liora, Yoni, Ari, Ilan, and Jasmine.

References

Ahmann, E. (1998). Review and commentary: Two studies regarding giving "bad news". *Pediatric Nursing, 24*, 554–556.

Altarac, M., & Strobino, D. (2002). Abuse during pregnancy and stress because of abuse during pregnancy and birth weight. *Journal of the American Medical Women's Association Fall, 57*, 208–214.

Bacchus, L., Mezey, G., & Bewley, S. (2004). Domestic violence: Prevalence in pregnant women and associations with physical and psychological health. *European Journal of Obstetrics & Gynecology and Reproductive Biology, 11*, 6–11.

Backenstrass, M., Joest, K., Rosemann, T., & Szecsenyi, J. (2007). The care of patients with subthreshold depression in primary care: Is it all that bad? A qualitative study on the views of general practitioners and patients. *BMC Health Services Research, 21*, 7–190.

Baile, W. F., Buckman, R., Lenzi, R., Glober, G., Beale, E. A., & Kudelka, A. P. (2000). SPIKES-A six-step protocol for delivering bad news: Application to the patient with Cancer. *Oncologist. 2000, 5*, 302–311.

Bailey, H., Semenenko, I., Pilipenko, T., Malyuta, R., & Thorne, C. (2010). Factors associated with abandonment of infants born to HIV-positive women: Results from a Ukrainian birth cohort. *AIDS Care, 6*, 1–10.

Baird, G., McConachie, H., & Scrutton, D. (2000). Parents' perceptions of disclosure of the diagnosis of cerebral palsy. *Archives of Disease in Childhood, 83*, 475–480.

Bensing, J. M., Kerseens, J. J., & van-der Pasch, M. (1995). Patient-directed gaze as a tool for discovering and handling psychosocial problems in general practice. *Journal of Nonverbal Behavior, 19*, 223–242.

Bohn, D. K., Tebben, J. G., & Campbell, J. C. (2004). Influences of income, education, age, and ethnicity on physical abuse before and during pregnancy. *Journal of Obstetric, Gynecologic, and Neonatal Nursing, 33*, 561–571.

Booton, P., & Collerton, J. (1998). Diagnosis and patient management in general practice. In A. Stephenson (Ed.), *A textbook of general practice* (pp. 47–59). London, UK: Arnold.

Bridges, K., & Goldberg, D. (1985). Somatic presentation of DSM-III psychiatric disorders in primary care. *Journal of Psychosomatic Research, 29*, 563–569.

Bowen, E., Heron, J., Waylen, A., & Wolke, D. (2005). ALSPAC study team. Domestic violence risk during and after pregnancy: Findings from a British longitudinal study. *BJOG: An International Journal of Obstetrics and Gynaecology, 112*, 1083–1089.

Boy, A., & Salihu, H. M. (2004). Intimate partner violence and birth outcomes: A systematic review. *International Journal of Fertility and Women's Medicine, 49*, 159–164.

Buckman, R. (1984). Breaking bad news: Why is it still so difficult?. *British Medical Journal (Clinical Research Ed), 288*, 1597–1599.

Bui, T. H., Cavanagh, H. D., & Robertson, D. M. (2010). Patient compliance during contact lens wear: Perceptions, awareness, and behavior. *Eye and Contact Lens: Science and Clinical Practice, 36*, 334–339.

Bullock, L. F., & McFarlane, J. (1989). The birth-weight/battering connection. *American Journal of Nursing, 89*, 1153–1155.

Butler, A. C., Chapman, J. E., Formen, E. M., & Beck, A. T. (2006). The empirical status of cognitive-behavioral therapy: A review of meta-analyses. *Clinical Psychology Review, 26*, 17–31.

Cape, J., & McCulloch, Y. (1999). Patients' reasons for not presenting emotional problems in general practice. *British Journal of General Practice, 49*, 875–879.

Chesney, M. A., Morin, M., & Sherr, L. (2000). Adherence to HIV combination therapy. *Social Science and Medicine, 50*, 1599–1605.

Chhabra, S., Palaparthy, S., & Mishra, S. (2009). Social issues around advanced unwanted pregnancies in rural single women. *Journal of Obstetrics and Gynecology, 29*, 333–336.

Cohen, J. (2010). Reducing HIV infection and abandonment of babies. *Science, 329* (5988), 172.

Copsey Spring, T., Yanni, L., & Levenson, J. (2007). A shot in the dark: Failing to recognize the link between physical and mental illness. *Journal of General Internal Medicine, 22*, 677–680.

Cuddihy, M. T., Amadio, P. C., Gabriel, S. E., Pankratz, V. S., Kurland, R. L., & Melton, L. J. (2004). A prospective clinical practice intervention to improve osteoporosis management following distal forearm fracture. *Osteoporosis International, 15*, (3rd ed.) 695–700.

Cuevas, S., Blanco, J., Juárez, C., Palma, O., & Valdez-Santiago, R. (2006). Violence and pregnancy in female users of Ministry of Health care services in highly deprived states in Mexico. *Salud Publica, 48*, Suppl. 2 S239–S249.

Curry, M. A. (1998). The interrelationships between abuse, substance use, and psychosocial stress during pregnancy. *Journal of Obstetric, Gynecologic, and Neonatal Nursing, 27*, 692–699.

Donovan, J. L. (1995). Patient decision making. The missing ingredient in compliance research. *International Journal of Technology Assessment in Health Care, 11*, 443–455.

Dosanjh, S., Barnes, J., & Bhandari, M. (2001). Barriers to breaking bad news among medical and surgical residents. *Medical Education, 35*, 197–205.

Durant, T., Colley., Gilbert, B., Saltzman, L., & Johnson, C. (2000). Opportunities for interventions discussing physical abuse during prenatal care visits. *American Journal of Preventive Medicine, 19*, 238–244.

Dye, T. D., Tollivert, N. J., Lee, R. V., & Kenney, C. J. (1995). Violence, pregnancy and birth outcome in Appalachia. *Paediatric and Perinatal Epidemiology, 9*, 35–47.

Ezechi, O. C., Kalu, B. K., Ezechi, L. O., Nwokoro, C. A., Ndububa, V. I., & Okeke, G. C. (2004). Prevalence and pattern of domestic violence against pregnant Nigerian women. *Journal of Obstetrics and Gynecology, 24*, 652–656.

Fallowfield, L., & Jenkins, V. (2004). Communicating sad, bad, and difficult news in medicine. *Lancet, 363*, 312–319.

Farvolden, P., McBride, C., Bagby, R. M., & Ravitz, P. (2003). A Web-based screening instrument for depression and anxiety disorders in primary care. *Journal of Medical Internet Research, 5*, e23.

Fisher, M., Yassour., Borochowitz, D., & Neter, E. (2003). Domestic abuse in pregnancy results from a phone survey in Northern Israel. *Israel Medical Association Journal, 5*, 35–39.

Friedrichsen, M., & Milberg, A. (2006). Concerns about losing control when breaking bad news to terminally ill patients with cancer: Physicians' perspective. *Journal of Palliative Medicine, 9*, 673–682.

Gallagher, A., Arber, A., Chaplin, R., & Quirk, A. (2010). Service users' experience of receiving bad news about their mental health. *Journal of Mental Health, 19*, 34–42.

Gask, L., Rogers, A., Oliver, D., May, C., & Roland, M. (2003). Qualitative study of patients' perceptions of the quality of care for depression in general practice. *British Journal of General Practice, 53*, 278–283.

Gazmararian, J., Lazorick, S., Spitz, A., Ballard, T., Saltzman, L., & Marks, J. (1996). Prevalence of violence against pregnant women. *JAMA: The Journal of the American Medical Association, 275*, 1915–1920.

Gelles, R. (1988). Violence and pregnancy: Are pregnant women at greater risk of abuse? *Journal of Marriage and Family*, 841–847.

Gold, D. T., & McClung, B. (2006). Approaches to patient education: Emphasizing the long-term value of compliance and persistence. *American Journal of Medicine, 119*, Suppl. 1 S32–S37 Review.

Goldberg, D., & Huxley, P. (1992). *Common mental disorders*. London, UK: Routledge.

Gondolf, E., & Fisher, E. (1988). *Battered women as survivors: An alternative to treating learned helplessness*. Lexington, MA: Lexington Books.

Goodwin, M., Gazmararian, J., Johnson., Gilbert, B., & Saltzman, L. (2000). Pregnancy intendedness and physical abuse around the time of pregnancy, findings from the pregnancy risk assessment monitoring system 1996–97. *Maternal Child Health, 4*, 85–92.

Greenberg, E. M., McFarlane, J., & Watson, M. G. (1997). Vaginal bleeding and abuse: Assessing pregnant women in the emergency department. *MCN. The American Journal of Maternal Child Nursing, 22*, 182–186.

Harlap, S., & Shiono, P. (1980). Alcohol smoking and incidence of spontaneous abortions in the first and second trimester. *Lancet, 2*, 173–176.

Heaman, M. I. (2005). Relationships between physical abuse during pregnancy and risk factors for preterm birth among women in Manitoba. *Journal of Obstetric, Gynecologic, and Neonatal Nursing, 34*, 721–731.

Hedin, L. (2000). Postpartum also a risk period for domestic violence. *European Journal of Obstetrics, Gynecology, and Reproductive Biology, 89*, 41–45.

Helton, A., McFarlane, J., & Anderson, E. (1987). Battered and pregnant: A prevalence study. *American Journal of Public Health, 77*, 1337–1339.

Hickie, I., Davenport, T., Scott, E., Hadzi-Pavlovic, D., Naismith, S., & Koschera, A. (2001). Unmet need for recognition of common mental disorders in Australian general practice. *Medical Journal of Australia, 6*, S18–S24.

Hilliard, P. (1985). Physical abuse in pregnancy. *Obstetrics & Gynecology, 66*, 185–190.

Hornberger, J. C., Gibson, C. D. Jr., Wood, W., Dequeldre, C., Corso, I., Palla, B., & Bloch, D. A. (1996). Eliminating language barriers for non-English-speaking patients. *Medical Care, 34*, 845–856.

Ishaque, S., Saleem, T., Khawaja, F. B., & Qidwai, W. (2010). Breaking bad news: Exploring patient's perspective and expectations. *Journal of the Pakistan Medical Association, 60*, 407–411.

Jewkes, R., PennKekana, L., Levin, J., Ratsaka, M., & Schrieber, M. (2001). Prevalence of emotional physical and sexual abuse of women in three South African Provinces. *South African Medical Journal, 91*, 421–428.

Johnson, J. K., Haider, F., Ellis, K., Hay, D. M., & Lindow, S. W. (2003). The prevalence of domestic violence in pregnant women. *BJOG: An International Journal of Obstetrics and Gynaecology, 110*, 272–275.

Kaye, D. K., Mirembe, F. M., Bantebya, G., Johansson, A., & Ekstrom, A. M. (2006). Domestic violence during pregnancy and risk of low birthweight and maternal complications: A prospective cohort study at Mulago Hospital, Uganda. *Tropical Medicine & International Health, 11*, 1576–1584.

Keeling, J., & Birch, L. (2004). The prevalence rates of domestic abuse in women attending a family planning clinic. *Journal of Family Planning and Reproductive Health Care, 30*, 113–114.

Kinnersley, P., Edwards, A., Hood, K., Ryan, R., Prout, H., Cadbury, N., ... Butler, C. (2008). Interventions before consultations to help patients address their information needs by encouraging question asking: Systematic review. *British Medical Journal, 337*, a485.

Kline, J., Shrout, P., Stein, Z., Susser, M., & Warburton, D. (1980). Drinking during pregnancy and spontaneous abortion. *Lancet, 2*, 176–180.

Kunkel, K. A. (2007). Safe-haven laws focus on abandoned newborns and their mothers. *Journal of Pediatric Nursing, 22*, 397–401.

Lau, Y. (2005). Does pregnancy provide immunity from intimate partner abuse among Hong Kong Chinese women? *Social Science and Medicine, 61*, 365–377.

Lau, Y., Keung., Wong, D. F., & Chan, K. S. (2008). The impact and cumulative effects of intimate partner abuse during pregnancy on health-related quality of life among Hong Kong Chinese women. *Midwifery, 24*, 22–37.

Lester, H., Tritter, J., & Sorohan, H. (2005a). Patients' and health professionals' views on primary care for people with serious mental illness: Focus group study. *British Medical Journal, 14*, 1122.

Lester, H., Tritter, J. Q., & Sorohan, H. (2005b). Patients' and health professionals' views on primary care for people with serious mental illness: Focus group study. *British Medical Journal, 330*, 1122.

Leung, W. C., Leung, T. W., Lam, Y. Y., & Ho, P. C. (1999). The prevalence of domestic violence against pregnant women in a Chinese community. *International Journal of Gynecology and Obstetrics, 66*, 23–30.

Lombas, C., Hakim, C., & Zanchetta, J. R. (2001). Compliance with alendronate treatment in an osteoporosis clinic. Presented at the American Society for Bone and Mineral Research (ASBMR) 23rd Annual Meeting, October 12–16. Phoenix, AZ.

Ludermir, A. B., Lewis, G., Valongueiro, S. A., de Araújo, T. V., & Araya, R. (2010). Violence against women by their intimate partner during pregnancy and postnatal depression: A prospective cohort study. *Lancet, 376*, 903–910.

Maguire, P. (1985). Barriers to psychological care of the dying. *British Medical Journal, 291*, 1711–1713.

Martin, S., Macie, I., Kupper, L., Buescher, P., & Moracco. (2001). Physical abuse of women before during and after pregnancy. *JAMA: The Journal of the American Medical Association, 285*, 1628–1630.

McFarlane, J., Campbell, J. C., Sharps, P., & Watson, K. (2002). Abuse during pregnancy and femicide urgent implications for women's health. *Obstetrics and Gynecology, 100*, 27–36.

McFarlane, J., Parker, B., Soeken, K., & Bullock, L. (1992). Assessing for abuse during pregnancy. *JAMA: The Journal of the American Medical Association, 267*, 3176–3178.

McNair, B., Highet, N., Hickie, I., & Davenport, T. A. (2002). Exploring the perspectives of people whose lives have been affected by depression. *Medical Journal of Australia, 20*, Suppl. 176 S69–S76.

Means-Christensen, A. J., Sherbourne, C. D., Roy-Byrne, P. P., Craske, M. G., & Stein, M. B. (2006). Using five questions to screen for five common mental disorders in primary care: Diagnostic accuracy of the Anxiety and Depression Detector. *General Hospital Psychiatry, 28*, 108–118.

Melnikow, J., & Kiefe, C. (1994). Patient compliance and medical research: Issues in methodology. *Journal of General Internal Medicine, 9*, 96–105.

Moraes, C. L., & Reichenheim, M. (2002). Domestic violence during pregnancy in Rio De Janeiro Brazil. *International Journal of Gynecology and Obstetrics, 79*, 269–277.

Mueller, J., & Sherr, L. (2009). Abandoned babies and absent policies. *Health Policy, 93* (2–3) 157–164.

Muhajarine, N., & D'Arcy, C. (1999). Physical abuse during pregnancy prevalence and risk factors. *CMAJ: Canadian Medical Association journal, 160*, 1007–1011.

O'Campo, P., Gielen, A. C., Faden, R. R., & Kass, N. (1994). Verbal abuse and physical violence among a cohort of low-income pregnant women. *Womens Health Issues, 4*, 29–37.

O'Connor, A. M., Bennett, C. L., Stacey, D., Barry, M., Col, N. F., Eden, K. B., . . . & Rovner, D. (2009). Decision aids for people facing health treatment or screening decisions. *Cochrane Database Syst, 8*, CD001431.

Orgel, E., McCarter, R., & Jacobs, S. (2010). A failing medical educational model: A self-assessment by physicians at all levels of training of ability and comfort to deliver bad news. *Journal of Palliative Medicine, 13*, 677–678.

Palmer, S. C., & Coyne, J. C. (2003). Screening for depression in medical care: Pitfalls, alternatives, and revised priorities. *Journal of Psychosomatic Research, 54*, 279–287.

Parker, B., McFarlane, J., Soeken, K., Torres, S., & Campbell, D. (1993). Physical and emotional abuse in pregnancy: A comparison of adult and teenage women. *Nursing Research, 42*, 173–178.

Plichta, S. B., Duncan, M., & Plichta, L. (1996). Spouse abuse patient physician communication and patient satisfaction. *American Journal of Preventive Medicine, 12*, 297–303.

Purwar, M. B., Jeyaseelan, L., Varhadpande, U., Motghare, V., & Pimplakute, S. (1999). Survey of physical abuse during pregnancy GMCH Nagpur India. *Journal of Obstetrics and Gynecology Research, 25*, 165–171.

Quirk, M., Mazor, K., Haley, H. L., Philbin, M., Fischer, M., Sullivan, K., & Hatem, D. (2008). How patients perceive a doctor's caring attitude. *Patient Education and Counseling, 72*, 359–366.

Ramsay, J., Carter, Y., Davidson, L., Dunne, D., Eldridge, S., Feder, G., . . . Warburton, A. (2009). Advocacy interventions to reduce or eliminate violence and promote the physical and psychosocial well-being of women who experience intimate partner abuse. *Cochrane Database of Systematic Reviews, 8*, CD005043.

Sahin, H. A., & Sahin, H. G. (2003). An unaddressed issue: Domestic violence and unplanned pregnancies among pregnant women in Turkey. *European Journal of Contraception and Reproductive Health Care, 8*, 93–98.

Saltzman, L. L., Johnson, C., Gilbert, B., & Goodwim, M. (2003). Physical abuse around the time of pregnancy an examination of prevalence and risk factors in 16 states. *Maternal Child Health Journal*, 131–143.

Sammons, M. (1981). Battered and pregnant. *American Journal of Maternal and Child Nursing, 6*, 246–250.

Sandelowski, M., Voils, C. I., Chang, Y., & Lee, E. J. (2009). A systematic review comparing antiretroviral adherence descriptive and intervention studies conducted in the USA. *AIDS Care, 21*, 953–966.

Savona Ventura, C., Savona Ventura, M., Drengsted, Nieldsen. S., & Johansen, K. (2001). Domestic abuse in a central Mediterranean pregnant population. *European Journal of Obstetrics, Gynecology, and Reproductive Biology, 98*, 3–8.

SCOPE. (2003). *Right from the start template: Good practice in sharing the news.* London, UK: Department of Health 8.

Schei, B., & Bakketeig, L. S. (1989). Gynaecological impact of sexual and physical abuse by spouse; a study of a random sample of Norwegian Women. *British Journal of Obstetrics and Gynaecology, 96*, 1379–1383.

Sherr, L., Mueller, J., & Fox Z. (2009). Abandoned babies in the UK – A review utilizing media reports. Child: Care, Health and Development, *35*, 419–430.

Sherman, S. E. (2002). Review: Screening for depression reduces persistent depression. *ACP Journal Club, 137*, 100.

Sigel, P., & Leiper, R. (2004). GP views of their management and referral of psychological problems: A qualitative study. *Psychology and Psychotherapy, 77*, 279–295.

Smedslund, G., Dalsbø, T. K., Steiro, A. K., Winsvold, A., & Clench-Aas, J. (2007). Cognitive behavioural therapy for men who physically abuse their female partner. *Cochrane Database of Systematic Reviews, 18*, CD006048.

Smith, C. J., Phillips, A. N., Dauer, B., Johnson, M. A., Lampe, F. C., Youle, M. S., . . . Staszewski, S. (2009). Factors associated with viral rebound among highly treatment-experienced HIV-positive patients who have achieved viral suppression. *HIV Medicine, 10*, 19–27.

Spitzer, R. L., Kroenke, K., & Williams, J. B. W. (1999). Patient health questionnaire primary care study group. Validation and utility of a self-report version of PRIME-MD. *JAMA: The Journal of the American Medical Association, 282*, 1737–1744.

Stenson, K., Heimer, G., Lundh, C., Nordstrom, M., Saarinen, H., & Wenker, A. (2001). The prevalence of violence investigated in a pregnant population in Sweden. *Journal of Psychosomatic Obstetrics and Gynecology,* 21(4) 189–197.

Stewart, C. (1992). *Abuse in pregnancy.* Canadian Study Paper, Presented at the Annual SRIP Conference, Glasgow.

Stewart, D. E., & Cecutti, A. (1993). Physical abuse in pregnancy. *CMAJ: Canadian Medical Association journal, 149*, 1257–1263.

Tiwari, A., Chan, K. L., Fong, D., Leung, W. C., Brownridge, D. A., Lam, H., . . . Ho, P. C. (2008). The impact of psychological abuse by an intimate partner on the mental health of pregnant women. *BJOG: An International Journal of Obstetrics and Gynaecology, 115*, 377–384.

Tiwari, A., Leung, W. C., Leung, T. W., Humphreys, J., Parker, B., & Ho, P. C. (2005). A randomized controlled trial of empowerment training for Chinese abused pregnant women in Hong Kong. *BJOG: An International Journal of Obstetrics and Gynaecology, 112*, 1249–1256.

Tsui, J., & Alward, W. L. M. (2010). Patient Non-Compliance: Physician responsibility. Eye-Rounds.org. Retrieved January 24, 2010, from http://www.EyeRounds.org/cases/106-Patient-Noncompliance.htm.

Urquhart, J. (1996). Patient non-compliance with drug regimens: Measurement, clinical correlates, economic impact. *European Heart Journal, 17*, Suppl. A 8–15.

Valladares, E., Peña, R., Persson, L. A., & Högberg, U. (2005). Violence against pregnant women: Prevalence and characteristics. A population-based study in Nicaragua. *BJOG: An International Journal of Obstetrics and Gynaecology, 112*, 1243–1248.

van der Hulst, L. A., Bonsel, G. J., Eskes, M., Birnie, E., van Teijlingen, E., & Bleker, O. P. (2006). Bad experience, good birthing: Dutch low-risk pregnant women with a history of sexual abuse. *Journal of Psychosomatic Obstetrics and Gynecology, 27*, 59–66.

Varma, D., Chandra, P. S., Thomas, T., & Carey, M. P. (2007). Intimate partner violence and sexual coercion among pregnant women in India: Relationship with depression and post-traumatic stress disorder. *Journal of Affective Disorders, 102*, 227–235.

Vasquez-Barquero, J. L. (1990). Mental health in primary care settings. In D. Goldberg & D. Tantam (Eds.), *The public health impact of mental disorder* (pp. 35–44). Toronto, ON: Hogrefe.

Verhaak, P. F. M. (1993). Analysis of mental health problems by general practitioners. *British Journal of General Practice, 43*, 203–208.

Vermeire, E., Hearnshaw, H., Van Royen, P., & Denekens, J. (2001). Patient adherence to treatment: Three decades of research. A comprehensive review. *Journal of Clinical Pharmacy and Therapeutics*, Oct, *26*, 331–342 Review.

Walker, L. (1984). *The battered woman syndrome*. New York, NY: Springer.

Webster, J., Sweett, S., & Stolz, T. A. (1994). Domestic violence in pregnancy. A prevalence study. *The Med Journal of Australia, 161*, 466–470.

Wenrich, M. D., Curtis, J. R., Shannon, S. E., Carline, J. D., Ambrozy, D. M., & Ramsey, P. G. (2001). Communicating with dying patients within the spectrum of medical care from terminal diagnosis to death. *Archives of Internal Medicine, 161*, 868–874.

West, S. G., Friedman, S. H., & Resnick, P. J. (2009). Fathers who kill their children: An analysis of the literature. *Journal of Forensic Sciences, 54*, 463–468.

Yang, M. S., Yang, M. J., Chou, F. H., Yang, H. M., Wei, S. L., & Lin, J. R. (2006). Physical abuse against pregnant aborigines in Taiwan: Prevalence and risk factors. *International Journal of Nursing Studies, 43*, 21–27.

Yost, N. P., Bloom, S. L., McIntire, D. D., & Leveno, K. J. (2005). A prospective observational study of domestic violence during pregnancy. *Obstetrics & Gynecology, 106*, 61–65.

Zabina, H., Kissin, D., Pervysheva, E., Mytil, A., Dudchenko, O., Jamieson, D., & Hillis, S. (2009). Abandonment of infants by HIV-positive women in Russia and prevention measures. *Reproductive Health Matters, 17*, 162–170.

Zantinge, E. M., Verhaak, P. F., Kerssens, J. J., & Bensing, J. M. (2005). The workload of GPs: Consultations of patients with psychological and somatic problems compared. *British Journal of General Practice, 55*, 609–614.

Zuckerman, B., Frank, D., & Hingson, R. (1989). Effects of maternal marijuana and cocaine use on fetal growth. *New England Journal of Medicine, 320*, 762–768.

Cognitive Psychology and Medical/Therapeutic Care

Mindfulness and Healthcare Professionals

Shauna L. Shapiro and Caitlin L. Burnham

Santa Clara University, Santa Clara, CA, USA

Healthcare professionals often face the challenge of maintaining their own health and well-being under the intense demands inherent in their work. The stress involved in the helping professions can result in deleterious consequences for the practitioner as well as for their patients. Lack of self-care and ability to manage stress often inhibits professionals' ability to deliver quality and empathic care to patients. It is essential to confront this issue within the healthcare profession to enhance quality of life and well-being for those who are receiving *and* giving care.

This concern has been identified in the literature, and clinician self-care has been suggested as an essential component of training programs for those in the helping professions (Shapiro & Carlson, 2009). Mindfulness training has been examined and discussed as an effective means of promoting self-care and clinician effectiveness (see Christopher et al., 2010; Dobkin & Hutchinson, 2009; Gokhan, Meehan, & Peters, 2010; Shapiro et al., 2007). Shapiro and Carlson (2009) suggest mindfulness can be incorporated into the helping professions for purposes of both maintaining clinician self-care and enhancing the quality of patient care. Mindfulness can be taught from the lens of self-care and personal stress management (Shapiro & Carlson, 2009), as well as from the lens of how to enhance clinical skill and therapeutic outcome (Grepmair & colleagues', 2007).

Germer, Fulton, and Siegel (2005), suggest three pathways through which mindfulness can be integrated into clinical work. One path is for the clinician to establish his or her own mindfulness practice to increase attention, empathy, and presence in clinical work (referred to as the *mindful therapist*). A second avenue is to allow therapy to be informed by mindfulness teachings and theory, using mindfulness to guide one's theoretical orientation in clinical work (*mindfulness-informed therapy*). Finally, mindfulness skills and practices can be explicitly taught to patients in formal manualized interventions as well as individually tailored therapy (*mindfulness-based therapy*).

This chapter will focus on these three dimensions of incorporating mindfulness into the healthcare professions, drawing on recent research to support the efficacy of this approach to improve the quality of care for both therapist and patient. First, the potential of mindfulness to inform clinician self-care will be examined. Next, the role of incorporating mindfulness in the therapeutic context will also be explored, examining potential pathways of a *mindfulness-oriented psychology* (Germer, Fulton, & Siegel, 2005) for enhancing patient care. Finally, we offer future suggestions for implementing mindfulness-based training into clinical program curricula to maximize its benefits for both trainees and their patients.

Mindfulness as a Self-Care Technique

The Problem of Clinician Stress and Burnout

The literature is replete with evidence that the stress inherent in the helping professions has deleterious consequences for professionals and trainees including burnout, substance abuse, decreased quality of life, anxiety, depression, and suicide (Braun et al., 2010; Dyrbye et al., 2008; Fothergill, Edwards, & Burnard, 2004).

Burnout has been characterized by three dimensions: Emotional exhaustion, an indifferent or cynical attitude towards clients (depersonalization), and reduced personal accomplishment (Maslach, Jackson, & Leiter, 1996). Physician burnout has been associated with poorer quality of care, patient dissatisfaction, increased medical errors, lawsuits, and decreased ability to express empathy (Crane, 1998; Haas et al., 2000; Shanafelt, Sloan, & Haberman, 2003; Shanafelt, West, Zhao, et al., 2005). It has been reported that up to 60% of practicing physicians report symptoms of burnout (Shanafelt, Bradley, Wipf, & Back, 2002). As healthcare professionals are constantly drawing on their own resources to relieve the suffering of others, they often fail to adequately tend to their own needs to maintain a sense of meaning and satisfaction in their careers and lives.

Characteristics of one's career such as the type of specialty (mental health) and work setting (rehabilitation centers) have been associated with greater risk of negatively impacting one's well-being (Prins et al., 2010). Stress-related psychological problems are especially found among healthcare providers working with patients who suffer from particular emotional disturbances, such as those who have experienced abuse (Cunningham, 2003) or trauma (Bride, 2007; Collins & Long, 2003), and those with personality disorders (Linehan et al., 2000).

Substance abuse has also revealed itself as a problem among healthcare professionals. The American Psychological Association (APA, 2006) reported that substance abuse was "one of the most researched areas for professional psychologists" (p. 9). Cicala (2003) reports between 8% and 12% of physicians (more than the population in general), will develop a substance abuse problem at some point during their career (Boisaubin & Levine, 2001; Brewster, 1986), and 1 out of every 14 practicing physicians are active substance abusers (Talbott, Gallegos, & Angres, 1998).

The literature reports significant links between healthcare professional stress and increases in depression, emotional exhaustion and anxiety (Gilroy, Carroll, & Murra, 2001, 2002; Radeke & Mahoney, 2000; Tyssen et al., 2001), social distancing and isolation (Baranowski, 2006), disrupted personal relationships (Meyers, 2001), loneliness (Lushington & Luscri, 2001), and reduced self-esteem (Butler & Constantine, 2005).

Research also reports significant effects on physical well-being including decreased physical health including suffering from fatigue, insomnia, heart disease, obesity, hypertension, infection, carcinogenesis, diabetes, and premature aging (Melamed, Shirom, Toker, Berliner, & Shapira, 2006; Melamed, Shirom, Toker, & Shapira, 2006; Spickard, Gabbe, & Christensen, 2002) and decreases in professional effectiveness, specifically citing decreased attention and concentration (Braunstein-Bercovitz, 2003; Mackenzie, Smith, Hashner, Leach, & Behl, 2007; Skosnik, Chatterton, Swisher, & Park, 2000), weakened decision-making and communication skills (Shanafelt, Bradley, Wipf, & Back, 2002), decreased empathy (Beddoe & Murphy, 2004; Thomas et al., 2007), reduced patient trust in healthcare providers (Meier, Back, & Morrisson, 2001), and reduced abilities of the professional to engage in meaningful patient relationships (Enochs & Etzbach, 2004).

The negative effects of stress for healthcare professionals and the quality of care for their patients requires significant attention. Thus, we now turn to self-care interventions to offer alternative means of coping with the myriad of stressors surrounding the effective delivery of health care.

Mindfulness Practice and Self-Care

What is Mindfulness?

According to Shapiro and Carlson (2009), mindfulness can be defined as "the awareness that arises through intentionally attending in an open, kind, and discerning way" (p. 15). Mindfulness can be understood as both an inherent, ever present awareness (mindful awareness), and a series of specific practices designed to enhance mindful attention and awareness (mindful practice). *Mindful awareness* "is fundamentally a way of being – a way of inhabiting one's body, one's mind, one's moment-by-moment experience ... It is a deep awareness; a knowing and experiencing of life as it arises and passes away each moment. (p. 5). This awareness involves an open receptive attention, however it also is a discerning, clear seeing attention, which invites insight (Shapiro & Carlson, 2009). This awareness is characterized by an accepting, nonstriving, caring attention, allowing what is here, as opposed to wanting things to be different.

Mindful practice involves a more formal set of exercises that are designed to train the cultivation of intentionally attending to one's present moment experience with openness, acceptance, and curiosity. Cultivating this type of attention is contrasted with "mindlessness" (Kangas & Shapiro, 2011), or one's engagement in "inner chatter" as described by McCollum and Gehart (2010) often dwelling on past events, preoccupation with thoughts or opinions about what is currently happening, or a focus on what could potentially happen in the future. When engaged in these ways of thinking, we miss the moment that is here before us right now. Mindfulness practice aims to center us back in this moment, allowing a state of "fluid attention" to emerge, rather than focusing on any specific object or sensation (Irving, Dobkin, & Park, 2009). The thoughts, emotions, and body sensations that arise during this practice are accepted as they come, but viewed from a certain distance without allowing oneself to get caught in them and carried away.

Mindfulness as a Health Intervention

A large body of research has explored the many health benefits associated with mindfulness practice. For example, research on mindfulness interventions have demonstrated salutary effects in the areas of smoking cessation (Bowen & Marlatt, 2009), substance use disorders (Dakwar & Levin, 2009), anxiety and mood disorders (Hofmann, Sawyer, Witt, & Oh, 2010), cardiovascular health (Low, Stanton, & Bower, 2008), general pain sensitivity (Perlman, Salomons, Davidson, & Lutz, 2010), and cancer patients (Speca, Carlson, Goodey, & Angen, 2000; Foley et al., 2010) to name a few. More recent research has begun to explore the benefits of mindfulness practice for healthcare professionals and trainees for managing stress and promoting self-care, in addition to the benefits for their patients (see Irving, Dobkin, & Park, 2009; Shapiro & Carlson, 2009 for a review of empirical studies). In a recent study by Gokhan et al. (2010), students in an undergraduate clinical field placement showed enhanced self-care, attention to well-being, self-awareness, empathy, compassion, and increased skills of directing and focusing attention after participating in mindfulness training in relation to a comparison group.

Additionally, numerous studies evaluating the effectiveness of Mindfulness-Based Stress Reduction (MBSR) have found decreased anxiety, depression, rumination and stress, and increased empathy, self-compassion, spirituality, and positive mood states among premedical students, nursing students, and therapists-in-training after completion of the MBSR program (Beddoe & Murphy, 2004; Jain et al., 2007; Shapiro et al., 1998). Research suggests healthcare professionals are also benefitting from MBSR interventions. Healthcare workers in hospital settings have showed reduced stress and emotional exhaustion, and increased mood, quality of life, and self-compassion after 8 weeks of MBSR training (Shapiro & colleagues, 2005; Galantino et al., 2005).

Studies with nurses and doctors have revealed similar findings. Practicing nurses have reported significant improvements in aspects of burnout (personal accomplishment and emotional exhaustion) after MBSR training (Cohen-Katz, Wiley, Capuano, Baker, & Shapiro, 2004, 2005; Cohen-Katz, Wiley, Capuano, Baker, Deitrick, et al., 2005), and primary-care doctors have showed improvements in burnout, depersonalization, empathy, total mood disturbance, consciousness, and emotional stability after an 8-week mindfulness course and a 10-month maintenance phase (2.5 hours/month) (Krasner et al., 2009). These doctors also showed improvements in their attitudes towards patient-centered care. It is because of such data that the proposition to teach mindfulness-based skills in helping profession training programs is supported.

Incorporating Mindfulness into Clinical Training Programs

Despite the growing body of research suggesting the beneficial effects of mindfulness interventions for healthcare professionals, efforts toward explicitly including mindfulness as part of clinical training programs are few. And yet, pioneering programmatic research is beginning to explore the potential benefits. For example, Hassed, de Lisle, Sullivan, and Pier (2009) evaluated the effectiveness of a mindfulness-based Health Enhancement Program (HEP) among 148 first year undergraduate medical students in Australia. Using a pre, post, follow-up design, results revealed a significant effect for time, significant improvements on the depression and hostility scales, in addition to improvements in psychological and physical health. The results of this study also show improvements in student well-being during the pre-exam period, a time typically characterized by a decline in student well-being. This finding optimistically suggests this health decline during the pre-exam period for medical students could potentially be avoidable.

A recent study by Gokhan et al. (2010), found similar results in a population of undergraduate psychology students. The intervention consisted of a 12-week mindfulness-based training as a part of a course while concurrently offering services to individuals with psychiatric and developmental disabilities as a part of an on-site field placement within a hospital setting. Students kept journals to reflect on their physical, behavioral, emotional, and cognitive reactions to their field placement experience. Quantitative and qualitative findings in this study were both consistent with the idea that mindfulness can increase through practice. Trained students showed increased scores on the mindfulness attention and awareness scale in relation to a comparison group that lacked mindfulness training. Students also spoke to qualitative themes of self-care, emotion regulation, self-awareness, compassion, and reference to mindfulness skills in their journals when describing their experience throughout the course and field placement. Statements were made such as, "When F. acted out, I found that concentrating on my breathing helped me to become less anxious" (emotion regulation), or "Even at home, I find I am aware of my listening skills and it has improved my relationship with my sister" (reference to skills). The students also stated that mindfulness-based methods helped them acquire the clinical target skills, including basic proficiencies such as listening, focusing, and reflecting, more efficiently through heightened attention to their personal reactions (p. 462). In addition to self-care, this finding suggests that mindfulness training served to enhance the students' learning, allowing them to develop core skills with greater mastery.

Another recent study by McCollum and Gehart (2010) supports the usefulness of mindfulness meditation in clinical training with pre practicum students in graduate level marriage and family therapy (MFT) programs. Students were taught mindfulness meditation as a component of their coursework, and then recorded very specific information about their experiences (in response to prompts by investigators) in journal entries. One of the significant findings was the way the students described a shift in their *modes of mind*. Segal and colleagues' (2002) make a distinction between the doing mode of mind and the being mode of mind. The doing mode is primarily concerned with planning and resolving discrepancy between our idea of how things should be versus how they actually are. In contrast, the being mode could be described as simply being present with whatever is occurring in the present, without feeling a need to change it. McCollum and Gehart point out that no one mode is better or more "right" than another, though they may vary in appropriateness given time and place. It is important for students to recognize that therapy utilizes both of these modes, whereas the assumption tends to be made that therapy operates almost solely on "doing," with the hope of planning to enact change in one's clients. One of the students' journal entries reflected an account of this shift in modes of mind.

It is astounding to me how sometimes just backing off in the therapy room ... creates new opportunity for movement. It is almost like for some clients, putting energy
in the room becomes an artificial barrier that they have to surmount, in addition to
any other challenges they bring with them. Only when I become still enough to feel
what is in the room am I able to accurately discern whether or not I should use more
or less of my own energy during the session (McCollum & Gehart, 2010, p. 355).

Another student spoke of his increasing awareness of both himself and his client during a therapy session as a result of mindfulness training. This awareness of himself in relation with another illustrates how the therapeutic relationship is brought to life in the midst
of the session.

One of my male clients had just woken up and had "bed head." When he demonstrated shame for looking the way he did, I was able to bring it to light, instead of
simply telling him that I didn't care how he looked. I was able to say, "I'm wondering
if it makes you really uncomfortable to be sitting there, across from me, in a non-per-
fect state." Then I was able to hear his answer without fixing. We were then not only
able to process his difficulty trusting women with who he really is, but our therapeutic
relationship along those lines as well. The conversation flowed and I was not nervous
in bringing so much unspoken truth to light (McCollum & Gehart, 2010, p. 352).

McCollum and Gehart suggest mindfulness practice helped these students develop
qualities of what they term therapeutic presence. They share detailed instances in which
the students described direct applicability of mindfulness training to their lives and work.

The students did not report vague claims of "being less stressed" or "more empathetic" but instead claimed that mindfulness was used in highly stressful client-ther-
apist interactions, moments of extreme personal vulnerability, and situations where
they would typically react otherwise. Their ability to ground their descriptions of the
impact of their mindfulness practice in specific day-to-day experience suggests to us
that they were not simply parroting back generalities learned in class (McCollum &
Gehart, 2010, p. 357).

McCollum and Gehart offer suggestions for the implementation of mindfulness training into graduate program curricula. They suggest the personal practice of the supervisor
to remain consistent and act as a guide to help students. Requiring practice has also been a
request of the students, and it helps them take the concept of self-care more seriously.
However, the frequency and length of time of mindfulness practice needs to be further
explored for maximum effectiveness.

McCollum and Gehart further suggest that the group process is a means of enhancing
student learning, allowing them to share individual experiences with one another
and receive the support and insight of each other. Finally, the authors suggest a "down-
to-earth" style in teaching mindfulness, an awareness of ethical concerns and careful

use of language to avoid students feeling pressured to adhere to a particular religious practice (p. 358).

Another recent study by Christopher and colleagues' (2010) reports on the effectiveness of teaching mindfulness to graduate students in counseling and psychotherapy. Sixteen students previously attending the "Mind/Body Medicine & the Art of Self-Care" as a part of their graduate coursework were interviewed. Interviews were conducted 2 to 6 years after the course to examine the long-term effects of completing this mindfulness-based course. The findings in this study were consistent with previous literature, reporting the benefits of mindfulness training for students, however it is the first study to demonstrate long-term changes as a result of mindfulness training. For example, 13 of the 16 participants reported they still engage in some type of formal mindfulness practice, and the majority of students conveyed the course helped them realize the importance of continuing to practice mindfulness throughout their lives.

The findings of Christopher et al. support the direct applicability of these terms in clinical work and training.

> Within the domain of their professional lives as counselors, the long-term impact of mindfulness training reported by our participants included (a) positive changes in the counselors' experience of themselves while in the role of being a counselor, (b) positive changes in the therapeutic relationship, and (c) changes in the way they practiced clinically (Christopher et al., 2010, p. 22).

Incorporating Mindfulness in Therapy
The Mindful Therapist

The therapeutic relationship has been shown to be the strongest predictor of therapeutic outcomes, with an emphasis on empathy, unconditional positive regard, and congruence between therapist and client (Bohart, Elliott, Greenberg, & Watson, 2002). Given the existence of research on mindfulness and the promotion of these positive qualities and skills of relating to self and others, it is not surprising that mindfulness is becoming viewed as a common factor for successful therapy, regardless of therapists' theoretical orientation (Germer, Fulton, & Siegel, 2005; Martin, 1997; Shapiro & Carlson, 2009).

In theory, the "mindful therapist" enhances the therapeutic relationship and thus improves therapy outcomes by practicing mindfulness in his or her own life. This theory was tested empirically by Grepmair and colleagues' (2007a) through conducting a nonrandomized sequential cohort pilot study comparing the outcomes of 196 patients treated by therapists-in-training. Some of these trainees were practicing Zen meditation, and the researchers determined the clients of these trainees reported better understanding of their own internal processes, difficulties, and goals. They also reported better progress overcoming their problems and symptoms, and developing new adaptive behaviors to use in their daily lives.

Brenner (2009) proposes the use of Zen in training clinical social workers after conducting an exploratory study with 10 Zen practitioners who are also practicing clinical social workers with MSW degrees. Results from these practitioners' semi-structured interviews suggest their work is characterized by a present focus, systemic view of the client in context rather than isolation, lack of discrimination between oneself and his or her client, open mindedness and comfort with not knowing, and a basic sense of confidence. Each of these aspects of practice reflect an overarching awareness which is foundational to the work of the clinician.

Grepmair and colleagues' also conducted a second study (2007b) in which 18 therapists-in-training were randomly assigned to learn Zen meditation in comparison to a control group which lacked this training. One hundred and four patients with mood and anxiety disorders were randomly assigned to work with these therapists in individual and group-therapy sessions. Without knowing which therapists were meditating, the patients rated the quality of the therapy and assessed their overall well-being before and after treatment. Therapeutic processes of "clarification" and "problem solving" were rated higher by patients with meditating therapists, and they reported a better understanding of the structure and characteristics of their problems. They also reported a better understanding of the potential and goals for their development, and greater improvements in symptoms of anxiety, depression, hostility, somatization, and obsessions and compulsions.

Attention and Presence

It's a very old story, told all around the world. A stranger comes to a little community that's been under great stress, where food is scarce, and where people have drawn away from each other and are looking out for themselves. The stranger manages to borrow a cooking pot and starts making soup. He begins with a "magic" ingredient, a stone, maybe a button, or even a nail. The community members become interested in what he's doing, and each secretly comes for a look at the pot. The stranger stirs and tastes. "Ah, it's coming along nicely," he says. "But it would be really wonderful if it had just a little something extra, like a potato, maybe…," he says to one visitor in just the way that she needs to hear it. She goes off inspired to find something to offer. "…like a carrot," he says in his just-right way to another. Later, "…a cabbage," and then "…some beans." And soon there's a shy parade of community folks bringing ingredients and standing around a pot that's now aswim with good things – enough for everyone. They share a meal. There's even a little music. Someone sings; another finds his fiddle; there's dancing into the night. And the stranger has already gone, picking up a new "magic" stone on his way to the next community.

Although this story is usually called "stone soup" or maybe "button borscht," nothing in the story happens because of the "magic" ingredient. It happens because of the stranger's presence – more, his ability to be present to everyone. That is the marvel and mystery attending co-creation. The stranger simply coaxes out what is already in the individuals and community. The stranger does not require much to do his work: a pot, a fire, a stone; faith, knowledge, and caring: faith that the people of the community always have what is needed; knowledge of how the world (meaning people) works; and caring in a way that supports and inspires others.

So, in teaching mindfulness as a professional, you are the stranger. The world ultimately depends on you, on who you are as a person. You enter the little community of participants with nothing, not even a pot. You meet them just as they are, just as you are. Your faith is exposed, as is your knowledge, and your caring, because to teach mindfulness is to practice it, and to practice means to bring all that you are to every moment. And all that you are is all that is needed; the real you really is sufficient" (McCown, Reibel, Micozzi, 2010, p. 91).

This story illustrates the importance of attention and presence as essential skills to therapy. The healing relationship relies on the healthcare professional to simply be present with the patient, as a method of healing in of itself. Cultivating presence within oneself is in contrast with constantly striving to "fix" and "heal" each problem presented by a patient.

The "stranger" in this story may also represent the role of the supervisor as described by McCollum and Gehart (2010). As Kabat-Zinn (1990) says, "The supervisor's personal experience with the challenges of mindfulness and contemplative practices is considered prerequisite to effectively teaching the practice." The most effective way to teach the skill of presence is to embody this way of being oneself. Someone maintaining this presence is able to help and serve others with this quality alone.

Researchers found greater cortical thickening in areas of the brain associated with sustained attention and awareness in practitioners experienced in mindful meditation, compared to nonmeditating participants (Lazar et al., 2005). Additionally, improvements were found in overall attention after novice meditators were trained in mindfulness meditation for 8 weeks, and more experienced meditators participated in a month-long retreat, as measured by response times on the Attention Network Test (ANT; Jha, Krompinger, & Baime, 2007). Mindfulness training has also been shown to enhance control over the distribution of attention to avoid the focus of attention on one stimulus at the expense of ignoring another (see e.g., Slaghter et al., 2007). This skill can be especially useful in attending to an array of information presented by the patient.

The type of attention cultivated through mindfulness practice is important to note and distinguish from attention which is cold and hard, hindering the therapeutic relationship. Attention characterized by acceptance, letting-go, nonattachment, nonstriving, nonjudging, patience, trust, warmth, friendliness, and kindness results from mindfulness practice (Kabat-Zinn, 1990; Segal et al., 2002; Shapiro & Schwartz, 2000). These qualities of attention enhance the therapeutic relationship as the patient feels safe to self-disclose when met with such openness and receptivity from the therapist.

Self-Compassion

Self-compassion is described by Neff (2003a) as a self-orientation with three components: mindful awareness, belief in common humanity, and self-kindness. Compassion incorporates both the ability to empathize with the suffering of oneself or others, and the desire to act upon this empathy to reduce the suffering (Kangas & Shapiro, 2011). Ying (2009) looked at how self-compassion related to competence and mental health in social work students. Sixty-five master's of social work (MSW) students were surveyed, and their self-compassion was measured by Neff's (2003b) six self-compassion subscales. Results showed self-compassion was positively correlated with a sense of coherence (a stable trait associated with mental health), and negatively correlated with depressive symptoms. Implications of this research further support the importance of self-care methods particularly focused on increasing compassion. Mindfulness practice is one way of pursuing its cultivation. Central to mindfulness is learning to let go of self-judgment, and to relate to oneself with compassion and kindness. Through mindfulness meditation, we begin to see that our personal suffering is not unique but part of the universality of being human (Shapiro & Carlson, 2009).

Loving-kindness meditation is a particular mindfulness meditation practice aimed at helping one develop greater self-compassion. (see Kornfield, 2008; Shapiro & Carlson, 2009). As a part of this meditation, participants repeat four or five phrases of well-wishing including "May I be peaceful and happy. May I be healthy." Participants are asked to feel the quality of loving-kindness in the body and heart as they recite these phrases. Love for oneself can be established after continuing to repeat these words. Then this same loving-kindness is extended to others, including family, friends, and eventually difficult people.

The relationship between mindfulness and increased self-compassion is supported by research. Shapiro and colleagues (2005) conducted a randomized controlled study of healthcare professionals working in a Veteran's Hospital. Mindfulness training showed a significant increase in self-compassion compared to pre-training. Another study with counseling psychology graduate students showed that MBSR led to significant improvements in self-compassion pre-to-post intervention, compared to a matched control group (Shapiro, Brown, & Biegel, 2007).

Empathy

Empathy, another vital skill in effective therapy, has also been shown to increase in the individual after mindfulness training. In a study by Lesh (1970), counseling psychology students showed significantly more empathy after a Zen meditation intervention, compared to a waitlist control group. The students' empathy was measured by their ability to accurately determine emotions expressed by a videotaped patient. Medical and pre-medical students also showed increased empathy after an 8-week MBSR intervention, compared to a control group, in a randomized controlled trial by Shapiro and colleagues (1998). Another study with counseling psychology graduate students revealed that 8-weeks of MBSR training significantly increased empathic concern for others pre-to-post intervention (Shapiro et al., 2007). Even further, increases in mindfulness correlated with increases in empathy, suggesting greater mindfulness led to greater empathic concern for others.

Emotional Regulation

Emotional regulation is an extremely important aspect of effective therapy. The therapist must be able to tolerate intense emotions and be comfortable knowing when to contain his or her own emotions and avoid expressing them to patients. The therapeutic relationship is enhanced when the therapist is able to act as a container to hold intense and emotionally charged experiences which may arise in the therapy room.

McCartney (2004) and Shapiro and Carlson (2009) have emphasized the importance of mindfulness training to help practitioners tolerate and hold emotions, and to prevent emotional reactivity to what the patient presents. Mindfulness has also been shown to benefit patients with emotion regulation disorders such as Borderline Personality Disorder and Major Depression (Linehan, 1993a, 1993b; Segal et al., 2002).

Mindfulness-Informed Therapy

Mindfulness-informed therapy refers to integrating mindfulness themes and teachings into psychotherapy, without instructing patients in formal meditation or mindfulness practices (Germer, Fulton, & Siegle, 2006). It offers a framework for integrating wisdom and insights from Buddhist literature, the psychological mindfulness literature, and/or the therapist's personal mindfulness practice into clinical work (Kangas & Shapiro, 2011). To date, there are no explicit instructions or manuals for how to develop a mindfulness-informed health care practice, nor is there research explicating the relationship between mindfulness-informed care and clinical outcomes for patients. However, numerous texts have been written articulating major themes and providing case examples of how insights and teachings of mindfulness can be incorporated into clinical practice (Shapiro & Carlson, 2009, Kornfield, 2008). Such themes include present moment awareness, impermanence, acceptance of what is, no self, essential goodness, and interdependence (see Shapiro and Carlson, 2009, Chapter 3, for further details).

Mindfulness-Based Therapy

Mindfulness-based therapy refers to therapies in which formal mindfulness meditation practices are explicitly taught to clients as part of the therapeutic intervention. In recent decades, treatment approaches have been developed to specifically integrate formal mindfulness practices as a central part of the intervention. These include mindfulness-based stress reduction (MBSR; Kabat-Zinn, 1990), mindfulness-based cognitive therapy (MBCT; Segal, Williams & Teasdale, 2002), dialectical behavior therapy (DBT; Linehan, 1993a, 1993b), and acceptance and commitment therapy (ACT; Hayes, 2005; Hayes, Strosahl, & Wilson, 1999). (See Baer, 2006, for a guide to evidence base and applications of numerous mindfulness-based treatment approaches.)

MBSR is the most widely used mindfulness-based therapy. This 8-week program of up to 35 participants meets weekly for 2.5 to 3 hours. Additionally, a 6-hour silent meditation retreat is incorporated between classes 6 and 7. Through MBSR, participants are taught meditation practices such as body scanning, sitting meditation, and walking meditation. (For details, see Kabat-Zinn, 1990, and Shapiro & Carlson, 2009.) In-class practice is accompanied by a requirement that participants practice meditation and gentle yoga at home for 45 minutes, 6 days per week. Mindfulness attitudes of nonjudging, patience, acceptance, beginner's mind, non-striving, letting go, nonattachment, and trust are interwoven throughout the course. A number of controlled studies highlight the efficacy of MBSR with clinical populations. Many studies have used MBSR interventions with patients suffering from chronic pain and illness such as cancer, depression, and generalized anxiety. Other studies have looked at the impact of mindfulness-based therapies on healthy populations to minimize stress and enhance well-being. (See Shapiro and Carlson, 2009, for an overview of these studies.)

MBCT was developed by John Teasdale, Mark Williams, and Zindel Segal, who are experts on treating depression using cognitive behavioral therapy (CBT; Segal, Williams & Teasdale, 2002). MBCT integrates CBT and MBSR, and is especially helpful in avoiding relapse in those who are recovering from depression. The treatment is conducted over 8 weeks, and works with a group of up to 12 participants. Like MBSR, MBCT utilizes the body scan, sitting meditation, walking meditation and informal daily mindfulness practices. However, loving kindness meditation is not included in the course, and there is more focus on understanding depression than the stress response, as in MBSR. It also includes a "3-minute breathing space" technique as well as other elements of cognitive therapy. (See Segal, Williams, & Teasdale, 2002, and Shapiro & Carlson, 2009, for more detailed discussions of these techniques.) Two randomized clinical trials provide strong empirical support for the efficacy of MBCT for the treatment of depression relapse (Teasdale et. al., 2000; Ma & Teasdale, 2004). Smaller research studies have also shown MBCT's effectiveness in treating people with bipolar disorder and unipolar MDD (Williams et al., 2008) and generalized anxiety disorder (Evans, 2008).

Other applications of MBCT are also being investigated. Some of these therapies include mindfulness-based eating awareness training (Kristeller, Bear, & Quillian-Wolever, 2006), mindfulness-based relapse prevention (Marlatt & Gordon, 1985; Marlatt & Witkiewitz, 2005), mindfulness-based relationship enhancement (Carson, Carson, Gil, & Baucom, 2006), and mindfulness-based art therapy (Monti et. al. 2005). (See Shapiro and Carlson, 2009, for a review of existing research on these therapies.)

Future Directions and Conclusion

Mindfulness has a variety of useful applications for healthcare providers including personal care, professional effectiveness, and specific therapeutic interventions. Numerous future directions and research paths merit attention in how to effectively integrate mindfulness into the healthcare profession. Below we discuss directions, focusing on each of the three avenues outlined previously: The mindful therapist, mindfulness-informed therapy, and mindfulness-based therapy.

One important research avenue that merits continued investigation is the extent to which training in mindfulness can help health professionals develop core clinical skills such as attention, presence, empathy and self-compassion. The next step will be to determine if training in mindfulness for the *clinician* results in clinically meaningful outcomes for the *patient*, as preliminarily supported by Grepmair and colleagues (2007).

Toward this end, research across a broad range of measures including patient self-report, behavioral observation, and clinician rating scales (Grepmair, Mitterlehner, Loew, Bachler, et al., 2007; Grepair, Mitterlehner, Loew, & Nickel, 2007) is needed. Finally, it will be important to investigate the mechanisms through which beneficial effects occur.

Another avenue of future research is to empirically test the effectiveness of mindfulness-informed therapy. Apart from clinical anecdotes, we know little of how mindfulness-informed therapy benefits patients. Studies investigating the outcomes associated with mindfulness-informed therapy are needed. In addition, more theory and guidance can be developed regarding how treatment providers can use ideas and teachings from Buddhism and other mindfulness literature to inform their clinical work.

Third, mindfulness-based therapy will require continued investigation, particularly studies which empirically validate newly developed mindfulness-based interventions. In addition, the continued integration of mindfulness into previously existing treatments for specific disorders, to enhance and expand the interventions is encouraged.

Finally, the potential of mindfulness as a means of teaching self-care to healthcare professionals seems an especially important avenue for future research, both in terms of protecting practitioners' own health and well-being, and for optimizing patient outcomes. Controlled clinical trials, which include long-term follow up of the effects of mindfulness training in educational programs, and in continuing education programs for professionals, is needed. This includes directing attention towards the integration of mindfulness training into higher education curricula (Shapiro & Carlson, 2009). The benefits of incorporating this practice into such programs could be far-reaching, when we become comfortable with our psyches, we become better able to explore our patients' inner worlds (Shapiro & Carlson, 2009).

Mindfulness has tremendous implications for healthcare professionals in terms of clinical effectiveness and self-care. Continued research and exploration will benefit healthcare professionals, and those whose lives they touch. We believe that cultivating mindfulness – the ability to intentionally attend in an open, caring and discerning way – is an essential ingredient to the health and healing of both professionals and patients alike.

References

American Psychological Association (2006, February 10). *Advancing colleague assistance in professional psychology.* Retrieved July 30, 2010, from http://www.apa.org/practice/acca_monograph. html.

Baer, R. A. (Ed.) (2006). *Mindfulness-based treatment approaches: Clinician's guide to evidence base and applications.* San Diego: Elsevier.

Baranowski, K. P. (2006). *Stress in pediatric palliative and hospice care: Causes, effects, and coping* strategies. NHPCO (National Hospice and Palliative Care Organization). Children's Project on Palliative/Hospice Services (CHIPPS). CHIPPS Newsletter, March 2006.

Beddoe, A. E., & Murphy, S. O. (2004). Does mindfulness decrease stress and foster empathy among nursing students? *Journal of Nursing Education, 43*, 305–312.

Bien, T. (2006). *Mindful therapy: Guide for therapists and helping professionals.* Boston: Wisdom Publications.

Bohart, A. C., Elliott, R., Greenberg, L. S., & Watson, J. C. (2002). Empathy. In J. C. Norcross (Ed.), *Psychotherapy relationships that work: Therapist contributions and responsiveness to patients* (pp. 89–108). New York: Oxford University Press.

Boisaubin, E. V., & Levine, R. E. (2001). Identifying and assisting the impaired physician. *American Journal of Medical Science, 322*, 31–36.

Bowen, S., & Marlatt, A. (2009). Surfing the urge: Brief mindfulness-based intervention for college student smokers. *Psychology of Addictive Behaviors, 23*, 666–671.

Braun, M., Schonfeldt-Lecuona, C., Freudenmann, R. W., Mehta, T., Hay, B., Kachele, H., & Beschoner, P. (2010). Depression, burnout and effort-reward imbalance among psychiatrists. *Psychotherapy and Psychosomatics, 79*, 326–327.

Braunstein-Bercovitz, H. (2003). Does stress enhance or impair selective attention? The effects of stress and perceptual load on negative priming. *Anxiety, Stress and Coping, 16*, 345–357.

Brenner, M. J. (2009). Zen practice: A training method to enhance the skills of clinical social workers. *Social Work in Health Care, 48*, 462–470.

Brewster, J. M. (1986). Prevalence of alcohol and other drug problems among physicians. *Journal of the American Medical Association, 255*, 1913–1920.

Bride, B. E. (2007). Prevalence of secondary traumatic stress among social workers. *Social Work, 52*, 63–70.

Butler, S. K., & Constantine, M. G. (2005). Collective self-esteem and burnout in professional school counselors. *Professional School Counseling, 9*, 55–62.

Carlson, L. E., Ursuliak, Z., Goodey, E., Angen, M., & Speca, M. (2004). The effects of a mindfulness meditation-based stress reduction program on mood and symptoms of stress in cancer outpatients: 6-month follow-up. *Supportive Care in Cancer, 9*, 112–123.

Carson, J. W., Carson, K. M., Gil, K. M., & Baucom, D. H. (2006). Mindfulness-based relationship enhancement. *Behavior Therapy, 35*, 471–494.

Chiesa, A., & Serretti, A. (2009). Mindfulness-based stress reduction for stress management in healthy people: A review and meta-analysis. *The Journal of Alternative and Complementary Medicine, 15*, 593–600.

Christopher, J. C., Chrisman, J. A., Trotter-Mathison, M. J., Shure, M. B., Dahlen, P., & Christopher, S. B. (2010). Perceptions of the long-term influence of mindfulness training on counselors and psychotherapists: A qualitative inquiry. *Journal of Humanistic Psychology, 20*, 1–32.

Cicala, R. S. (2003). Substance abuse among physicians: What you need to know. *Hospital Physician, 39*, 39–46.

Cohen-Katz, J., Wiley, S., Capuano, T., Baker, D. M., Deitrick, L., & Shapiro, S. (2005). The effects of mindfulness-based stress reduction on nurse stress and burnout: A qualitative and quantitative study, part III. *Holistic Nursing Practice, 19*, 78–86.

Cohen-Katz, J., Wiley, S., Capuano, T., Baker, D. M., & Shapiro, S. (2004). The effects of mindfulness-based stress reduction on nurse stress and burnout: A qualitative and quantitative study. *Holistic Nursing Practice, 18*, 302–308.

Cohen-Katz, J., Wiley, S., Capuano, T., Baker, D. M., & Shapiro, S. (2005). The effects of mindfulness-based stress reduction on nurse stress and burnout: A quantitative and qualitative study. *Holistic Nursing Practice, 18*, 302–308.

Collins, S., & Long, A. (2003). Working with the psychological effects of trauma: Consequences for mental health-care workers: A literature review. *Journal of Psychiatric and Mental Health Nursing, 10*, 417–424.

Crane, M. (1998). Why burned-out doctors get sued more often. *Medical Economics, 75*, 210–212, 215–218.

Cunningham, M. (2003). Impact of trauma work on social work clinicians: Empirical findings. *Social Work, 48*, 451–459.

Dakwar, E., & Levin, F. R. (2009). The emerging role of meditation in addressing psychiatric illness, with a focus on substance use disorders. *Harvard Review of Psychiatry, 17*, 254-267.

Di Pellegrino, G., Fadiga, L., Fogassi, L., Gallese, V., & Rizzolatti, G. (1992). Understanding motor events: A neurophysical study. *Experimental Brain Research, 91*, 176-180.

Dobkin, P. L., & Hutchinson, T. A. (2009). Primary prevention for future doctors: Promoting well-being in trainees. *Journal of Medical Education, 44*, 224–226.

Dyrbye L. N., Thomas M. R., Massie F. S., Power, D. V., Eacker, A., Harper, W., . . . Shanafelt, T. D. (2008). Burnout and Suicidal Ideation among US Medical Students. *Annals of Internal Medicine, 149*, 334–341.

Enochs, W. K., & Etzbach, C. A. (2004). Impaired student counselors: Ethical and legal considerations for the family. *The Family Journal, 12*, 396–400.

Evans, S., Ferrando, S., Fidler, M., Stowell, C., Smart, C., & Haglin, D. (2008). Mindfulness-based cognitive therapy for generalized anxiety disorder. *Journal of Anxiety Disorders, 22*, 716–721.

Foley, E., Baillie, A., Huxter, M., Price, M., & Sinclair, E. (2010). Mindfulness-based cognitive therapy for individuals whose lives have been affected by cancer: A randomized control trial. *Journal of Consulting and Clinical Psychology, 78*, 72–79.

Fothergill, A., Edwards, D., & Burnard, P. (2004). Stress, burnout, coping and stress management in psychiatrists: Findings from a systematic review. *International Journal of Social Psychiatry, 50*, 54–65.

Galantino, M. L., Baime, M., Maguire, M. Szapary, P. O., & Farrar, J. T. (2005). Short-communication: association of psychological and physiological measures of stress in health-care professionals during and 8-week mindfulness meditation program: Mindfulness in practice. *Stress and Health, 21*, 255–261.

Germer, C. K., Siegel, R. D., & Fulton, P. R. (2005). *Mindfulness and psychotherapy.* New York: Guilford Press.

Gilroy, P. J., Carroll, L., & Murra, J. (2002). A preliminary survey of counseling psychologists' personal experiences with depression and treatment. *Professional Psychology: Research and Practice, 33*, 402–407.

Gokhan, N., Meehan, E. F., & Peters, K. (2010). The value of mindfulness-based methods in teaching at a clinical field placement. *Psychological Reports, 106*, 455–466.

Goldenberg, D. L., Kaplan, K. H., Nadeau, M. G., Brodeur C., Smith S., & Schmid H. C. (1994). A controlled study of a stress-reduction, cognitive-behavioral treatment program in fibromyalgia. *Journal of Musculoskeletal Pain, 2*, 53–66.

Goldstein, J. (1993). *Insight meditation: The practice of freedom.* Boston: Shambhala.

Goodman, T. A., & Greenland, S. K. (2008). Mindfulness with children: Working with difficult emotions. In F. Didonna (Ed.), *Clinical handbook of mindfulness* (pp. 417–430). New York: Springer.

Grepmair, L., Mitterlehner, F., Loew, T., Bachler, E., Rother, W., & Nickel, M. (2007). Promoting mindfulness in psychotherapists in training influences the treatment results of their patients: A randomized, double-blind, controlled study. *Psychotherapy and Psychosomatics, 76*, 332–338.

Grepmair, L., Mitterlehner, F., Loew, T., & Nickel, M. (2007). Promotion of mindfulness in psychotherapists in training: Preliminary study. *European Psychiatry, 22*, 485–489.

Haas, J. S., Cook, E. F., Puopolo, A. L., Burstin, H. R., Cleary, P. D., & Brennan, T. A. (2000). Is the professional satisfaction of general internists associated with patient satisfaction? *Journal of General Internal Medicine, 15*, 140–141.

Hassed, C., de Lisle, S., Sullivan, G., & Pier, C. (2009). Enhancing the health of medical students: outcomes of an integrated mindfulness and lifestyle program. *Advances in Health Sciences Education: Theory and Practice, 14*, 387–398.

Hayes, S. C. (2005, July 2). *Training*. Retrieved February 10, 2009, from Association for Contextual Behavioral Science website: http://www.contextualpsychology.org/act_training.

Hayes, S. C., Strosahl, K., & Wilson, K. G. (1999). *Acceptance and commitment therapy*. New York: Guilford Press.

Hofmann, S. G., Sawyer, A. T., Witt, A. A., & Oh, D. (2010). The effect of mindfulness-based therapy on anxiety and depression: A meta analytic review. *Journal of Consulting and Clinical Psychology, 78*, 169–183.

Irving, J. A., Dobkin, P. L., & Park, J. (2009). Cultivating mindfulness in health care professionals: A review of empirical studies of mindfulness-based stress reduction. *Complementary Therapies in Clinical Practice, 15*, 61–66.

Jain, S., Shapiro, S. L., Swanick, S. Roesch, S. C., Mills, P. J., Bell, I., & Schwartz, G. (2007). A randomized control trial of mindfulness meditation versus relaxation training: Effects on distress, positive states of mind, rumination, and distraction. *Annals of Behavioral Medicine, 33*, 11–21.

Jha, A. P., Krompinger, J., & Baime, M. J. (2007). Mindfulness training modifies subsystems of attention. *Cognitive, Affective & Behavioral Neuroscience, 7*, 109–119.

Kabat-Zinn, J. (1990). *Full catastrophe living: Using the wisdom of your body and mind to face stress, pain and illness*. New York: Delacourt.

Kabat-Zinn, J., Wheeler, E., Light, T., Skillings, A., Scharf, M. S., Cropley, T. G., ... Bernhard, J. D. (1998). Influence of a mindfulness meditation-based stress reduction intervention on rates of skin clearing in patients with moderate to severe psoriasis undergoing phototherapy (UVB) and photochemotherapy (PUVA). *Psychosomatic Medicine, 60*, 625–632.

Kangas, N. L., & Shapiro, S. L., (2011). Mindfulness-based training for health care professionals. In McCracken, L. M. (Ed.), *Mindfulness and Acceptance in Behavioral Medicine* (pp. 303–340). Oakland: New Harbinger Publications.

Kaplan, K. H., Goldenberg, D. L., & Galvin, N. M. (1993). The impact of a meditation-based stress reduction program on fibromyalgia. *General Hospital Psychiatry, 15*, 284–289.

Kornfield, J. (2008). *The wise heart: A guide to the universal teachings of Buddhist psychology*. New York: Bantam Books.

Krasner, M. S. , Epstein, R. M., Beckman, H., Suchman, A. L., Chapman, B., Mooney, C. J., & Quille, T. E. (2009). Association of an educational program in mindful communication with burnout, empathy, and attitudes among primary care physicians. *The Journal of the American Medical Association, 302*, 1284–1293.

Kristeller, J. L., Baer, R. A., & Quillian-Wolever, R. (2006). Mindfulness-based approaches to eating disorders. In R. A. Baer (Ed.), *Mindfulness-based treatment approaches: Clinician's guide to evidence base and applications* (pp. 75–91). London: Academic Press.

Lazar, S. W., Kerr, C. E., Wasserman, R. H., Gray, J. R., Greve, D. N., Treadway, M. T., ... Fischl, B. (2005). Meditation experience is associated with increased cortical thickness. *Neuroreport, 16*, 1893–1897.

Lesh, T. V. (1970). Zen meditation and the development of empathy in counselors. *Journal of Humanistic Psychology, 10*, 39–74.

Linehan, M. M. (1993a). *Cognitive-behavioral treatment of borderline personality disorder*. New York: Guilford Press.

Linehan, M. M. (1993b). *Skills training manual for treating borderline personality disorder*. New York: Guilford Press.

Linehan, M. M., Cochran, B. N., Mar, C. M. Levensky, E. R., & Comtois, K. A. (2000). Therapeutic burnout among borderline personality disordered clients and their therapists: Development and evaluation of two adaptations of the Maslach Burnout Inventory. *Cognitive and Behavioral Practice, 7,* 329–337.

Low, C. A., Stanton, A. L., & Bower, J. E. (2008). Effects of acceptance-oriented versus evaluative emotional processing on heart rate recovery and habituation. *Emotion, 8,* 419–424.

Lushington, K., & Luscri, G. (2001). Are counseling students stressed? A cross-cultural comparison of burnout in Australian, Singaporean and Hong Kong counseling students. *Asian Journal of Counseling, 8,* 209–232.

Ma, S. H., & Teasdale, J. D. (2004). Mindfulness-based cognitive therapy for depression: Replication and exploration of differential relapse prevention effects. *Journal of Consulting and Clinical Psychology, 72,* 31–40.

Mackenzie, C. S., Smith, M. C., Hasher, L. Leach, L., & Behl, P. (2007). Cognitive functioning under stress: Evidence from informal caregivers of palliative patients. *Journal of Palliative Medicine, 10,* 749–758.

Marlatt, G. A., & Gordon, J. R. (Eds.). (1985). *Relapse prevention: maintenance strategies in the treatment of addictive behaviors.* New York: Guilford Press.

Marlatt, G. A., & Witkiewitz, K. (2005). Relapse prevention for alcohol and drug problems. In G. A. Marlatt & D. M. Donovan (Eds.), *Relapse prevention* (pp. 1–44). New York: Guilford Press.

Martin, J. R. (1997). Mindfulness: A proposed common factor. *Journal of Psychotherapy Integration, 7,* 291–312.

Maslach, C., Jackson, S. E., & Leiter, M. P. (1996). *Maslach Burnout Inventory Manual.* Palo Alto: Consulting Psychologists Press.

McCartney, L. (2004). *Counsellors' perspectives on how mindfulness meditation influences counsellor presence within the therapeutic relationship.* Unpublished Master's thesis, University of Victoria, British Columbia, Canada.

McCollum, E. E., & Gehart, D. R. (2010). Mindfulness meditation to teach beginning therapists therapeutic presence: A qualitative study. *Journal of Marital and Family Therapy, 36,* 347–360.

McCown, D., Reibel, D. C. & Micozzi, M. S. (2010). *Teaching mindfulness: A practical guide for clinicians and educators.* New York: Springer.

Meier, D. E., Back, A., & Morrison, S. (2001). The inner life of physicians and the care of the seriously ill. *The Journal of the American Medical Association, 286,* 3007–3014.

Melamed, S., Shirom, A., Toker, S. Berliner, S., & Shapira, I. (2006). Burnout and risk of cardiovascular disease: Evidence, possible causal paths, and promising research directions. *Psychological Bulletin, 32,* 327–353.

Melamed, S., Shirom, A., Toker, S., & Shapira, I. (2006). Burnout and risk of type 2 diabetes: A prospective study of apparently healthy employed persons. *Psychosomatic Medicine, 68,* 863–869.

Meyers, M. F. (2001). The well-being of physician relationships. *Western Journal of Medicine, 174,* 30–33.

Monti, D. A., Peterson, C., Kunkel, E. J., Hauck, W. W., Pequignot, E., Rhodes, L., & Brainard, G. C. (2005). A randomized, controlled trial of mindfulness-based art therapy (MBAT) for women with cancer. *Psycho-Oncology, 15,* 363–373.

Neff, K. D. (2003a). Self-Compassion: An alternative conceptualization of a healthy attitude toward oneself. *Self and Identity, 2,* 85–101.

Perlman, D. M., Salomons, T. V., Davidson, R. J., & Lutz, A. (2010). Differential effects on pain intensity and unpleasantness of two meditation practices. *Emotion, 10,* 65–71.

Prins, J. T., Hoekstra-Weebers, J. E. H. M., Gazendam-Donofrio, S. M., Dillingh, G. S., Bakker. A. B., Huisman. M., Jacobs, B., & van der Heijden, F. M. M. A. (2010). Burnout and engagement among resident doctors in the Netherlands: A national study. *Medical Education, 44,* 236–247.

Radeke, J. T., & Mahoney, M. J. (2000). Comparing the personal lives of psychotherapists and research psychologists. *Professional Psychology: Research and Practice, 31,* 82–84.

Randolph, P. D., Caldera, Y. M., Tacone, A. M., & Greak, M. L. (1999). The long-term combined effects of medical treatment and a mindfulness-based behavioral program for the multidisciplinary management of chronic pain in West Texas. *Pain Digest, 9*, 103–112.

Segal, Z. V., Williams, M. G., & Teasdale, J. D. (2002). *Mindfulness-based cognitive therapy for depression: A new approach to preventing relapse.* New York: Guilford Press.

Shanafelt, T. D., Bradley, K. A., Wipf, J. E., & Back, A. L. (2002). Burnout and self-reported patient care in an internal medicine residency program. *Annals of Internal Medicine, 136*, 358–367.

Shanafelt, T. D., Sloan, J. A., & Haberman, T. M. (2003). The well being of physicians. *American Medical Journal, 114*, 513–517.

Shanafelt, T. D., West, C., Zhao, X., Novotny, P., Kolars, J., Habermann, T., & Sloan, J. (2005). Relationship between increased personal well-being and enhanced empathy among internal medicine residents. *Journal of General Internal Medicine, 20*, 559–564.

Shapiro, S. L., Astin, J. A., Bishop, S. R., & Cordova, M. (2005). Mindfulness-based stress reduction for health care professionals: Results from a randomized trial. *International Journal of Stress Management, 12*, 164–176.

Shapiro, S. L., Brown, K. W., & Biegel, G. M. (2007). Teaching self-care to caregivers: Effects of mindfulness-based stress reduction on the mental health of therapists in training. *Training and Education in Professional Psychology, 1*, 105–115.

Shapiro, S. L., & Carlson, L. E. (2009). *The art and science of mindfulness: Integrating mindfulness into psychology and the helping professions.* Washington, DC: American Psychological Association.

Shapiro, S. L., & Izette, C. (2008). Meditation: A universal tool for cultivating empathy. In D. Hick & T. Bien (Eds.), *Mindfulness and the therapeutic relationship* (pp. 161–175). New York: Guilford Press.

Shapiro, S. L., & Schwartz, G. E. (2000). Intentional systemic mindfulness: An integrative model for self-regulation and health. *Advances in Mind-Body Medicine, 16*, 128–134.

Shapiro, S. L., Schwartz, G. E., & Bonner, G. (1998). Effects of mindfulness-based stress reduction on medical and pre-medical students. *Journal of Behavioral Medicine, 21*, 581–599.

Skosnik, P. D., Chatterton, R. T., Swisher, T., & Park, S. (2000). Modulation of attentional inhibition by norepinephrine and cortisol after psychological stress. *International Journal of Psychophysiology, 36*, 59–68.

Slaghter, H. A., Lutz, A., Greischar, L. L., Francis, A. D., Nieuwenhuis, S., Davis, J. M., & Davidson, R. J. (2007). Mental training affects distribution of limited brain resources. *PLoS Biology, 5*, e138.

Speca, M. Carlson, L. E., Goodey, E., & Angen, M. (2000). A randomized, wait-list controlled clinical trial: The effect of a mindfulness meditation-based stress reduction program on mood and symptoms in cancer outpatients. *Psychosomatic Medicine, 62*, 613–622.

Spickard, A., Gabbe, S. G., & Christensen, J. F. (2002). Mid-career burnout in generalist and specialist physicians. *Journal of the American Medical Association, 288*, 1447–1450.

Talbott, G., Gallegos, K., & Angres, D. (1998). Impairment and recovery in physicians and other health professionals: Alcohol and drug use in the workplace. *Principles of Addiction Medicine*, 1263–1279.

Teasdale, J. D., Segal, Z. V., Williams, J. M., Ridgeway, V. A., Soulsby, J. M., & Lau, M. A. (2000). Prevention of relapse/recurrence in major depression by mindfulness-based cognitive therapy. *Journal of Consulting and Clinical Psychology, 68*, 615–623.

Thomas, M. R., Dyrbye, L. N., Huntington, J. L., Lawson, K. L., Novotny, P. J., Sloan, J. A., & Shanafelt, T. D. (2007). How do distress and well-being relate to medical student empathy? A multicenter study. *Journal of General Internal Medicine, 22*, 1525–1497.

Tyssen, R., Vaglum, P., Gronvold, N. T., & Ekeberg, O. (2001). Suicidal ideation among medical students and young physicians: A nationwide and prospective study of prevalence and predictors. *Journal of Affective Disorders, 64*, 69–79.

Williams, J. M., Alatiq, Y., Crane, C., Barnhofer, T., Fennell, M. J., Duggan, D. S., . . . Goodwin, M. (2008). Mindfulness-based cognitive therapy (MBCT) in bipolar disorder: Preliminary evaluation of immediate effects on between-episode functioning. *Journal of Affective Disorders, 107*, 275–279.

Williams, J. M. G., Teasdale, J. D., Segal, Z., & Soulsby, J. (2000). Mindfulness-based cognitive therapy reduces over general autobiographical memory in formerly depressed patients. *Journal of Abnormal Psychology, 109*, 150–155.

Ying, Y. (2009). Contribution of self-compassion to competence and mental health in social work students. *Journal of Social Work Education, 45*, 2, 309–321.

Medical Health Care

Cognitive Psychologists' Contribution

Michael W. Eysenck

Roehampton University, Royal Holloway University of London, UK

When we consider effective ways of treating disease and chronic health conditions, the enormous contribution made by doctors and surgeons is obvious. However, the central thesis of this chapter is that cognitive factors are also very important, and that medical health care can benefit substantially when it takes account of relevant cognitive processes.

Some of the earliest psychological research on human cognition focused on individual differences in intelligence, with those having high IQs possessing superior cognitive skills to those with low IQs. As we will see, intelligence is important in predicting the ability to make maximal use of health care.

Intelligence and Cognition

There are various types of intelligence. One is fluid intelligence, which involves a rapid understanding of novel relationships. There is also crystallized intelligence, which depends on knowledge and expertise. Unsworth (2010) found that working memory capacity (involving the ability to process and store information concurrently) was strongly related to fluid intelligence. Unsworth and Spillers (2010) put forward a dual-component model of working memory capacity: Attentional control was one component and long-term memory was the other. Long-term memory is important because measures of working memory capacity involve the retrieval of information from long-term memory. As predicted, individuals high in working memory capacity have superior long-term memory to those of low capacity (e.g., Unsworth, Spillers, & Brewer, 2010).

Unsworth and Spillers (2010) obtained several measures of attentional control, long-term memory, and fluid intelligence. What did they find? Attentional control and long-term memory were both moderately strongly associated with working memory capacity, with the contribution of long-term memory being somewhat greater. In addition, individual differences in fluid intelligence were associated with attentional control, long-term memory, and working memory capacity.

Health Literacy

What links together intelligence, working memory capacity, and health is health literacy – the ability to read and make sense of information about healthcare, and then to use that information to make appropriate decisions. Not surprisingly, levels of health literacy are greater among highly intelligent and well-educated individuals than those who are less intelligent and poorly educated (Gottfredson & Deary, 2004). For example, Australians who left school by the age of 15 are 8 times more likely than well-educated ones to have inadequate health literacy (Adams et al., 2009).

Evidence that health literacy is strongly related to cognitive ability was reported by Levinthal, Morrow, Tu, Wu, and Murray (2008). They found that cognitive ability in terms of working memory and processing accounted for 24% of the variance in health literacy scores.

Individual differences in health literacy partially determine hospitalized patients' level of satisfaction patients with the quality of communication they experienced with physicians (Kripalani et al., 2010). Patients low in health literacy gave significantly lower ratings than those high in health literacy to general clarity, explanation of care processes, and responsiveness to patient concerns. These findings suggest that communication difficulties impair the medical health care received by patients having low health literacy.

Does health literacy matter in terms of health outcomes? It is easy to imagine that most of the information provided by doctors and others involved in medical health care is simple and easy to use, so that nearly everyone has adequate health literacy for most purposes. In fact, that is simply not the case. In the early 1990s, it was estimated that a total of 1.8 billion prescriptions were handed out in the United States every year. Of those receiving prescriptions, about 30–50% failed to take their medicine properly, causing the deaths of approximately 125,000 Americans each year. When all hospital admissions for those over the age of 65 are considered, almost 30% of them are due to medication non-adherence.

It is important to note that the limited cognitive abilities and poor health literacy of millions of individuals mean that they have great difficulty in adhering to even apparently very simple medical instructions. For example, Williams et al. (1995) found that 65% of those deemed to have "inadequate health literacy" didn't understand the instructions for taking medicine on an empty stomach! In addition, 40% could not work out from an appointment slip when their next appointment was due. The respective figures for those with adequate health literacy were 24% and 5%. In another study (Deary et al., 2009), individuals at risk of developing peripheral vascular disease were investigated. Those at risk were instructed to take medication consisting of 100 mg of aspirin every day. Even though it was extremely easy to comply with this request, those with the lowest IQs were 2½ times more likely than those with the highest IQs to stop taking the medication within 2 years.

More dramatic evidence of the importance of health literacy comes from research on diabetic patients taking insulin daily (Williams, Baker, Parker, & Nurss, 1998). Almost unbelievably, 50% of those with inadequate health literacy did not know that feeling sweaty, shaky, and nervous strongly suggested their blood glucose level was too low.

Of these same patients, 62% did not know they should respond to that situation by eating some form of sugar.

In view of the evidence considered so far, it is unsurprising that health literacy is an important factor in determining longevity. Batty et al. (2009) conducted a large-scale study on one million Swedish men. Each 15-point decrease in IQ (strongly correlated with health literacy) was associated with a 32% increase in mortality by middle age.

Everyone can be regarded as a manager of his/her own health. That task is becoming progressively more complex. As a consequence of the ready availability of the Internet, most people have far more access than at any time in human history to information about the meanings of symptoms, how to diagnose disease, and so on. There has been a dramatic increase in the range of treatments available for many diseases, which means it is more time consuming than before to work out what to do for the best. The increasing complexity of health issues may help to explain why the gap in mortality rate is increasing between those belonging to the higher and lower social classes (Gottfredson & Deary, 2004).

Cognitive Factors in Poor Health Literacy

So far as health literacy is concerned, individuals with inadequate health literacy tend to have relatively low IQs and so are limited in their cognitive and intellectual functioning. It is worth considering the issue of health literacy in a broader context. As Shaw, Huebner, Armin, Orzech, and Vivian (2009) pointed out, poor communication between patients and doctors and poor compliance by patients can be due to factors such as socio-economic status and culture that are only partially related to health literacy.

How can patients with low health literacy be helped to ensure that they derive maximal benefit from health care? Shaw et al. (2009) pointed out that the American Medical Association has started to address this problem in a serious fashion, but only relatively modest progress has been achieved to date. One promising approach would be to start by identifying the main differences between individuals high and low in health literacy. Wister, Malloy-Weir, Rootman, & Desjardins (2010) did precisely this in a study on older adults. Individuals with high health literacy had a higher educational level, and devoted more time to self-study (e.g., of books and journals), to the Internet, to leisure reading of books, and made more use of libraries. Thus, individuals low in health literacy spend far less time than those high in health literacy engaged in developing language skills related to reading comprehension.

We can relate the findings of Wister et al. (2010) to those of cognitive psychologists who have studied language comprehension in individuals high and low in working memory capacity. Given that individuals low in working memory capacity tend to have poor health literacy, it is reasonable to predict that they will have poor language comprehension. This finding was reported by Daneman and Merikle (1996) in a meta-analysis of 77 studies.

It could be concluded on the basis of studies such as that of Wister et al. (2010) that the optimal way of enhancing health outcomes for patients low in health literacy is to provide health information in a simpler, more readable, fashion. Wilson and Wolf (2009) argued that two kinds of factors determine the cognitive demands imposed by health-related text. First, there are intrinsic factors (e.g., the conceptual complexity of the material). Second, there are extrinsic factors (e.g., format, word choice, use of white space). Wilson and Wolf identify several ways in which comprehension for health-related text can be improved for patients low in health literacy.

There is some validity in the notion that simplifying health-related communications will benefit individuals low in health literacy. However, it represents a gross oversimplification because individuals low in health literacy have a range of cognitive limitations in addition to impaired language comprehension. As was discussed earlier, individuals low in working memory capacity (a dimension of individual differences related to health literacy) have poor attentional control and impaired long-term memory (Unsworth & Spillers, 2010). Waldrop-Valverde, Jones, Gould, Kumar, and Ownby (2010) studied cognitive processes in patients who were HIV-positive. Those who were low in health literacy exhibited poorer executive skills, verbal memory, and planning than those who possessed high health literacy.

In sum, research suggests that there are several reasons why patients having low health literacy have substantially poorer health outcomes than those with high health literacy. That means that interventions designed to enhance health outcomes in patients with deficient health literacy should be multifaceted. More specifically, such interventions need to incorporate components focusing on attentional control, executive functioning, planning, long-term memory, and language comprehension.

Emotion Regulation

Patients suffering from a very wide range of diseases and health problems experience greater negative affect (e.g., anxiety, depression, anger) than healthy individuals. Cognitive psychologists and cognitive neuroscientists have made progress in the past few years in identifying some of the most successful strategies for emotion regulation, in which deliberate processes are used to "override people's spontaneous emotional responses" (Koole, 2009, p. 6). Emotion-regulation strategies can be used by patients with physical illnesses to enhance their psychological well-being.

Gross and Thompson (2007) put forward a process model that provides a reasonably comprehensive basis for categorizing emotion-regulation strategies. According to this model, different emotion-regulation strategies can be used at various points in time. More specifically, five types of strategies were identified. First, there are strategies involving situation selection. Patients can select situations most likely to trigger positive emotions and try to avoid those situations (perhaps those associated with their health problems) that activate negative emotional states. Second, there are strategies involving situation modification. Third, there are strategies involving attention deployment, for example, having pleasant distracting thoughts when experiencing pain from an injury. Fourth, there are emotion-regulation strategies involving cognitive change (e.g., interpreting one's symptoms in a less negative fashion). Fifth, there are strategies involving response modulation.

All five categories of emotion-regulation strategies can reduce negative emotional states (see Koole, 2009, for a review). However, most research has focused on two categories: Attention deployment and cognitive change. There is a large literature showing that cognitive change (e.g., appraisal and reappraisal) can have a considerable impact on the intensity and nature of emotional experience (Power & Dalgleish, 2008). Augustive and Hemenover (2009) carried out a meta-analysis combining the findings from numerous studies. Reappraisal and distraction were on average the most effective strategies for reducing negative affect. We will consider these two strategy types in turn.

Distraction

It is often claimed that negative mood states can be reduced by means of distraction or attending to something else. Much evidence supports that claim (Augustive & Hemenover, 2009; Van Dillen & Koole, 2007). How does distraction reduce negative affect? According to Van Dillen and Koole, the working memory system (involved in the processing and storage of information) plays a central role. The working memory system has strictly limited capacity. As a consequence, if most of the capacity of working memory is devoted to processing distracting stimuli, there is little capacity left to process negative emotional information.

Van Dillen and Koole (2007) tested the above working memory hypothesis. Participants were presented with photographs varying in their emotional negativity. After that, they performed an arithmetic task making high or low demands on working memory. Participants' mood state following presentation of strongly negative photographs was less negative when they had been performing a task with high working memory demands.

Van Dillen, Heslenfeld, and Koole (2009) replicated the findings of Van Dillen and Koole (2007). In addition, they compared brain activity when task demands were high or low. The more demanding task was associated with greater activation in the prefrontal cortex (involved in working memory) but less activity in the amygdala (involved in fear and other negative emotions). The more demanding task produced more activation within the working memory system, which led to a dampening of negative emotion at the physiological (i.e., amygdala) and experiential (i.e., self-report) levels.

Cognitive Change: Reappraisal

One of the main ways in which an individual can regulate his/her emotional state is by means of cognitive reappraisal (Augustive & Hemenover, 2009). This involves "reinterpreting the meaning of a stimulus to change one's emotional response to it" (Ochsner & Gross, 2005, p. 245).

In recent years, brain-imaging studies have clarified *how* cognitive reappraisal influences emotional states. Ochsner and Gross (2008) reported a view of this literature focusing on two types of cognitive reappraisal. First, there is reinterpretation, which involves changing the way in which the context is interpreted (e.g., imagining an aversive picture has been faked). Second, there is distancing, which involves adopting a detached perspective.

The prefrontal cortex and the anterior cingulate (brain areas associated with executive processing) were consistently activated with both reinterpretation and distancing. Thus, cognitive reappraisal involves executive processes. Reappraisal strategies designed to reduce negative emotional reactions to stimuli produced reduced activation in the amygdale (strongly implicated in emotional responding). This is as predicted given that reappraisal reduces self-reported negative emotional experience. Further details concerning the patterns of brain activation associated with distancing are provided by Koenigsberg et al., 2010).

In one study (McRae et al., 2010), participants were presented with very negative pictures. They were instructed to use reappraisal (reinterpret the pictures to make themselves feel less negative about it) or distraction (focus on remembering a six-letter string). Both strategies reduced amygdala activation and negative affect, but reappraisal was more effective in reducing negative affect. Reappraisal was associated with greater increases in activation than distraction in the medial prefrontal cortex and anterior temporal regions, which are associated with processing affective meaning. Reappraisal was likely more effective than distraction because it was associated with more cognitive control of the individual's emotional state.

In sum, progress has been made in understanding why reappraisal is effective in reducing negative emotional states. Higher cognitive control processes associated with the prefrontal cortex are used rapidly and are followed by reduced emotional responses within the amygdala. Thus, cortical and subcortical processes are both heavily involved in successful reappraisal. The precise pattern of brain activation varies across cognitive strategies, which suggests that emotion regulation is complex and involves more different cognitive processes than previously assumed.

Cognitive Factors in Pain Perception

There are two main reasons for devoting a section of this chapter to pain perception and to methods of reducing pain. First, pain is a symptom associated with a myriad of health problems and diseases, with tens of millions of individuals around the world suffering from pain on a daily basis. Second, there is clear-cut evidence that cognitive factors play an important role in pain perception.

The starting point for discussing the relevance of cognitive factors to pain perception is to distinguish between nociception and pain (Van Damme, Legrain, & Crombez, 2010). In essence, nociception refers to the transfer of information from damaged tissue to the brain via specialized nerves. In contrast, pain refers to the perception or subjective experience that an individual has in a given set of circumstances. While it is indisputable that nociception is typically of major importance in determining pain perception, the consensual view is that pain perception is also influenced by various other factors. For example, consider a review of the literature by Gatchel, Peng, Peters, Fuchs, and Turk (2007). They argued with supporting evidence in favor of a biopsychosocial approach in which pain perception depends on biological, psychological, and social factors.

Here we will focus on various cognitive factors (especially cognitive biases). Relevant context is provided by research on individuals varying in their level of trait anxiety (a personality dimension relating to the extent to which anxiety is experienced). Much of the difference in the experience of anxiety between those high and low in trait anxiety is due to three cognitive biases (see Eysenck, 1997, for a review). First, there is attentional bias, which is the tendency to allocate attentional resources to threat-related rather than neutral stimuli (Bar-Haim, Lamy, Pergamin, Bakermans-Kranenburg, & van Yzendoorn, 2007). Second, there is interpretive bias, which is the tendency to interpret ambiguous stimuli and events in a threatening fashion. Third, there is memory bias, which is the tendency to recall disproportionately many negative or threat-related memories rather than neutral or positive ones.

Pincus and Morley (2001) applied the above theoretical approach to chronic pain. They argued that patients with chronic pain exhibit attentional, interpretive, and memory biases. These biases are especially strong in those patients whose self-schema becomes enmeshed with their pain and illness schemas. Of the three types of cognitive bias, attentional bias (also known as hypervigilance) has most often been found to be associated with chronic pain, although the findings have been somewhat inconsistent.

How can we account for the inconsistent nature of findings with respect to attentional bias in pain patients? What is important in determining whether an attentional bias is observed are the individual's current goals or motives (Van Damme et al., 2010)? For example, someone who is highly motivated to achieve a task goal (e.g., completing urgent work) is less likely to attend to his/her pain than someone who is not (e.g., sitting on a train staring into space).

Cognitive Treatment for Pain

We have seen that attentional processes are of major importance with respect to the experience of pain. A plausible implication is that an effective cognitive approach to the management and/or reduction of pain might involve attempts to re-direct attention from nociception to some alternative task or goal. This implication in turn depends on the assumption that attentional resources possess strictly limited capacity, an assumption for which the evidence is compelling (Eysenck & Keane, 2010).

Several studies have considered the effects of various forms of distraction on the experience of pain. The findings have been somewhat inconsistent. This inconsistency probably results in part from a failure in many studies to ensure that the distracting stimuli or tasks were actually capturing attention as expected (Van Damme et al., 2010). However, more promising findings have been obtained in recent studies, a few of which are discussed below.

Hoffman et al. (2006) argued that immersive virtual reality (provided by a head-mounted display) might provide a powerful distraction that would significantly reduce the experience of pain. They manipulated the distraction power of the virtual reality Snow World by using either a 60° field of view or a 35° field of view as participants received a thermal pain stimulus. In the 60° condition, 65% of the participants reported a clinically significant reduction in pain compared to only 29% of participants in the 35° condition.

Hoffman et al., (2008) carried out a study on patients with burn wounds undergoing debridement (surgical removal of dead, infected, or damaged tissue). Each patient spent 3 min in a distraction condition involving immersive virtual reality and 3 min in a control condition with no distraction. There were two main findings. First, the mean "worst pain" ratings on a 10-point scale dropped from 7.6 ("severe") in the control condition to 5.1 ("moderate") in the distraction condition. Those patients who felt most strongly that they had entered fully into the virtual world (and who were thus most distracted) reported a drop from a mean pain rating of 7.2 in the control condition to only 3.7 ("mild pain") in the distraction condition.

Fibromyalgia

Fibromyalgia is a chronic musculoskeletal pain syndrome in which there is widespread pain and tenderness in at least 11 of the so-called tender points. In addition, fibromyalgia patients very often report experiencing fatigue, morning stiffness, disrupted sleep patterns, affective distress, and some of the symptoms of irritable bowel syndrome.

Patients with fibromyalgia typically experience more pain than other patients with conditions producing chronic pain. When patients with fibromyalgia were compared with other patients with chronic pain, it was found that they reported greater vigilance to pain (hypervigilance) and more extreme catastrophic thinking about their pain and their condition generally (Crombez, Eccleston, van den Broeck, Goubert, & van Houdenhove, 2004).

The fact that especially severe chronic pain is found in patients with fibromyalgia suggests that it is likely to be a condition that it is difficult to treat. That is, indeed, the case, and no treatment so far developed approximates to being fully effective. For example, drug therapies (e.g., those involving analgesics or antidepressants) often alleviate some of the symptoms of fibromyalgia, but any beneficial effects generally disappear rapidly following drug cessation (see van Koulil et al., 2007, for a review).

The most used forms of therapy for fibromyalgia are cognitive behavior therapy and exercise training. In one meta-analysis (Goldenberg, Burckhardt, & Crofford, 2004), the beneficial effects of both kinds of therapeutic intervention were relatively modest. In addition, there were large individual differences in terms of the effectiveness of any given form of therapy. More promisingly, however, there were greater reductions in symptomatology when cognitive behavior therapy and exercise training were combined.

Van Koulil et al. (2007) reviewed studies in which patients with fibromyalgia had been treated with cognitive behavior therapy and/or exercise training. There was much diversity within each form of treatment. For example, cognitive behavior therapy was either single-method of multi-method. The former often consisted solely of an educational program (e.g., active self-management, relaxation), whereas the latter typically involved components such as cognitive restructuring, pain-coping skills, and increasing activity levels. Exercise training could involve aerobic exercise (e.g., cycling), strength training, flexibility exercises, and hydrotherapy.

Chronic Fatigue Syndrome

Chronic fatigue syndrome is a condition that is characterized by severe fatigue that lasts for more than 6 months and that leads to disability and inability to function effectively. Several factors (e.g., physiological, cognitive) play a role in producing the syndrome. However, the evidence suggests that cognitive factors (rather than behavioral responses) are of special importance in perpetuating the condition (Knoop, Prins, Moss-Morris, & Bleijenberg, 2010). One of these cognitive factors relates to the way in which fatigue is perceived, which depends in part on the widespread activation of illness schemas or packages of information. Other cognitive factors concern beliefs about the effects of fatigue on behavior and also on the individual's ability to perform and the extent to which attention is directed to the symptoms of fatigue.

Patients with chronic fatigue syndrome typically exhibit discrepancies between their actual and perceived levels of performance, muscular strength, sleep, problems, and pain (Knoop et al., 2010). All these discrepancies represent interpretive biases because they are all in the direction of perceptions or beliefs being more negative than more objective measures. Relevant evidence was reported by Mahurin et al. (2004). They compared cognitive processing in pairs of monozygotic twins discordant with respect to chronic fatigue syndrome. Mahurin et al. found that there was no difference in cognitive performance between twins with and without chronic fatigue syndrome. However, twins with the syndrome reported being more cognitively impaired than their co-twins.

One of the major forms of treatment for chronic fatigue syndrome is cognitive behavior therapy, which involves attempts to reduce attentional and interpretive biases for fatigue and to increase levels of physical activity. Another major form of treatment is graded exercise therapy in which the focus is on producing a gradual increase in the amount of physical exercise taken by patients with chronic fatigue syndrome. A meta-analysis carried out by Chambers, Bagnall, Hempel, and Forbes (2006) indicated that cognitive behavior therapy and graded exercise therapy are both effective in reducing fatigue and disability. However, the balance of the evidence suggests that cognitive behavior therapy is somewhat more effective.

One of the criticisms that has been offered of cognitive behavior therapy as a form of treatment for chronic fatigue syndrome is that it sometimes produced a significant deterioration (rather than amelioration) in symptoms. This issue was addressed by Heins et al. (2010), who considered the effects of treatment on various symptoms including fatigue, pain, psychological distress, and functional impairment. The frequency of symptom deterioration ranged between 2% and 12% in patients treated with cognitive behavior therapy and between 7% and 17% in control patients. None of the symptoms assessed showed significantly greater frequency in patients receiving cognitive behavior therapy than in control patients. In similar fashion, the severity of symptoms deterioration was broadly comparable between the two groups. Thus, there was no evidence that cognitive behavior therapy produced an increase in the frequency or severity of symptom deterioration.

The intervention studies on chronic fatigue syndrome discussed so far have been limited. It is highly desirable for therapists who are developing an intervention or therapy designed to reduce the symptoms of a condition such as chronic fatigue syndrome to proceed through two stages. First, it needs to be established that the intervention or therapy in question is effective. This first stage has been accomplished successfully in several therapeutic studies.

Second, but very often neglected or ignored, it is very important to develop an understanding of the mechanisms responsible for the beneficial effects of any therapy. That is especially important when considering forms of intervention or therapy (e.g., cognitive behavior therapy) that consist of several different components. More specifically, what is required are mediational analyses designed to identify the mechanisms responsible for any beneficial effects. The reason why such mediational analyses are potentially of major value is that identification of the "active ingredients" in any given intervention or therapy provides a solid foundation for modifying that intervention or therapy so as to make it more effective in the future.

Wiborg, Knoop, Stulemeijer, Prins, and Bleijenberg (2010) discovered in three different randomized trials that cognitive behavior therapy had a significantly positive effect on fatigue and disability in patients suffering from chronic fatigue syndrome. Increased physical activity is a major component of therapy, and so Wiborg et al. used actigraphy to assess physical activity before and after treatment. When they considered the mediation effect of physical activity, they found that it accounted for only 1% of the total treatment effect. In other words, increased levels of physical activity were almost completely unrelated to the beneficial effects of treatment. Two mediating effects that were important were a reduced attentional focus on fatigue coupled with an increased focus on physical activity. Thus, cognitive behavior therapy achieved symptom reduction via cognitive rather than specifically behavioral mediating mechanisms.

Moss-Morris, Sharon, Tobin, and Baldi (2005) used a randomized controlled trial to assess the effects of graded exercise over a 12-week period on sufferers from chronic fatigue syndrome. There was a significant reduction in fatigue after the intervention compared to prior to the intervention. Mediational analysis revealed that increased physical fitness did not mediate the beneficial effects. The most important mediating factor identified by Moss-Morris et al. was a decreased focus on the patient's symptoms.

Summary and Conclusions

We have seen in this chapter that there are two major ways in which the insights of cognitive psychology can contribute towards medical health care. First, the effects of medical health care often depend to a much greater extent than was realized until comparatively recently on individual differences in health literacy. More specifically, patients with deficient health literacy are substantially less likely than those with adequate health literacy to understand the advice provided by doctors, to take medicine at the times and doses recommended, and so on. There is a reasonably strong association between health literacy on the one hand and intelligence and cognitive ability on the other hand. As a consequence, attempts to improve the adherence to prescribed treatments of patients low in health literacy should be based on our current understanding of the cognitive limitations of such individuals.

Second, cognitive factors play a significant role in determining the number and nature of symptoms experienced by patients with a wide range of conditions including chronic pain, fibromyalgia, and chronic fatigue syndrome. It follows that cognitive interventions (e.g., cognitive behavior therapy) designed to reduce such symptoms hold considerable promise.

What needs to be done in the future? This question is addressed below first with respect to health literacy. After that, we will briefly consider future directions with respect to cognitively based forms of treatment.

Enhancing Health Literacy

Several cognitive deficiencies associated with poor health literacy have been identified. For example, there are deficiencies in working memory capacity, in attentional control and other executive abilities, in long-term memory, in language comprehension, and in planning. There are two major ways in which interventions might be devised to respond to these deficiencies. First, it would be possible to devise training programs designed to enhance all these cognitive skills in individuals having poor health literacy. A disadvantage with this approach is that it would be very time-consuming to implement training programs that produced significant improvements in all the deficient cognitive abilities.

Second, it would be possible for health psychologists to devise ways of changing patient-health practitioner communications so as to minimize the extent to which patients need high-level cognitive skills. Such an approach, which would necessarily involve regular monitoring to ensure that it was being implemented successfully, offers the most promise for the future.

Enhancing Cognitively Based Treatment

Earlier in the chapter, we considered some of the studies carried out to assess the effects of cognitive behavior on various health conditions (e.g., chronic fatigue syndrome, chronic pain, fibromyalgia). As we have seen, cognitive behavior therapy is a moderately effective form of treatment for various health conditions. However, most intervention studies are limited in several ways. At a general level, the most important limitation is that it is often difficult (or even impossible) to interpret the outcomes of such studies in an unequivocal fashion. At the risk of oversimplifying a complex reality, what happens too often in treatment studies is that cognitive behavior therapy consists of a complex package of components delivered to all the patients. The main findings consist of a comparison of the treated and one or more control groups on various measures of improvement. With such studies, the precise reasons why the treated group shows more improvement than the control group(s) cannot be determined.

What should be done in future treatment studies? First, it would be highly desirable (but undeniably expensive and hard to implement) to try to establish the effectiveness of the separate components of any treatment package. That would involve having several treatment conditions in which specific components were systematically included or excluded.

Second, it is important to identifying the mediating mechanisms underlying the effectiveness of treatment. Some such studies were discussed earlier, but much remains to be done. What is needed is to assess a range of cognitive, physiological, and behavioral measures at several points during treatment in order to establish which ones are predictive of final outcome.

Third, more account needs to be taken of individual differences among patients. For example, Bazelmans, Prins, and Bleijenberg (2006) classified patients with chronic fatigue syndrome as being relatively active or relatively passive in their everyday lives. Forms of treatment that are suitable for one group of patients are unlikely to be suitable for the other group.

References

Adams, R. J., Appleton, S. L., Hill, C. L., Dodd, M., Findlay, C., & Wilson, D. H. (2009). Risks associated with low functional health literacy in an Australian population. *Medical Journal of Australia, 191*, 530–534.

Augustive, A. A., & Hemenover, S. H. (2009). On the relative effectiveness of affect regulation strategies: A meta-analysis. *Cognition & Emotion, 23*, 1181–1220.

Bar-Haim, Y., Lamy, D., Pergamin, L., Bakermans-Kranenburg, M. J., & van Yzendoorn, M. H. (2007). Threat-related attentional bias in anxious and non-anxious individuals: A meta-analytic study. *Psychological Bulletin, 133*, 1–24.

Batty, G. D., Wennerstad, K. M., Smith, G. D., Gunnell, D., Deary, I. J., Tynelius, P., & Rasmussen, F. (2009). IQ in early adulthood and mortality by middle age: Cohort study of one million Swedish men. *Epidemiology, 20*, 100–109.

Bazelmans, E., Prins, J. B., & Bleijenberg, G. (2006). Cognitive behavior therapy for relatively active and for passive chronic fatigue syndrome patients. *Cognitive and Behavioral Practice, 13*, 157–166.

Chambers, D., Bagnall, A., Hempel, S., & Forbes, C. (2006). Interventions for the treatment, management and rehabilitation of patients with chronic fatigue syndrome/myalgic encephalomyelitis: An updated systematic review. *Journal of the Royal Society of Medicine, 99*, 506–520.

Crombez, G., Eccleston, C., van den Broeck, A., Goubert, L., & van Houdenhove, B. (2004). Hypervigilance to pain in fibromyelitis: The mediating role of pain intensity and catastrophic thinking about pain. *Clinical Journal of Pain, 98*–102.

Daneman, M., & Merikle, P. M. (1996). Working memory and language comprehension: A meta-analysis. *Psychonomic Bulletin & Review, 3*, 422–433.

Deary, I. J., Gale, C. R., Stewart, M. C. W., Fowkes, F. G. R., Murray, G. D., Batty, G. D., & Price, J. F. (2009). Intelligence and persisting with medication for two years: Analysis in a randomized controlled trial. *Intelligence, 37*, 607–612.

Eysenck, M. W. (1997). *Anxiety and cognition: A unified theory.* Hove, UK: Psychology Press.

Eysenck, M. W., & Keane, M. T. (2010). *Cognitive psychology: A student's handbook.* Hove, UK: Psychology Press.

Gatchel, R. J., Peng, Y. B., Peters, M. L., Fuchs, P. N., & Turk, D. C. (2007). The biopsychosocial approach to chronic pain: Scientific advances and future directions. *Psychological Bulletin, 133*, 581–624.

Goldenberg, D. L., Burckhardt, C., & Crofford, L. (2004). Management of fibromyalgia syndrome. *Journal of the American Medical Association, 229*, 2388–2395.

Gottfredson, L. S., & Deary, I. J. (2004). Intelligence predicts health and longevity, but why? *Current Directions in Psychological Science, 13*, 1–4.

Gross, J. J., & Thompson, R. A. (2007). Emotion regulation: Conceptual foundations. In J. J. Gross (Ed.), *Handbook of emotion regulation.* New York, NY: Guilford Press.

Heins, M. J., Knoop, H., Prins, J. B., Stulemeijer, M., van der Meer, J. W. M., & Bleijenberg, G. (2010). Possible detrimental effects of cognitive behavior therapy for chronic fatigue syndrome. *Psychotherapy and Psychosomatics, 79*, 249–256.

Hoffman, H. G., Patterson, D. R., Seibel, E., Soltani, M., Jewett-Leahy, L., & Sharar, S. R. (2008). Virtual reality pain control during burn would debridement in the hydrotank. *Clinical Journal of Pain, 24*, 299–304.

Hoffman, H. G., Seibel, E. J., Richards, T. L., Furness, T. A., Patterson, D. R., & Sharar, S. R. (2006). Virtual reality helmet display quality influences the magnitude of virtual reality analgesia. *Journal of Pain, 7*, 843–850.

Knoop, H., Prins, J. B., Moss-Morris, R., & Bleijenberg, G. (2010). The central role of cognitive processes in the perpetuation of chronic fatigue syndrome. *Journal of Psychosomatic Research, 68*, 489–494.

Koenigsberg, H. W., Fan, J., Ochsner, K. N., Liu, X., Guise, K., Pizzarello, S., . . . Siever, L. J. (2010). Neural correlates of using distancing to regulate emotional responses to social situations. *Neuropsychologia, 48*, 1813–1822.

Koole, S. (2009). The psychology of emotion regulation: An integrative review. *Cognition & Emotion, 23*, 4–41.

Kripalani, S., Jacobson, T. A., Mugalia, I. C., Cawthon, C. R., Niesner, K. J., & Vaccarino, V. (2010). Health literacy and the quality of physician-patient communication during hospitalization. *Journal of Hospital Medicine, 5*, 269–275.

Levinthal, B. R., Morrow, D. G., Tu, W. Z., Wu, J. W., & Murray, M. D. (2008). Cognition and health literacy in patients with hypertension. *Journal of General Internal Medicine, 23*, 1172–1176.

Mahurin, R. K., Claypoole, K. H., Goldberg, J. H., Arguelles, L., Ashton, S., & Buchwald, D. (2004). Cognitive processing in monozygotic twins discordant for chronic fatigue syndrome. *Neuropsychology, 18*, 232–239.

McRae, K., Hughes, B., Chopra, S., Gabrieli, J. D. E., Gross, J. J., & Ochsner, K. N. (2010). The neural bases of distraction and reappraisal. *Journal of Cognitive Neuroscience, 22*, 248–262.

Moss-Morris, R., Sharon, C., Tobin, R., & Baldi, J. C. (2005). A randomized controlled graded exercise trial for chronic fatigue syndrome: Outcomes and mechanisms of change. *Journal of Health Psychology, 10*, 245–259.

Ochsner, K. N., & Gross, J. J. (2005). The cognitive control of emotion. *Trends in Cognitive Sciences, 9*, 242–249.

Ochsner, K. N., & Gross, J. J. (2008). Cognitive emotion regulation: Insights from social cognitive and affective neuroscience. *Current Directions in Psychological Science, 17*, 153–158.

Pincus, T., & Morley, S. (2001). Cognitive-processing bias in chronic pain: A review and integration. *Psychological Bulletin, 27*, 599–617.

Power, M., & Dalgleish, T. (2008). *Cognition and emotion: From order to disorder* (2nd ed.). Hove, UK: Psychology Press.

Shaw, S. J., Huebner, C., Armin, J., Orzech, K., & Vivian, J. (2009). The role of culture in health literacy and chronic disease screening and management. *Journal of Immigrant and Minority Health, 11*, 460–467.

Unsworth, N. (2010). On the division of working memory and long-term memory and their relation to intelligence: A latent variable approach. *Acta Psychologica, 134*, 16–28.

Unsworth, N., & Spillers, G. J. (2010). Working memory capacity: Attentional control, secondary memory, or both? A direct test of the dual-component model. *Journal of Memory and Language, 62*, 392–406.

Unsworth, N., Spillers, G. J., & Brewer, G. A. (2010). The contribution of primary and secondary memory to working memory capacity: An individual differences analysis of immediate free recall. *Journal of Experimental Psychology: Learning, Memory, & Cognition, 36*, 240–247.

Van Damme, S., Legrain, V., & Crombez, G. (2010). Keeping pain in mind: A motivational account of attention to pain. *Neuroscience and Biobehavioral Reviews, 34*, 204–213.

Van Dillen, L. F., Heslenfeld, D. J., & Koole, S. L. (2009). Turning down the emotional brain: An fMRI study of the effects of cognitive load on the processing of affective images. *Neuroimage, 45*, 1212–1219.

Van Dillen, L. F., & Koole, S. L. (2007). Clearing the mind: A working-memory model of distraction from negative mood. *Emotion, 7*, 715–723.

Van Koulil, S., Effting, M., Kraaimaat, F. W., van Lankveld, W., van Helmond, T., Cats, H., . . . Evers, A. V. M. (2007). Cognitive-behavioral therapies and exercise programs for patients with fibromyelitis: State of the art and future directions. *Annals of the Rheumatic Diseases, 66*, 571–581.

Waldrop-Valverde, D., Jones, D. L., Gould, F., Kumar, M., & Ownby, R. L. (2010). Neurocognition, health-related reading literacy and numeracy in medication management for HIV infection. *Aids Patient Care and Studies, 24*, 477–484.

Wiborg, J. F., Knoop, H., Stulemeijer, M., Prins, J. B., & Bleijenberg, G. (2010). How does cognitive behavior therapy reduce fatigue in patients with chronic fatigue syndrome? The role of physical activity. *Psychological Medicine, 40*, 1281–1287.

Williams, M. W., Baker, D. W., Parker, R. M., & Nurss, J. R. (1998). Relationship of functional health literacy to patients' knowledge of their chronic disease: A study of patients with hypertension and diabetes. *Archives of Internal Medicine, 158*, 166–172.

Williams, M. V., Parker, R. M., Baker, D. W., Pirikh, N. S., Pirkin, K., Costes, W. C., & Nurss, J. R. (1995). Inadequate functional health literacy among patients at two public hospitals. *Journal of the American Medical Association, 274*, 1677–1682.

Wilson, E. A. H., & Wolf, M. S. (2009). Working memory and the design of health materials: A cognitive factors' perspective. *Patient Education and Counseling, 74*, 318–322.

Wister, A. V., Malloy-Weir, L. J., Rootman, I., & Desjardins, R. (2010). Lifelong educational practices and resources in enabling health literacy among older adults. *Journal of Aging and Health, 22*, 827–854.

Humor and Other Positive Interventions in Medical and Therapeutic Settings

Willibald Ruch,[1] Frank A. Rodden,[2] and René T. Proyer[1]

[1]University of Zurich, Switzerland
[2]University of Tübingen, Christian Hospital of Quakenbrück, Germany

No matter what the setting, humor and laughter can make life easier, particularly in the kinds of distressing situations endemic to medical and therapeutic settings. Despite the fact humor and laughter are at risk when people face adversity, for example, traumatic events, bereavement, physical illness, or prolonged unemployment, they are also available, on the long term, when humans need them most. The fact is: Among people with pronounced senses of humor, the frequency of humor increases when they face adversity, and, of course, humor seems to elevate moods. Laughter binds people together, leads to relaxation, and enhances pain tolerance – but humor and laughter also represent a double-edged sword. They can be offensive when used as sarcasm and ridicule hurt. Humor can be used to put others down (ingratiating) and laughing *at* others obviously has different effects than laughing *with* others. Patients sometimes avoid talking about their vulnerabilities because of their fear of ridicule. Knowledge of the benefits – as well as the untoward side effects of humor and laughter – are not optional for the healthcare professional, they are vital. Just as every powerful pill has its "therapeutic range," so is it also with humor. Unfortunately, the potential benefits of humor in both diagnostics and treatment have been frequently overlooked.

For the past 30 years "evidence based" research on fundamental and applied issues with respect to health care has been burgeoning. The disciplines involved in humor research span the range from psychology, anthropology, sociology, and education to physiology, medicine, nursing, and health care. The international society of humor studies (www.hnu.edu/ishs/) unites several hundred researchers from these disciplines and the Association of Applied and Therapeutic Humor (www.aath.org) is an international community of health professionals involved in the use of humor and laughter in healing. In addition to these international organizations, there are also national (e.g., in Germany, Japan, and Switzerland) humor societies promoting basic and applied research. Most recently, the "Positive Psychology" movement has concerned itself with basic human powers and, among these, humor and laughter have become mainstream topics. In fact, the considered use of the positive, perhaps even virtuous, components of humor seem to be coalescing into potent instruments for the health professional.

Introduction to Key Concepts in Humor and Laughter

Empirical research on the elements of humor is relatively new and, unfortunately, its practitioners have yet to reach a consensus on a common terminology. Some key concepts have not even been properly defined, much less rendered valid, and/or reliable. Nevertheless, as is the case with any new discipline, rapid progress has been made and this will be reviewed.

Humor: The "This is Funny" Sensation and Its Various Meanings

The core experience of humor is the sensation that something is "funny," "ludicrous" or "witty" (i.e., the so-called "humor response," an expression coined by McGhee, 1971). This sensation is a distinct experiential quality requiring a comparison: an incongruity either between objects, elements of an object, or between an event and an expectation (Ruch, 2008). Noticing incongruity may cause us to engage in its playful processing: we feel the "lightness" involved in amusement.

There are, however, "second meanings" for these basic terms (e.g., funny and comical). Things that are "funny" may not be "funny: ha-ha" but rather "funny-novel" (e.g., *peculiar*, *strange*, or *odd*) or even "funny-suspicious ("There was something funny about this offer"). This calls to mind that not all incongruities are light hearted. There are also serious incongruities.

In the humorous genre of "funny," the information we process is not serious; it does not require an immediate and appropriate response: This is recognized as a form of play. A "funny joke" is something radically other than a "funny car deal." In a "funny joke" there is no need to upgrade our knowledge inasmuch as the information we received only has an "as if" character; it is playing with sense and nonsense (Ruch, 2008).

Humor: Smiling and Laughter

Smiling is the most frequent response to funny stimuli. "Smiling," however, is a very mixed category and there are approximately 20 different kinds of smiles that can be distinguished on the basis of strict anatomical criteria (Ruch, 2008). Only one of these smiles reflects enjoyment of humor. When individuals genuinely enjoy humor they show the facial configuration called the *Duchenne display*: This refers to the joint contraction of the *zygomatic major* and *orbicularis oculi* muscles (pulling the corners of the lip backwards and upwards and raising the cheeks to cause wrinkles lateral to the eyes). Typically these contractions are roughly symmetrical and their typical duration is between one half and 4–5 s (Ekman & Rosenberg, 2005). Smiles not meeting these criteria are unlikely to reflect the genuine enjoyment of humor.

It is, of course, important for the practitioner to remember that smiling does not necessarily reflect amusement. Smiles can be involved in blends of emotions (e.g., when enjoying a disgusting or frightening film) or they can be masking negative emotions (e.g., pretending enjoyment when actually sadness or anger is felt). In phony smiles, one pretends to be amused but actually does not experience any enjoyment (of, say, a joke). There are also smiles of: misery, flirting, sadism, embarrassment, compliance, coordination, contempt, etc., (for definitions see Ekman & Rosenberg, 2005). *Cave*: not all smiles should be seen as indicative of the enjoyment of humor.

Whereas the basic physiological expressions of smiling and laughter are innate, learned behavior guides the intensity and the "when and to whom" enjoyment is exhibited. Display rules alter facial actions and attempts to dampen, control, or suppress smiling (e.g., Ekman & Rosenberg, 2005). The intensity of laughter, for example, can be accomplished by hiding the mouth behind a hand.

Higher levels of enjoyment typically accompany laughter rather than mere smiling but there are individual differences in expressivity among individuals (Ruch, 2007). Darwin (1872) gave a comprehensive and, in many ways, remarkably accurate description of laughter in terms of facial action, respiration, vocalization, gesture, and posture. For Darwin, smiling and laughter were on a single continuum. He stated that a graduated series can be followed from "... violent to moderate laughter, to a broad smile, to a gentle smile, and to the expression of mere cheerfulness" (p. 206). The contraction of the muscles forming the *Duchenne smile* also represent the core of the facial expression during laughter, thus the smooth transitions between smiling and laughter. The exact number of additional muscles involved in laughter is not yet known, but electromyographic studies suggest that several additional muscles are involved (Ruch & Ekman, 2001).

Whereas morphologically based taxonomies exist for smiling, nothing comparable has been achieved for the more complex behavior laughter. Dictionaries distinguish between, for example: hearty and derisive laughter, or between a guffaw, chuckle or chortle. These distinctions however, have not yet been rigorously identified in terms of physiology or acoustics. In a recent pilot study (Huber, Drack, & Ruch, 2009) actors performed 23 "kinds" of laughter: Acoustic analyses of these laughters distinguished among mocking laughter, or hearty laughter or laughter induced by tickling (e.g., Szameitat, 2007).

Enjoyment of Humor/Amusement

Research on humor came into being during the last decades of the 20th century, a time when cognitive psychology was a domineering force and at that time the "humor response" (i.e., denoting the perception that something is funny; McGhee, 1971) was interpreted primarily in terms of its cognitive nature. Later, the emotional elements of responses to humor were explored and it was argued that the response of an individual to humor is not restricted to her/his perception of a stimulus (e.g., "this is funny"), but rather that humor can also influence her/his "feeling" state (e.g., "I am amused"), or behavioral tendencies (e.g., "I feel like laughing") (Ruch, 1993).

The subjective, experiential level of emotion is, of course, accompanied by behavioral changes (smiling, laughter) and changes in basic physiology via the peripheral and central nervous systems. There is not yet agreement on how to label the emotion(s) associated with humor. Amusement is one of 16 pleasurable emotions distinguished by Ekman (2003) and it is the term that emotion researchers perhaps most often use in studies of humor (Ruch, 2008, 2009): "Mirth" or "hilarity" have often been used when studying (humor-induced) laughter. The only explicit emotion associated with humor that has been discussed in detail is *"Erheiterung"*, a German noun that emphasizes the uplifting of the subject into a cheerful state (German *heiter* = cheerful).

At the present state of the art/science, among the most important lessons that have been learned are that the enjoyment of humor is associated not only with the very specific *Duchenne* display (with or without vocalization) but also with a variety of other mental and physiological alterations discussed in the following sections.

Cognitive Processes

Numerous theories have been proposed to explain the perceived funniness of humor, with cognitive approaches being the most prominent together with arousal and superiority theories (for a review of theories, see Martin, 2007). Cognitive theories typically analyze either the structural properties of humorous stimuli or the way they are processed (Ruch, 2008). Already for a long time incongruity was considered to be a necessary condition for humor. From this perspective, humor involves the bringing together of two normally disparate ideas, concepts, or situations in a surprising or unexpected manner. While there is widespread agreement that incongruity is a necessary condition for humor, it was argued that it is not a sufficient one. Sheer incongruity may also lead to puzzlement and even to aversive reactions and therefore such variables as the resolution of the incongruity, appropriateness of the incongruity, the acceptance of unresolvable incongruity, or the "safeness" of the context in which the incongruity is processed have been proposed (Ritchie, 2010). Others emphasized the importance of the distinction between possible and impossible incongruities and between complete and incomplete resolutions. This is important, as only possible incongruities can be resolved completely while for an impossible incongruity only a partial resolution is possible, and a residue of incongruity is left (Ritchie, 2010).

How are jokes cognitively processed? It is plausible to distinguish three stages. The perceiver finds his expectation about the text disconfirmed by the ending of the joke (in the punch line); that is, he or she encounters an incongruity. As a next step, the perceiver engages in a form of problem solving to find a cognitive rule which makes the punch line follow from the main part of the joke and reconciles the incongruous parts (Suls, 1983). However, unlike after real problem solving, the recipient is aware that the fit of the solution is a pseudo-or "as if"-fit; what makes sense for a moment is subsequently abandoned as not really making sense (Ruch, 2008). At a meta-level we experience that we have been fooled; our ability to make sense, to solve problems, has been misused.

Motivational Processes

Some theorists argue that the cognitive-structural aspects in jokes are peripheral, as one may respond more to the connotative elements involved. Sexual themes are apparently one of the most prominent contents in humor and other topics like scatological ones (bathroom humor), violence and aggression, sick, black, ethnic groups, blondes, or Scottish or Irish people, etc., come into mind when one does an intuitive classification and those are all content-related. We seem to enjoy mishaps happening to others more, if we feel negatively predisposed to them.

Several theories tried to explain the favorite topics and targets (see Martin, 2007). Mostly, two models serve as a theoretical framework for predicting appreciation of tendentious content in humor. Freud (1905) argued that repressed impulses find relief in a disguised form in jokes as well as in dreams. The basic idea is that the "id" serves as a reservoir for desires and drives. As society and parental influence (represented in the super ego) do not permit direct expression of sexual and hostile impulses, gratification can only be achieved in an indirect way. From the Freudian perspective, one might derive the postulate that individuals repressing their sexuality or aggression would display a preference for sexual humor of an aggressive nature. Such a model would have implications for health professionals, especially in the domain of psychotherapy.

The salience theory (Goldstein, Suls, & Anthony, 1972) states that salience of certain themes (e.g., aggression) leads to exaggerated attention to such themes, to a better availability of the information necessary to comprehend the joke and finally to enhanced funniness of humor of that content. One can also make "harmless" topics salient (by presenting them repeatedly), such as cars or music, and this has been demonstrated to lead to enhanced funniness of subsequently presented humor relating to automobiles or music (Goldstein et al., 1972). Salience theory was also extended to the study of individual differences. It was hypothesized that sexual topics are habitually more salient for individuals with higher libido, more positive attitudes toward sex, and a higher degree of sexual satisfaction. The possibility of assaying a patient's taste in "dirty" jokes or cartoons in order to estimate psychological realms which he/she might be reluctant to discuss would be an obvious application of this theory.

Disparagement/superiority theory also may be used to explain preference of aggressive content and other preferred targets in humor. According to disparagement theory, funniness of humor depends on the identification of the recipient with the person (or group) that is being disparaging and with the victim of the disparagement. It was claimed that humor appreciation varies inversely with the favorableness of the disposition toward the agent or the entity being disparaged, and varies directly with the favorableness of the disposition toward the agent or the entity disparaging it (Zillmann & Cantor, 1976). This theory is in the tradition of a line of thinking that also involved, for example, Thomas Hobbes (1651/1987). Who stated that the passion of laughter is nothing else but some sudden glory arising from some sudden conception of some eminence in ourselves, by comparison with the infirmity of others, or with our own formerly. Laughter is thought to result from a sense of superiority derived from the disparagement of another person or of one's own past blunders or foolishness. Clearly, laughing at others should be distinguished from laughing with them as it has adverse effects on humans. "Laughing at" typically elicits anger and shame, not joy amongst the targets.

Mood States and Frame of Mind

The display of humor is facilitated or impaired by various types of mood and frames of mind. This is incorporated in everyday language. Phrases such as "to be in good humor", "in the mood for laughing," "out of humor," "ill-humored," "in a serious/playful mood or frame of mind," etc., refer to such states of enhanced or lowered readiness to respond to humor or act humorously. Humans are inclined to appreciate, initiate, or laugh at humor more at given times and less at others ("temporal specificity"). Therefore, humor research proposes a need to consider and measure actual dispositions for humor; internal states and moods that vary over time (Deckers, 2007).

A state-trait model of cheerfulness, seriousness, and bad mood was formulated and subsequently scales for their assessment were created (Ruch & Köhler, 2007; Sommer & Ruch, 2009). State cheerfulness was considered to be composed of cheerful mood and hilarity. The former is more calm and composed and the latter is more arousing and contains items relating to action tendencies (e.g., *I feel the urge to laugh*). In high state cheerfulness, individuals display a heightened readiness to respond to a humor stimulus with enjoyment. It turned out that most interventions to increase appreciation of humor only worked for those being in a cheerful state (Ruch & Köhler, 2007). Two different states of humorlessness are distinguished: *State seriousness* (composed of earnestness, pensiveness, soberness) and *state bad mood* (composed of sadness/melancholy, ill-humor). While both serious individuals and those in a bad mood may be perceived as humorless, the reasons are generally quite different. The state section of the State-Trait Cheerfulness Inventory (STCI-S; Ruch & Köhler, 2007) permits scoring of seven facets as well as the three scales and thus the hypotheses relating to different states of humorlessness can be empirically examined.

Laughter is preceded by a sudden annulment of seriousness, as laughter follows the buildup of strain or tension and its abrupt relief, and the incongruity inherent in humor needs to be processed in a "safe" (i.e., non-dangerous, non-serious) context. A play signal (McGhee, 1979) might help to shift a serious frame of mind to a playful one, and alcohol might raise our level of cheerful mood; both, in turn, might facilitate responding more favorably to humor. A reciprocal relationship is likely too; laughing a lot will boost the mood level and have an impact on the frame of mind. Thus, there is a feedback loop between actual states and moods or humor behavior (Deckers, 2007; Ruch, 2008). The STCI-S has been used in a variety of studies examining the effectiveness of humor interventions (Brutsche et al., 2008; Hirsch, Junglas, Konradt, & Jonitz, 2010).

Sense of Humor and Humor Styles and Traits

Everyday experience tells us that there are enduring differences among peoples' suscepti-bility to humor. Some people *habitually* tend to appreciate, initiate, or laugh at humor more often, or more intensively, than others do. In everyday language we typically ascribe a person to the possession of a "sense of humor." The sense of humor may be defined as a cognitive-affective style of dealing with situations and life in general that allows the der-ivation of a positive or light side in adverse and serious situations, to remain cheerful and composed, and even smile about them; that is, at least find them marginally amusing (Ruch, 2004). The term "humor" is here seen in opposition to other phenomena such as wit, ridicule, and fun and considered as stemming from a good heart. Humor accepts human weaknesses and it does not ostracize a target, in the same manner as ridicule or wit. In fact, recent research has shown that humor is predominantly related to the virtue of humanity (Beermann & Ruch, 2009).

"Sense of humor" covers the more benevolent forms of humor but this is not compre-hensive. Dictionaries typically contain various types of nouns (e.g., *cynic*, *wit*, and *wag*), trait-describing adjectives (e.g., *humorous*, *witty*, and *cynical*), and verbs (e.g., to tease, to joke, to humor or wind up someone) in attempts to define humor. This suggests that, at the present time, the notion of humor is nebulous. The simple fact is that humor, in its present meanings, is multidimensional and, up to how, research has not unraveled the number of dimensions that need to be distinguished and described. There are many facets of humor behavior (e.g., comprehension, enjoyment, creation, initiation, and entertainment), and they involve many domains of *psychic functioning* (e.g., perception, cognition, emotion, motivation, attitudes, and performance). Furthermore, different forms of humorlessness need to be distinguished as well. A variety of expressions have been proposed and they often refer to the same thing (e.g., *sense of humor*, *styles of humor*, *humorous tempera-ment*, *creation of humor*, *wit*, etc.) and frequently the same expression is used for totally unrelated aspects of humor. A review of the historical and current accounts and a survey of instruments (including self- and peer-evaluation techniques, and objective tests) can be found in a recent edited volume on the sense of humor (Ruch, 2007).

A few instruments should be mentioned here as well. Two instruments measure humor styles, namely the Humorous Behavior Q-sort Deck (Craik, Lampert, & Nelson, 1996) which assessed five bipolar styles (socially warm vs. cold, reflective vs. boorish, compe-tent vs. inept, earthy vs. repressed, and benign vs. mean-spirited) and the Humor Styles Questionnaire HSQ; Martin, Puhlik-Doris, Larsen, Gray, and Weir (2003) that provides results for affiliative, self-enhancing, aggressive, and self-defeating humor. The state-trait cheerfulness inventory (STCI-T; Ruch & Köhler, 2007) assesses the temperamental basis of humor with trait cheerfulness facilitating humor, and the dimensions trait seriousness and trait bad mood predisposing to humorlessness. Likewise, the PhoPhiKat-45 (Ruch & Proyer, 2009) measures one form of humorlessness, namely gelotophobia (i.e., the fear of being laughed at), and two further dimensions relate to the joy of being laughed at (i.e., gelotophilia) and the joy of laughing at others (i.e., katagelasticism). Finally, the Sense of

Humor Scale (SHS, McGhee, 2010) is perhaps less useful as a research metric but well suited to measure the effects of the humor training offered by Paul McGhee. In addition to the "sense of humor" (composed of the components of: enjoyment of humor, laughter, verbal humor, finding humor in everyday life, laughing at yourself, and humor under stress), also playfulness versus seriousness and positive versus negative mood are measured. There are further instruments that see humor as coping style, ability, virtue, attitude or world view, esthetic judgment, competence, or interaction style, etc. Most of the scales do overlap highly and indeed can be reduced to a significantly smaller number of factors (see Martin, 2007; Ruch, 2008).

Humor and Physical Health

The idea that humor is somehow conducive to good health is at least as old as the Bible: in Proverbs 17:22, one reads, "A cheerful heart is a good medicine, but a downcast spirit dries up the bones." From another direction, the notion that laughter brings good health has been around since classical Greek culture (Martin, 2007) and more recently it was popularized via the bestselling book, *The Anatomy of an Illness* (Cousins, 1979). This idea is still en vogue, and is probably even true – although the intersection of two such large and complex concepts as "humor" and "health" are prima vista problematical (Bennett & Lengacher, 2006, 2008).

One of the first collections of "evidence based" claims for the health-yielding properties of humor came from the pioneer humor-researcher William Fry published in 1963 (Fry, 1963). Many of these claims (that humor and/or laughter provided unique exercise for the lungs and heart, produced muscle relaxation, reduced pain, enhanced the immune system, etc.) were largely diluted or dismissed by a high quality if somewhat mood dampening review in 2001 (Martin, 2001) but since then, modest but reliable publications suggest that humor and/or laughter are at the very least correlated with "good health" (Taber, Redden, & Hurley, 2007).

The question of the direction of causality (Does humor produce good health or do healthy people have more robust senses of humor?) has not always been adequately addressed, nor has it been excluded that both humor and good health stem from some other extraneous variable.

In his book, *The Psychology of Humor*, Rod Martin lists five ways that humor and/or laughter might conceivably influence health (Martin, 2007): (1) through the (relatively modest) physiological effects of laughter itself (activation of the lungs, increased pulse rate, etc.), (2) through the beneficial effect of positive emotions associated with humor and laughter, (3) through cognative mechanisms – by ameliorating the adverse effects of stress on the body by assuming a more buoyant life stance, (4) indirectly through interpersonal mechanisms facilitated by close relationships that benefit from the potentially buffering effects of humor, and (5) by behavioral mechanisms associated with cheerful people who, because of their enjoyment of life will work harder to adopt more health-conscious strategies to prolong their life spans (quit smoking, eat moderately, etc.). It is obvious that rigorous associations between such global concepts as humor/laughter and any of these factors will be complex and difficult to measure in isolation. Given the limitations of the studies, a brief summary of recent research is provided below. Early reports of an increase in the activity of the immune system due to laughter have not been reproducible (Bennett & Lengacher, 2008). At least partly because of the complexity and multi-dimensionality of the immune system (and difficulties in defining what "strengthening" it might actually mean), the nature of associations between immunity and sense of humor (if there are any) remain unclear (Booth & Pennebaker, 2000). Although there appears to be an inverse relationship between sense of humor and coronary heart disease (Clark, Seidler, & Miller, 2001), the direction of causality in this study is questionable: The sense of humor was measured *after* patients had developed coronary heart disease and it may well be that people after heart attacks are less likely to exhibit high ratings on sense-of-humor scores. At a more modest level it has been recently confirmed that within moderate limits, laughter does increase the heart rate, respiratory rate, respiratory depth and oxygen consumption (Bennett & Lengacher, 2008). Mirthful laughter also increased flow-mediated vasodilation in one of the main arteries to the arm to an extent similar to that observed in aerobic exercise (Miller & Fry, 2009). The relevance of these results to the general circulatory system remains to be seen.

In well-designed experiments, the (rather moderate) pain-relieving effects of laughter have, however, been well documented (Stuber et al., 2009; Zweyer, Velker, & Ruch, 2004). Results of studies addressing the very basic question of whether people with greater senses of humor actually *are* healthier, or whether, due to their greater senses of humor, they merely endure ill-health with greater tranquility remain contradictory (Svebak, Martin, & Holman, 2004). In a recent cross-cultural study of populations in India and Canada (Hasan & Hasan, 2009), it was found that "a moderate" amount of reported laughter was correlated with the highest degree of health in both cultural settings. Both parameters (laughter and health) were determined by a questionnaire. Conversely, in the Canadian population, the *highest* frequency of laughter was negatively correlated with health – an effect the authors suggest was due to the higher prevalence of bronchial asthma in Canada (and the adverse effects of laughter in this diseased group). At present, the consensus seems to be that humor is probably good for one's health, but the nature of that effect has, so far, been difficult to operationalize much less to measure (Bennett & Lengacher, 2006, 2008).

Investigations on the correlation between humor and longevity are also small and inconclusive, and, unfortunately, so far most of the evidence seems disheartening. Most studies seem to indicate that cheerful people take worse care of themselves than their unhappier counterparts and thus die younger – albeit happier (Svebak et al., 2004). A newer study, however, suggests that a good sense of humor appears to increase the probability of survival to retirement, but that the effect disappears after age 65 (Svebak, Romundstadt, & Holmen, 2010).

In summary, not much has changed since Rod Martin's rather wet-blanket review on "Humor, laughter and physical health" in 2001. The going assumption is still that humor and laughter *must* be somehow good for us and that "In the case of physical illness, less of a toll on life satisfaction was found among those with the character strengths of bravery, kindness, and humor" (Peterson et al., 2006). So far, however, their measured salutary effects have not been dramatic.

There is a certain similarity between the presumed health benefits of laughter and the benefits of sex. Controlled, randomized, and placebo-controlled studies showing benefits associated with good sex are also lacking. Nonetheless, neither sex nor laughter is in danger of falling from the human repertoire – even if they were shown to be *detrimental* to health. Good health is good – but it isn't everything and, as the next section will show, in the realm of the spirit, humor and laughter are vital ingredients.

Humor and Mental Health

Exactly *why* evolution has given us the "humor response" and laughter remains unclear and the object of biological speculation (Gervais, 2005). What *is* clear is that they are basic elements of our human nature and their role in our lives has also been discussed since antiquity. In the Bible, Abraham named his long promised son "Isaac" – a form of the Hebrew word, "laughter." From the section above on "Humor and Physical Health," it seems unlikely that humor and laughter have evolved for reasons describable in terms of physiology – their effects there are simply too small: They make the heart beat a bit faster, they alleviate pain a bit and, they may tweak the immune system. These miniscule effects, however, would hardly outweigh the survival *dis*advantages of loud laughter, a phenomenon that interferes with normal breathing, makes the knees weak and results in the unambiguous announcement that "here is a group of relaxed people with their defenses down." As Gervais speculates (Gervais, 2005), the survival benefit(s) of humor and laughter seem more likely to lie in the dimensions of psychology and sociology than in personal physiology.

Humor and laughter (as well as music, dance, and language) can bind individuals together in numbers of magnitude greater than the largest band of apes. If one sought the "biological meaning" of language or music exclusively in the realm of parameters such as blood pressure, the immune system, or longevity – the results would surely be disappointing. Some of the greatest poets and musicians (and comedians) have had the shortest of lives and indeed displayed anxiety and depression and strong emotional mood swings above those of their less creative counterparts!

With respect to humor and laughter, at the personal level, the obvious has been unequivocally proven: they can positively influence one's mood (Ruch, 2008). A less obvious fact has also been proven: even "forced" or "voluntary" or "fake" smiling and laughter can induce the positive feelings of mirth (Neuhoff & Schaefer, 2002). The Indian physician and "guru of laughter," Dr. Madan Kataria has made something of a cottage industry out of this phenomenon in the form of "laughter clubs": groups of people that meet in order to laugh for no reason at all (Kataria, 2002). In the cold light of research, however, in a group of undergraduate students, "Laughter-induction exercises" over a period of six weeks, were shown to be less effective than "relaxation training" in reducing mood disturbances (White & Camarena, 1989). These results call into question (but certainly do not disprove) the long-term benefits of "Laughter Clubs."

The degree to which one's "sense of humor" can be developed remains unclear, but if it *can* be, a recent book by one of the world's foremost humor researchers suggests how (McGhee, 2010).

Evidence for longer term positive effects of humor and laughter on emotional well-being (realistically high self-esteem, lack of psychological disorders) has not been overwhelming (Martin, 2007). Studies using the HSQ have shown that there are even styles of humor that are *negatively* correlated with mental health (Martin, 2007). Self-defeating humor, for example, can be seen as a form of defensive denial (Marcus, 1990). Again a useful "diagnostic" indicator in medical contexts. Clinicians may identify specific forms of humor as an instrument to gain an understanding of underlying psychopathology.

It must be kept in mind that studies on "humor and emotional well-being" have all been correlational in nature, not causal. The observation that depressed people are prone to using self-defeating humor, and the observation that jolly people are prone to use self-enhancing humor – describe symptoms of psychological states. As symptoms, styles of humor are certainly interesting – none of the studies suggest that changing one's style of humor (if that is possible) would change one's personality.

The use of humor in patients with serious mental illness (depression, schizophrenia, and bipolar disorder) has recently been reviewed (Gelkopf, 2009) and the opinion of the author was that although a plethora of therapeutic approaches involving humor have been developed over the past two decades, few evidence-based studies have been carried out that might help the practicing physician decide what kind of humor to use with what kind of patient.

With respect to the notion that humor alleviates the debilitating effects of stress: "Nine studies found at least some significant stress-moderating effects, three obtained no significant results, and two produced results in the wrong direction ... it is difficult to discern from this research which particular uses of humor are beneficial for coping with which sorts of stressors to produce which types of outcomes" (Martin, 2007, p. 295). Once again, not all forms of humor are equivalent and different forms of humor may have different effects on the reduction of stress-induced pathologies.

Humor and Intervention, Can Humor Be Trained?

Humor research is not only interested in describing, explaining, and predicting behavior, but also in controlling it. Being able to change behavior is the ultimate proof for controlling it. As humor is a highly praised personal resource many adults are interested in developing their humor skills and in modifying the less appropriate social forms of humor. More recently, humor trainings became popular and they are applied in hospital, educational, and counseling settings. They most often are based on the assumption that humor is a set of skills those typically can be taught in group-settings during approximately 5–10 sessions (Hirsch et al., 2010).

McGhee developed a program that is both explicit and theoretically founded (e.g., McGhee, 2010). It is based on the assumption that playfulness forms the basis for the sense of humor, and the rediscovery of a playful attitude or outlook on life (that might have declined during education, school years, and work) is a key element for change. The set of skills to be taught during group meetings and "home play" is distributed across eight steps ordered in difficulty from simple (e.g., enjoying humor in everyday life) to difficult (e.g., laughing at yourself and laughing under stress) to acquire. To assess progress in the skills to be acquired the SHS is provided consisting of subscales that partly match these steps. Ruch, Stolz, and Rusch (manuscript in preparation) applied McGhee's program over a duration of two months to four groups. The adults who underwent the theoretical and practical part of the program yielded improved scores on the SHS in self-report, with some of those increases still prevailing for one month after completion of the intervention. Changes involved increases in the six scales measuring the skills (that comprise the sense of humor), in playfulness, in positive mood and there were also reductions in the seriousness and bad mood scales of the STCI. Also, life satisfaction was shown to increase.

Humor, Mental Health, and Life in the Hospital

If, as the above sections suggest, the effects of laughter and humor on the human body and on the individual human psyche are somewhat underwhelming, perhaps the evolutionary advantage we gain from them must be sought at the sociological level. As a species, humans did not survive because they were the fittest individuals in the jungle, but because they were the fittest *community* (see Brune's chapter in this book). Evolutionary psychologists are of one voice that close relationships among human beings are among the most important factors in the survival of the human species (Buss & Kendrick, 1998; Gervais, 2005). The life-and-death-stress-filled-lives of modern health professionals living under the anachronistically primitive, rigid structures of post-Napoleonic modern hospitals bear uncomfortable similarities to what life must have been like for *Australopithecus africanus*. The mini-effects that humor and laughter have on individual bodies and psyches are negligible compared with the binding and buffering effects that make survival in the setting of the 21st century hospital possible.

A recent article entitled, "The purpose and function of humor in health, health care, and nursing: A narrative review" (McCreaddie & Wiggins, 2008) identified 1,630 papers on the general subject of humor and laughter in the healthcare system. Perhaps the most obvious manifestation of humor and laughter in the hospital setting is the increasing presence of "clinic clowns." In the medical journal, *Pediatrics*, evidence based justification for "clown doctors" during the induction of anesthesia to children (Vagnoli, Caprilli, Robiglio, & Messeri, 2005) has been reported and critical models of therapeutic clinic clowning have been developed (Koller & Gryski, 2007).

Children's need for an atmosphere of light heartedness, laughter, and clowns seems obvious. But what about the other end of the spectrum: what about serious adults suffering from serious illnesses? What about cancer? In an article in the cancer-related journal, *The Oncologist*, the views of patients, nurses, social workers and doctors on the topic of humor and laughter during treatment were presented (Penson et al., 2005, p. 658). Such statements as these were reported, "The ability to laugh, for doctors to take a moment to detach themselves from medicine, is something that certainly is appreciated by patients" or "Humor is an important piece of my survival skills. Over time, if I took home the weight of everything that goes on every day here, I wouldn't be able to get out of bed in the morning". An oncology nurse said, "I find that being able to use humor goes a long way in helping many patients cope. We have a patient who wanted to help her grandchildren cope with her illness and she would joke with them. They were really concerned about her losing her hair and she didn't know how they would deal with that. She decided to make it fun. So she let them put press-on tattoos on her bald head ... Not only does it help her grandkids cope, it helps her grandkids and her join together."

Humor may help to relax the patient, acting as a "leveling agent" among the patient, family, and oncologist, as it can often relieve the tension caused by intimate questions or exams (Robinson, 1991). Of course, humor is a powerful element in human communication and it must be used as prudently as one would use dynamite! "When is it okay to joke with patients? When is it not okay to joke with patients?" one physician asked. "When is it okay to laugh about cancer? Have we as caregivers found ourselves in trouble by going a little too far over the line? ... Are there times when your sense humor might have broken the rules and gone down like a lead balloon with a patient?" Of course there are situations in which humor annoys patients (Dobson, 2003). Obviously, when bad news is being delivered, humor is utterly out of place (Penson et al., 2005). It is also obvious that the use of humor must be individually selected and delivered in appropriate doses.

The notion of "clinic clowns" would probably have seemed too bizarre even fifty years ago and no-one knows what the future holds ... but we live in the present, and perhaps every age has its preferred modality of coping. The "positive psychology movement" is exploring sources of strength that, up to now, were hardly acknowledged. Such titles as, "Humor, laughter and happiness in the daily lives of recently bereaved spouses" (Lund, Utz, Caserta, & de Vries, 2008) might have seemed like a bad joke only a few decades ago. In the modern hospital setting, humor and laughter are powerful forces that caregivers can scarcely afford to ignore. It is obvious that their use must be appropriate to the situation and their potency titrated to the need of the patient, but they can not only help heal patients (Gelkopf, 2009), they can help health professionals cope with the stresses of hospital life (Penson et al., 2005), reduce anxiety (Vagnoli et al., 2005), and provide comfort when things go badly (Lund et al., 2008). Laughter and humor may or may not be "the best medicines," but they can powerfully enhance hospital life for all concerned.

Positive Interventions

Positive psychology is a discipline within psychology that focuses on what is best in people (Seligman & Csikszentmihalyi, 2000). It criticizes the way that psychology has focused for a long time on almost exclusively studying pathology. The aim is to complete psychology in a sense that research topics from pathology to human flourishing are equally well represented. In this sense the scientific examination of talents, giftedness, virtuousness, well-being, positive emotions, character strengths, or other similar areas is positive psychology's prime mission. This is structured mainly around three major topics: (a) positive subjective experiences (e.g., happiness or pleasure); (b) positive individual traits (e.g., character strengths or talents); and (c) positive institutions (e.g., families or schools) (Peterson, 2006). Humor is a central topic within this framework, as it is a character-strength associated with the virtue "transcendence" (Peterson & Seligman, 2004; see also Beermann & Ruch, 2009).

Positive psychology has a strong focus on practical applications. Interventions focusing primarily on humor have already been presented: but in the past few years diverse studies have been conducted that have empirically tested the impact of positive interventions and which are worth briefly reviewing here. Positive interventions are "treatment methods or intentional activities that aim to cultivate positive feelings, behaviors, or cognitions" (Sin & Lyubomirsky, 2009). Sin and Lyubomirsky conducted a meta-analysis and found that those interventions are effective in significantly enhancing satisfaction with life and in attenuating depression. They also identified factors such as regular practice and working on a "record of positive strategies" (p. 483) or practicing multiple strategies that may contribute positively to the effectiveness of such trainings in practice. In total, 51 studies entered the meta-analysis. A few of these should be highlighted briefly. Michael Fordyce (1977) proposed fourteen fundamentals (e.g., keep busy and more active, spend more time socializing, develop positive, optimistic thinking, or become involved with meaningful work) that may strengthen a persons' well-being. In a series of studies, he found empirical evidence for the effectiveness of such programs. Seligman, Steen, Park, and Peterson (2005) tested various interventions in a placebo-controlled online study in which approximately 500 participants were randomly assigned to one out of five intervention groups or a placebo group. Participants completed measures for life satisfaction and a depression scale before the training started and in several follow-up sessions. Results suggested that the interventions of learning more about ones dominant character strengths (the so-called *signature strengths*; Peterson & Seligman, 2004) and of devoting more time in the following weeks for using them in different ways in daily life as well as taking time each day to note three good things[1] that happened to one-self that day (and to provide causal explanations for each good thing) yielded positive effects (enhanced well-being and alleviated depression) for up to a period of six months. Writing and delivering a gratitude letter in a gratitude visit (to someone who had been especially kind to the person but had never been properly thanked) had the same effects over a period of one month. Various other positive interventions have recently been tested empirically, for example, for the sense of beauty, gratitude, or for kindness (for an overview see Sin & Lyubomirsky, 2009). Other authors showed that (positive) changes in intentional activities (rather than circumstances; e.g., exercising regularly accentuating the positive) contribute to well-being

---

[1]   There is preliminary evidence from the first author's lab that asking participants to note the three funniest things that happened to them that day for a week yielded highly similar effects as the three good things intervention (Proyer, Gander, Ruch, & Wyss, 2011).

(Sheldon & Lyubomirsky, 2006). In Proyer, Ruch, and Buschor (2011) interventions in humor, curiosity, hope, gratitude, and zest led to a significant increase in life satisfaction in a 10-week program (compared to a control group and a group that trained strengths like love of learning, kindness, or creativity). King (2001) suggests that a program where students were asked to write for 20 min on four consecutive days about a traumatic event in their life, their best possible future self (i.e., life goals), or a combination of those two (or a non-emotional topic) led to positive outcomes among her participants. Overall, researchers and clinicians would do well to exploit the potential beneficial effects of humor in terms of health-related benefits.

Conclusion

It is only recently that the beneficial effects of humor and laughter (and other positive psychological interventions) have become the subjects of serious empirical investigation. At the cost of normal breathing, evolution seems to have provided us with laughter. To supplement simple simian sense, evolution has granted us humor. It is obvious that humor and laughter function as psychological balsams in the kinds of distressful situations that prevail in the quotidian life of medical and therapeutic settings.

More precise diagnostic and therapeutic tools that exploit the highly individual and profoundly human attributes of laughter and humor will, no doubt, be developed in the near future. The wave has begun and the invitation to ride it is open for all.

Acknowledgments

The completion of this chapter has been facilitated by a research grant from the Swiss National Science Foundation awarded to the Zurich-based authors (SNSF 100014-132512/1).

References

Beermann, U., & Ruch, W. (2009.) How virtuous is humour? What we can learn from current instruments. *The Journal of Positive Psychology, 4*, 528–539.

Bennett, M. P., & Lengacher, C. (2006). Humor and laughter may influence health. I. History and Background. *Evidence-Based Complementary and Alternative Medicine, 3*, 61–63.

Bennett, M. P., & Lengacher, C. (2008). Humor and laughter may influence health. IV. Humor and immune function. *Evidence-Based Complementary and Alternative Medicine, 6*, 159–164.

Booth, R. J., & Pennebaker, J. W. (2000). Emotions and immunity. In M. Lewis & J. M. Haviland-Jones (Eds.), *Handbook of emotions* (2nd ed., pp. 558–570) New York, NY: Guilford.

Brutsche, M. H., Grossman, P., Müller, R. E., Wiegand, J., Pello Baty, F., & Ruch, W. (2008). Impact of laughter on air trapping in severe chronic obstructive lung disease. *International Journal of COPD, 3*, 1–8.

Buss, D. M., & Kendrick, D. T. (1998). Evolutionary social psychology. In D. T. Gilbert, S. T. Fiske, & G. Lindzey (Eds.), *The handbook of social psychology* (4th ed., Vol. 2, pp. 982–1026). Boston, MA: McGraw-Hill.

Clark, A., Seidler, A., & Miller, M. (1996). Inverse association between sense of humor and coronary heart disease. *International Journal of Cardiology, 80*, 87–88.

Cousins, N. (1979). *Anatomy of an illness as perceived by the patient: Reflections on healing and regeneration.* New York, NY: W. W. Norton.

Craik, K. H., Lampert, M. D., & Nelson, A. J. (1996). Sense of humor and styles of everyday humorous conduct. *Humor: International Journal of Humor Research, 9*, 273–302.

Darwin, C. (1872). *The expression of the emotions in man and animals.* London, UK: Murray.

Deckers, L. (2007). Influence of mood on humor. In W. Ruch (Ed.), *The sense of humor: Explorations of a personality characteristic* (pp. 309–328). Berlin, Germany: Mouton de Gruyter.

Dobson, R. (2003). Enforced humor annoys patients. *British Medical Journal, 326*, 1418.

Ekman, P. (2003). *Emotions revealed: Recognizing faces and feelings to improve communication and emotional life.* New York, NY: Times Books.

Ekman, P., & Rosenberg, E. (2005). *What the face reveals. Basic and applied studies of spontaneous expression using the facial action coding system (FACS).* Oxford, UK: Oxford University Press.

Fordyce, M. W. (1977). Development of a program to increase personal happiness. *Journal of Counseling Psychology, 24*, 511–521.

Freud, S. (1905). *Der Witz und seine Beziehung zum Unbewussten* [Wit and its relation to the unconscious]. Wien: Deuticke.

Fry, W. (1963). *Sweet madness: A study of humor.* Palo Alto, CA: Pacific Books.

Gelkopf, M. (2009). The use of humor in serious mental illness. *Evidence-based Complementary and Alternative Medicine, 10*, 1–8.

Gervais, M. (2005). The evolution and functions of laughter and humor: A synthetic approach. *The Quarterly Review of Biology, 80*, 395–430.

Goldstein, J. H., Suls, J., & Anthony, S. (1972). Enjoyment of specific types of humor content: Motivation or salience. In J. H. Goldstein & P. E. McGhee (Eds.), *The psychology of humor: Theoretical perspectives and empirical issues* (pp. 159–171). New York, NY: Academic Press.

Hasan, H., & Hasan, T. F. (2009). Laugh yourself into a healthier person: a cross-cultural analysis of the effects of varying levels of laughter on health. *International Journal of Medical Sciences, 6*, 200–211.

Hirsch, R. D., Junglas, K., Konradt, B., & Jonitz, M. F. (2010). Humor therapy in the depressed elderly. Results of an empirical study. *Zeitschrift für Gerontologie und Geriatrie, 43*, 42–52.

Hobbes, T. (1651). Human nature. Reprinted in W. Molesworth (Ed.), The English works of Thomas Hobbes of Malmesbury (Vol. 4, pp. 1–76). London, UK: John Bohn.

Huber, T., Drack, P., & Ruch, W. (2009). Sulky and angry laughter: The search for distinct facial displays. In D. Peham & E. Bänninger-Huber (Eds.), *Proceedings of the FACS – Workshop 2007* (pp. 38–44). Innsbruck, Austria: Innsbruck University Press.

Kataria, M. (2002). *Laugh for no reason.* Mumbai, India: Madhuri International Publishers.

King, L. (2001). The health benefits of writing about life goals. *Personality and Social Psychology Bulletin, 27*, 798–807.

Koller, D., & Gryski, C. (2007). The life threatened child and the life enhancing clown: Towards a model of therapeutic clowning. *Evidence-Based Complementary and Alternative Medicine, 5*, 17–25.

Lund, D. A., Utz, R., Caserta, M. S., & de Vries, B. (2008). Humor, laughter & happiness in the daily lives of recently bereaved spouses. *Omega, 58*, 87–105.

Marcus, N. N. (1990). Treating those who fail to take themselves seriously: Pathological aspects of humor. *American Journal of Psychotherapy, 44*, 423–432.

Martin, R. A. (2001). Humor, laughter and physical health: Methodological issues and research findings. *Psychological Bulletin, 127*, 504–519.

Martin, R. A. (2007). *The psychology of humor: An integrative approach.* Burlington, MA: Elsevier Academic Press.

Martin, R. A., Puhlik-Doris, P., Larsen, G., Gray, J., & Weir, K. (2003). Individual differences in uses of humor and their relation to psychological well-being: Development of the humor styles questionnaire. *Journal of Research in Personality, 37*, 48–75.

McCreaddie, M., & Wiggins, S. (2008). The purpose and function of humor in health, health care and nursing: A narrative review. *Journal of Advanced Nursing, 61*, 584–595.

McGhee, P. E. (1971). Cognitive development and children's comprehension of humor. *Child Development, 42*, 123–138.

McGhee, P. E. (1979). *Humor: Its origin and development.* New York, NY: W. H. Freeman.

McGhee, P. E. (2010). *Humor as survival training for a stressed-out world – The 7 humor habits program.* Bloomington, IN: AuthorHouse.

Miller, M., & Fry, W. M. (2009). The effect of mirthful laughter on the human cardiovascular system. *Medical Hypotheses, 73*, 636–641.

Neuhoff, C. C., & Schaefer, C. (2002). Effects of laughing, smiling and howling on mood. *Psychological Reports, 91*, 1079–1080.

Penson, R. T., Partridge, R. A., Rudd, P., Seiden, V., Nelson, J. E., Chabner, B. A., & Lynch, T. L. (2005). Update: Laughter the best medicine? *The Oncologist, 10*, 651–660.

Peterson, C. (2006). *A primer in positive psychology.* New York, NY: Oxford University Press.

Peterson, C., Park, N., & Seligman, M. E. P. (2006). Greater strengths of character and recovery from illness. *The Journal of Positive Psychology, 1*, 17–26.

Peterson, C., & Seligman, M. E. P. (2004). *Character strengths and virtues: A handbook and classification.* Washington, DC: American Psychological Association.

Proyer, R. T., Gender, F., Ruch, W., & Wyss, T. (2011). *A replication and extension of the study by Seligman et al. (2005).* Manuscript in preparation.

Proyer, R. T., Ruch, W., & Buschor, C. (2011). *Strengths-based interventions: Targeting curiosity, gratitude, hope, humor, and zest to enhance satisfaction with life.* Manuscript submitted for publication.

Ritchie, G. (2010). Variants of incongruity resolution. *Journal of Literary Theory, 3*, 313–332.

Robinson, V. M. (1991). *Humor and the health professions: The therapeutic use of humor in health care.* Thorofare, NJ: SLACK.

Ruch, W. (1993). Exhilaration and humor. In M. Lewis & J. M. Haviland (Eds.), *The handbook of emotions* (pp. 605–616). New York, NY: Guilford.

Ruch, W. (2004). Humor. In C. P. Peterson & M. E. P. Seligman (Eds.), *Character strengths and virtues: A handbook and classification* (pp. 583–598). Washington, DC: American Psychological Association.

Ruch W. (Ed.), (2007). *The sense of humor: Explorations of a personality characteristic.* Berlin, Germany: Mouton de Gruyter.

Ruch, W. (2008). The psychology of humor. In V. Raskin (Ed.), *The primer of humor research* (pp. 17–100). Berlin, Germany: Mouton de Gruyter..

Ruch, W. (2009). Amusement. In Sander, D. & Scherer, K. (Eds.), *The Oxford companion to the affective sciences* (pp. 27–28). New York/Oxford: Oxford University Press.

Ruch, W., & Ekman, P. (2001). The expressive pattern of laughter. In A. W. Kaszniak (Ed.), *Emotion, qualia, and consciousness* (pp. 426–443). Tokyo: Word Scientific Publisher.

Ruch, W., & Köhler, G. (2007). A temperament approach to humor. In W. Ruch (Ed.), *The sense of humor: Explorations of a personality characteristic* (pp. 203–230). Berlin, Germany: Mouton de Gruyter.

Ruch, W., & Proyer, R. T. (2011). Extending the study of gelotophobia: On gelotophiles and katagelasticists. *Humor: International Journal of Humor Research, 22*, 183–212.

Ruch, W., Stolz, H., & Rusch, S. (2011). An evaluation of the 8 step program for the improvement of the sense of humor. Manuscript in preparation.

Seligman, M. E. P., & Csikszentmihalyi, M. (2000). Positive psychology: An introduction. *American Psychologist, 55*, 5–14.

Seligman, M. E. P., Steen, T., Park, N., & Peterson, C. (2005). Positive psychology progress: Empirical validation of interventions. *American Psychologist, 60*, 410–421.

Sheldon, K. S., & Lyubomirsky, S. (2006). Achieving sustainable gains in happiness: Change your actions not you circumstances. *Journal of Happiness Studies, 7*, 55–86.

Sin, N. L., & Lyubomirsky, S. (2009). Enhancing well-being and alleviating depressive symptoms with positive psychology interventions: A practice-friendly meta-analysis. *Journal of Clinical Psychology, 65*, 467–487.

Sommer, K., & Ruch, W. (2009). Cheerfulness. In S. J. Lopez (Ed.), *The encyclopedia of positive psychology* (pp. 144–148). Massachusetts, MA: Blackwell.

Stuber, M., Hilber, S. D., Mintzer, L. L., Castaneda, M., Glover, D., & Zeltzer, L. (2009). Laughter, Humor and pain perception in children: A pilot study. *Evidence-Based Complementary and Alternative Medicine, 6*, 271–276.

Suls, J. M. (1983). Cognitive processes in humor appreciation. In P. E. McGhee & J.H. Goldstein (Eds.), *Handbook of humor research* (Vol. 1, Basic Issues; pp. 39–57). New York, NY: Springer.

Svebak, S., Martin, R. A., & Holman, J. (2004). The prevalence of sense of humor in a large unselected county population in Norway: Relations with age, sex, and some health indicators. *Humor: International Journal of Humor Research, 17*, 121–134.

Svebak, S., Romundstadt, S., & Holmen, J. (2010). A 7-year prospective study of sense of humor and mortality in an adult county population: The hunt-2 study. *The International Journal of Psychiatry in Medicine, 40*, 125–146.

Szameitat, D. P. (2007). *Perzeption und akustische Eigenschaften von Emotionen in menschlichem Lachen* [Perception and acoustic characteristics of emotions in human laughter]. Leipzig: Max Planck Institute for Human Cognitive and Brain Sciences, 2007 (MPI Series in Human Cognitive and Brain Sciences; 91).

Taber, K. H., Redden, M., & Hurley, R. A. (2007). Functional anatomy of humor: Positive affect and chronic mental illness. *Journal of Neuropsychiatry Clinical Neurosciences, 19*, 358–362.

Vagnoli, L., Caprilli, S., Robiglio, A., & Messeri, A. (2005). Clown doctors as a treatment for preoperative anxiety in children: A randomized, prospective study. *Pediatrics, 116*, e563–e567.

White, S., & Camarena, P. (1989). Laughter as a stress reducer in small groups. *Humor: International Journal of Humor Research, 2*, 73–79.

Zillmann, D., & Cantor, J. R. (1976). A disposition theory of humour and mirth. In A. J. Chapman & H. C. Foot (Eds.), *Humour and laughter: Theory, research and applications* (pp. 93–115). London, UK: Wiley.

Zweyer, K., Velker, B., & Ruch, W. (2004). Do cheerfulness, exhilaration and humor production moderate pain tolerance? A FACS study. *Humor: International Journal of Humor Research, 17*, 85–119.

Literary and Economic Aspects
of Medicine

The Economic Dimensions of Medical Practice

Douglas McCulloch

University of Ulster, Newtownabbey, UK

Economics is the art of argument in the real world; significant decisions always involve resources, and their relationship to outcomes is key. It is not often realized that value judgments are important in economics; its contribution lies more often in choice clarification than in conflict resolution. Value judgments are the basis for all economic arguments, without exception.

Another difference with the relative certainties of science is the sheer size of the issues economists have to consider, in relation to the tools and the data available. Science proceeds by refining its questions, but the subject matter of economics is usually indivisible, and the real world is vastly complex. Reasonable conclusions often have to be found on the basis of very limited factual information, and the tools and the arguments of economics can seem to be abstract or remote. Unfortunately, they are often all we have, to deal with the hard choices of a complex, dynamic, and little-known world.

However, we can say that post-1945 medicine has been a great success story, if too successful for the viability of national health budgets. The extension of life has opened up new diseases and specialties, so that the dream of the 1940s, that ill-health could be eliminated, remains unrealizable. Greater longevity and successful interventions in later life are two of the main factors causing the financial crisis in health care throughout the developed world; this will not be relieved by the decline in the populations of the rich countries, because the supply of health personnel will also fall. The pressing need to prioritize has in turn led to the development of health economics, and to the implementation of government health technology guidelines, stating the requirements of the "fourth hurdle," cost-effectiveness, which new interventions must pass.

We begin with the essential ideas of scarcity and choice, on which most of health economics is built. The economic dimensions we then consider are prioritizing, health sector management, and the physician's role in prioritization. Maximizing the impact of health sector resources is the recurring theme; it is a challenge for every country in the world. While the author has had experience of prioritization in only three countries (England, Northern Ireland, and the Irish Republic), the nature of modern health care, and its delivery by specialized medicine, is common; the dimensions discussed appear to be global in nature, though the examples used to illustrate are necessarily taken from the author's experience.

Scarcity and Choice

Limitless wants and limited resources give rise to the necessity of choice. However, in any given context, we have to be aware of what the alternatives are, before the choice can be made. The economist's initial reaction to any situation is less often "how do I choose?" than "what are the alternatives, and what does each involve?"

Consider this example: A hospital has made efficiency gains, which allow it to adopt only one of the following alternatives:

(a) 40 more heart bypass operations,
(b) 120 more hip replacement operations,
(c) 3 more neonatal intensive care cots,
(d) a cancer screening program expected to save 12 lives per year.

Weighing benefits against costs, the hospital development committee agrees a ranking for the alternatives as follows:

First: 120 hip replacements,
Second: cancer screening,
Third: 40 bypasses,
Fourth: 3 neonatal intensive care cots.

We can easily imagine the reasons for these priorities; the eventual poor quality of life of premature infants, the remarkable impact of the bypass and the hip replacement on patient quality of life, the relatively few lives saved by cancer screening, and so on. The arguments are only that, arguments, but they determine people's lives. It may be that rhetorical rules could be established, which would enable such committees to avoid contradictions, or the expression of values that a majority of the committee might not endorse. There seems to be a fairly strong model in people's minds of what ideal rational decision-making might be like; judgments made over time are expected to be consistent, though one might expect human beings to understand both the possibility of human error, and the variations that are possible in circumstances which change over time. (The development of the Oregon experiment in prioritization is a salutary tale of the pitfalls involved.) Life and death issues of this kind are evidently very serious, but this does not in itself imply that the value judgments involved are required to be permanent. We have to accept failure as a fact of life, through human error, or through a lack of information, so justified post hoc criticism is unavoidable. Because of decisions made on the basis of one set of value judgments, one set of people may live, and another set may die; if these value judgments alter, different sets will live and die. This is a fact of the human condition.

Given the committee's priorities in our example, the spare money will be spent on the hip replacements; the cost of the hip replacements, therefore, is the screening program, the best alternative that would have been implemented if the hip replacements had not been chosen. Our usual focus, the money, is not relevant to the idea of cost when a specific choice is in view. Cost is therefore a matter of valuation; the development committee is valuing the health impact of the hips more highly than the health impact of the screening. We may or may not agree; values are like that. The committee's preferences are shown by its ranking of the alternatives, which determines the cost of their first choice; in fact, every budget's allocation of the available money is a statement of values.

The clarity of the choice depends on the information available. It is usual to suppose that information costs substantial resources, based on the expense of running a randomized controlled trial, or any other kind of research exercise. However, one could argue that providing accurate data regarding treatment and its effects is a duty of a member of any health insurance system (whether public, such as the UK's NHS, or private), and that data collection in the age of information technology is feasible. Such routine data collection would raise the issues of confidentiality and accuracy, but it seems foolish to tolerate our ignorance of prescription noncompliance, or of self-abuse, when relatively inexpensive technologies exist to monitor the health of patients, to check the accuracy of such monitoring, and therefore to check the compliance of patients with treatment regimes.

A national health database could also provide the means to make health insurance economic, because such data permits forecasts to be made of the life-time demands on health services by patients in different categories. Given such forecasts, general practitioners could be credited with expected expenditures for each category of patient, and allowed to retain the balance between the saved expenditure when patients successfully avoided the treatments expected, and the expenditures on treatments which were greater than expected.

Some choices are simply unarguable; we allow a degree of license in the advertising of food and alcohol that future generations will find insane. Advertising works; why do we allow it to cause resources to be wasted on the treatment of preventable diseases such as diabetes, obesity, and liver disease?

Prioritizing: Outcome Measurement and Cost-effectiveness Analysis

Introduction

Outcome measures clarify choices; we review outcome measurement approaches, including the quality-adjusted life year (QALY); by way of contrast, we also consider the lattice approach, to illuminate the nature of health sector choices.

Outcome Measurement Approaches

The first kind of outcome measure was devised by physicians, using observable variables such as blood pressure, numbers of falls, or red blood cell counts. This was followed by surveys of mental or physical health which assessed different dimensions of well-being, either on one dimension (e.g., to measure mental health), or on overall health, or "health-related quality of life" (hrqol). Taking the profile approach one step further, researchers have since the mid-1980s been developing an overall health summary measure, known as the "quality-adjusted life year" (QALY). In brief, this is a set of health states and their values, which are the outcome of a detailed and rigorous research process in which health states are described and valued in relation to full health on a scale from zero to one. This means that the responses of a patient to a questionnaire can deliver a figure which measures hrqol. The measure most commonly used in UK work is the EuroQol or the EQ-5D, though it has a recent rival in the Australian QALY (or Aqol – see the website, www.aqol.com.au) There is also the Disability Adjusted Life Year or DALY (Sassi, 2006), which has given rise to an umbrella acronym, the Health Adjusted Life Year or HALY (Gold, Stevenson, & Frynack, 2002); QALYs and DALYs are in widespread use in the medical and health economics literature.

For example, we might find that an existing drug increases survival by three years, and improves quality of life from 0.3 to 0.7; by comparison with no treatment, the drug delivers 3 years times 0.4, or 1.2 QALYs. If the new drug costs $30,000 per year, by comparison with no treatment, it delivers each additional QALY for a cost of $25,000. Are the extra QALYs worth it? This value judgement has to be made by the budget holder, not the economist. The UK's National Institute for Health and Clinical Excellence (NICE) sets the maximum acceptable cost of a QALY at £30,000, and this seems to be the "going rate." Its origins might be worth study, as it has no foundation in science.

Controversies about the different HALY approaches remain (Gold et al., 2002; Nord, 2009; Sassi, 2006); however large the sample of respondents and whatever the research method, the statements and values established cannot have objective status. The ideal is to establish a set of health states, and measure their values using questionnaires, in a detailed and rigorous scientific process. How is such a process to be justified? It seems that every possible process could be criticized, because there is no objective basis for the method adopted. There is never going to be an objective way of making the value judgments we require for health prioritization decisions.

Outcome Measurement: The Lattice Approach

We turn from what might be called the detailed and complex calculation of the HALY, to a minimal application of analysis, which can deliver meaningful results, albeit only in the case of small numbers of patients. In many health contexts, the understanding and sometimes the consent of patients and families is important, and the complexity of HALY procedures may render them opaque, and therefore unacceptable. Nowhere is this more true than in the care of the severely disabled, for which Hirst (1990) developed a lattice analysis approach to deal with prioritization issues.

Disablement is represented using binary descriptors, a series of statements which either do or do not apply to a particular individual. Patients are described using a set of zeros and ones, and comparisons are made, for example, with a view to allocating scarce respite care days.

Table 1.

Patient	Disabilities						
	A	B	C	D	E	F	G
1	0	1	0	0	1	1	0
2	1	1	0	1	0	1	0
3	1	0	1	0	1	1	1
4	0	1	0	1	1	1	0
5	1	1	0	1	0	1	1
6	0	0	1	0	0	0	1
7	0	1	0	0	1	1	0

For example, the binary states might be:

A: IQ under 90,
B: Speech disability,
C: Vision defective,
D: Hearing defective,
E: Epilepsy,
F: Unable to feed unaided,
G: Unable to dress unaided.

We would be able to describe patients using a matrix such as the one in Table 1: and so on.

This "condition mapping" enables a discussion of priorities which would take into account all of the available information (assuming there is agreement that all the important dimensions have been identified), and enable the identification of groups of patients who have the same set of states. There is no necessity for making once for all priority determinations, which would involve the resolution of the difficult methodological problems which continue to trouble the users and developers of QALYs. While the lattice approach can only be used with up to a maximum of about 20 patients, it does offer the meaningful setting of priorities which does not require complex analysis.

Cost-Effectiveness Analysis

Cost-effectiveness Analysis (CEA) measures the incremental cost of each intervention against its incremental health impact, such as greater years of survival, more falls avoided, or improvement in a numerical health index or group of indices, such as the Nottingham Health Profile. It can be shown that interventions (drugs as well as surgery) reliably have such impacts (expressed within confidence intervals). In any particular context, the identification of the costs and the impacts depend on a series of assumptions; the wider value of CEA lies in its exploration of the production space of health care, to show cost and outcome functions in relation to the number of cases.[1]

On the cost side, clinicians, economists, and managers operate with figures in mind which guide their everyday activities – the "average cost-per-case," "cost-per-bed-day," and so on. Useful as such figures are, they may not be the best information on which to base resource allocation decisions. A classic example was the "Care in the Community" measure adopted in the UK in the 1980s; briefly, the rationale was: "if the average cost of caring for a mentally ill patient is £x a week, releasing such a patient into the community for a cost to social services of £y per week will save the Exchequer £(x − y) per week." In fact, the physicians only released the patients who were best able to look after themselves, and who cost much less as in-patients than the average, so that the program achieved much less in terms of cost saving than the planners had expected.

The true incremental cost of a proposal is also relevant to the decision to expand the number of procedures in a facility. Some costs do not change as the number of procedures increases, until the capacity limit is reached, when greater numbers cannot be delivered without an expanded facility. For example, expanding the number of hip replacements from 2,000 to 2,100 per month may be possible without incurring any more costs other than staff overtime, drugs, hotel costs, and the cost of the metal hip joint. However, if the existing capacity limit is 2,400, the 2,401st procedure will cost much more than the preceding 400.

Cost-Effectiveness Analysis in Practice

As far as the achievement of maximum health impact is concerned, the first problem with CEA lies in the actual opportunity cost of the new treatment; a particular cost-per-QALY figure from a rigorous study has to be interpreted, rather as clinical trial results have to be carefully applied in other contexts. Some money costs may remain the same between different locations (in our example, the metal hip joints, or anesthetic drugs) but medical facilities inevitably differ in the quality of their staff and equipment. A particular "cost-per-QALY" figure from a particular location will only be valid elsewhere if the factors of production in use, and their productivity, are the same. Differences also arise between localities in the width of budgets; if (as in Oliver et al. (2002)) a central government ruling demands the acquisition and use of a new drug out of a fixed budget, different health authorities will have to give up different alternatives to buy it, depending on the production activities they are engaged in and their characteristics.

Finally, important diseases are not always amenable to conventional CEA based on clinical trials. The care of patients with Alzheimer's disease (AD) occurs in a variety of contexts, and other conditions and diseases are frequently present, so that scientific control

---

[1]   CEAs which use a QALY as an outcome measure are known as "cost-utility" studies; examples of all types of CEA are to be found in the NHS Economic Evaluation Database at www.crd.york.ac.uk.

in a research trial is difficult to achieve. To take one example, the difference between the average caregiver hrqol for a control group, and for those in a caregiver support program, was found to be 20% (Drummond, 1991), but because the sample was small, statistical significance could not be achieved. Of 146 caregiver-relative pairs, only 60 were eligible for the study; 178 in each group would have been required to reach statistical significance. This result might be considered favorable to the expansion of the caregiver support program, until the argument over resources begins; if a result is not statistically significant, it does not have standing, and those programs which do achieve a statistically significant benefit will take precedence. A budget committee is probably not the best place to begin an argument with another discipline about the validity or otherwise of accepted values for statistical significance levels.

AD is an interesting example; the "fourth hurdle" for new drugs to pass, that is, the achievement of cost-effectiveness, was introduced by governments in the mid-late 1990s, and the companies developing donepezil and rivastigmine had to adapt their multinational randomized controlled trials to meet it. The trials lasted six months, while the average survival was about five years; there was an imperative to calculate the hrqol impact so that it would take account of this survival period, and to show that the drugs were cost-effective, since the cost of care was an important burden to health services over the patients' lifespans.

In outline, the studies worked as follows:

1. At the beginning and end of the six-month trial (in a number of different countries) the Mini Mental State Examination scale (MMSE) was used to measure the impact of the drug on the AD patients.
2. The MMSE scores were used to calculate the "before" and "after" cost of care for each patient, using data from another study (in one country) which had established a relationship between the cost of care and MMSE score.
3. The trial results were "repeated," by assuming that the same progressions down the MMSE scale would occur in each of between four and twenty imaginary trials "lasting" a total of two years and five years, respectively. Survival functions or Markov analysis were used to estimate the total time of each patient at each MMSE level.
4. The analyses demonstrated cost-effectiveness, because the drugs increased the time spent by patients in the community, and reduced institutional care, so that the cost of care to health insurers (NHS or private) were reduced by a greater amount than the cost of the drugs.

There are (at least) four crucial assumptions:

1. Is the MMSE reliable and valid as measure of health outcome? Clinical measures do not often possess the rigor required for health outcome measurement, and the MMSE is at least debatable in this application.

2. Will England (one study) really have the same relationship between costs and MMSE scores as another country (such as Ireland) does?
3. Is this repetition valid? We do not know whether or not repetition will reduce or magnify the differences between the results and reality.
4. Are patient costs adequately considered? In one study (O'Brien, 1999), carer time was valued at two-thirds of the minimum wage; this is better than nothing, as in the other studies, but not much.

This example of CEA shows the evolution of statistical approaches in response to government pressures for economy, and illustrates the kinds of assumptions to look for in CEA studies. The CRD website mentioned above has examples of a wide array of CEA methods, all of which depend on assumptions for the validity of their conclusions; the contribution of CEA to health service economy throughout the world is not in doubt.

Health Sector Management

Introduction

The idea of health sector management is prompted by the observation that the defining characteristic of firms in other parts of the economy is the specialized technology they employ. This gives them their common views of cost functions, revenue possibilities, and even their corporate culture, particularly the strategic aims, what the firm values and strives towards. The medical specialties have common technologies, which define their structure, their costs, and their outcomes; hospitals are not firms, but exist as coalitions (more or less uneasy) comprised of the local branches of national firms, the specialties. Prioritization within a specialty can be achieved by defining procedures of diagnosis and treatment which are common in all branches of the "firm," on the basis of a common understanding of the relationships between costs and outcomes. While intra-hospital struggles over resources are important, they take place in an environment defined by the scientific progress and the resulting treatment criteria of the medical specialties.

How should we manage a health sector in its entirety, to maximize its impact on the health of society? Programmed Budgeting and Marginal Analysis (PBMA) is reportedly used to allocate resources throughout England and Wales. The idea is simple: If we have more to spend, what budgets should be increased by the available amount? If we have less, which budgets should be cut? Scientific evidence informs these decisions, but they may also be determined by managers' and practitioners' views of their local context. In principle, the PBMA approach involves the framing of alternative changes in budgets, and the discussion of the quantitative and qualitative impacts of each. Scientific evidence is important, but other kinds of consideration may be taken into account in the PBMA decision-making process.

Currently, in the UK, Primary Care Trusts have 23 budgetary headings for their overall expenditure, making it possible to compare spending totals on a specialty basis, taking into account population age distributions, and other health-related factors. The impact of the copious data provided by central government of course depends on the ability and the will of managers and other health professionals to use it; without an agreed decision-making framework for explicit priority setting, changes to budgets may be hard to implement.

Also, it remains a point for discussion, whether, without the control of a national specialty by its senior management, the production of health in all the regions of a country is carried out using identical technologies, that is, identical along the dimensions of cost and health impact. If we have reservations about the uniformity of production functions, the outcome or cost expectations of a national administration may not be valid. Here, we consider a database analysis approach to prioritization, and then consider the effects of trends in health care which have impacts on costs and outcomes, but which are difficult to analyze.

A Database Analysis Approach to Prioritization

Health sector management needs outcome measures as well as cost data, if the impact of health budgets is to be maximized; the average cost of a patient treated in a health sector (such as cardiac care) must include all of the outliers, those difficult and thus expensive cases which require more complex or longer term care than the average patient. The existence of such cases requires the use of database analysis to measure the health increments for the whole population, following Knaus et al. (1994).

The database approach involves collecting data from every patient, rather than from a random sample, establishing patient categories, and using multi-variable statistical techniques to determine the risk factors for each category of patient from the population studied. We can apply this approach to the treatment sectors of a region, so that they can be compared in terms of their health outcomes and costs, and so that scientific techniques can be used to establish the effectiveness and cost-effectiveness of treatment delivery.

Consider the collection of QALY data, at regular intervals, from each patient in a particular sector (such as the cardiac sector), updating relevant patient characteristics at the same time, and recording the date of decease if appropriate. This would permit the construction of the Mean Expected QALY Indicator (MEQI), based on the following assumptions:

1. Heart disease patients in the UK can be reliably identified, and registered as "cardiac sector" patients.
2. The costs of such a sector can be identified, for both its diagnoses and treatments.
3. QALY and clinical data can be collected from every such patient at least once a year.

The proposal is to monitor the sector's effectiveness by measuring the mean expected QALYs of these patients, to establish figures such as the fictional examples shown in Table 2.

As survival fluctuates, and the mean age changes, so the MEQI value will alter; its value will depend on treatment effectiveness, and on the incidence and severity of the disease. From the accumulated database, statistical analysis could determine what the trends

Table 2. Mean expected QALY indicator (MEQI) calculation

Mean survival of cardiac patients	59 years
Mean age of cardiac patients now	50 years
Mean patient life expectancy (1–2)	9 years
Mean patient QALY health state value	0.88
MEQI (= 9 × 0.88) in QALYs	7.92

in incidence are, and establish the case mix of patients (e.g., between "mild" and "severe" angina, and between "low" and "high" risk of a fatal heart attack), so that the expected change in the MEQI over time can be calculated. Given the trends established by publicly accessible findings, the MEQI value (adjusted as necessary) over time would indicate whether treatment effectiveness was rising or falling. After allowance had been made for changes in the case mix, and their effects on the MEQI value, increases in the adjusted MEQI would indicate greater effectiveness, and vice versa.

Such a measure would of course require judgment by experts in the interpretation of the database to discern the factors affecting the MEQI value. In particular, it would involve the application of econometric techniques, to analyze the time series of the value of the MEQI.

A sector-wide MEQI, calculated by a particular specialty, would conceal the performance of individual surgeons; observers of sector performance would be focused on the issues related to the trends in the incidence and severity of the disease, and the performance of the sector as a whole. Given the availability of the data proposed, and the physicians' common interest in a high MEQI value, senior clinicians might be more willing to agree treatment criteria.

Cost-Effectiveness

If the incidence and severity of cardiac disease remain unchanged, the value of the proposed MEQI variable should be constant over time; if its value increases, and expert (epidemiological and public health) opinion agrees that it should have remained constant, we can say that the sector's effectiveness is increasing. If the cost-per-patient, that is, the total cost of the sector, divided by the number of patients, is also constant, then a rise in the value of the MEQI implies that cost-effectiveness has also increased. The cost data for this calculation is already provided by the NHS, under the heading of each of the twenty-three budgets referred to above.

The MEQI in Other Sectors

Clearly, a similar approach, and similar surveys, could be applied to other sectors; a MEQI could be calculated for the population as a whole, and sector figures compared with it, as a measure of "need," shown by the fictional example in Table 3.

Table 3. Measuring "need": The expected QALY deficit (EQD)

Sector	Sector MEQI	Population MEQI	Difference	Number of patients	Expected QALY deficit
Cardiac	7.9	34.3	26.4	3,000	79,200
Arthritis	25.2	34.3	9.1	20,000	182,000
Renal	2.4	34.3	31.9	500	15,950

Such figures would not prove that a particular service should be funded; they will not bring arguments about resource allocation to an end. They do demonstrate need however, and enable discussions of the effectiveness of proposed interventions and the unmet need in each sector. We perhaps need to be explicit about such QALY deficits, for example, in respect of Alzheimer's disease; they indicate the need for research, as well as the need for treatment.

Structural Features of Health Services

The meaning of the data for health choices depends on contexts; there may also be unintended outcomes of CEA, which a strategic policy maker might need to take into account. For example, it is the mission of obstetricians to save the lives of infants with poor prospects of survival. Imagine that, at time t_1, they are able routinely to achieve an average 95% survival rate. Over time, the profession develops new techniques, which (after suitable trials and peer review, including cost-effectiveness analysis) become part of the required skills for qualified personnel, so that by time t_2, the average survival rate is increased to 97%.

Such neonates may not have full life expectancy, or an expected hrqol of 100%; let us suppose that the CEA took this into account, and that the new procedures are indeed cost-effective. What is the impact of this change on the profession? The new techniques become a necessary part of a consultant's training, and the minimum number of births for a training hospital increases, because the patients who now have a remedy for their condition are a very small proportion of all births. It follows that the minimum size of maternity hospital increases, and obstetric services become concentrated in fewer and fewer centers. This increases the risk to some pregnant women and their infants, who have to travel further for a hospital delivery, with effects on the health of infants and mothers.

Judging from other examples of cost-effectiveness analysis, it seems unlikely that a CEA would include the risk of the extra distances which mothers might have to travel to a maternity unit because of greater specialization resulting from the new procedure. These could be called "second order" effects, which do not result directly from the innovation analyzed, but for which the chain of cause and effect is undeniable.

As medicine develops, it has become more and more specialized, so that physicians' careers become focused on success in smaller and smaller fields. In itself, this seems innocuous; however, each specialty requires its support staff. It may be that escalating medical costs have as much to do with a scarcity of medical manpower as with profit-seeking companies and over-generous governments. At the least, we have to ask whether we may not be rewarding the production of new science more than the routine delivery of health care.

The Physician's Role in Resource Allocation

To state the obvious: doctors are trained to make judgments about patients' health on the basis of the signs and symptoms presented. Diagnosis is always a judgment, and all the evidence in the world will not make the cure of a particular case absolutely certain. Such judgments are what society expects of physicians; the means by which people access them are a separate issue, though of course people expect that doctors will at least safeguard their own interests, if not to over-reward themselves (whatever "over" might mean in this context), in a political process which seems to be beyond democratic understanding or control. In short, making judgments about health priorities is not part of a physician's responsibilities, though it is the role of the NICE. The judgments of NICE are subject to the caveats noted above regarding CEA; also, decisions about actual priorities cannot be decided "in principle." Specific choices are value judgments, and there is no apparent means for giving direct responsibility for them; in practice, the responsibility is exercised when Primary Care Trusts make their spending decisions. The reason for not making choices too explicit is the certainty of a legal action by someone whose relative may (apparently) have died because of the explicit spending decision.

Many articles have been written (by doctors as well as by economists) to urge physicians to become aware of scarcity and opportunity cost; the preceding words of this chapter will have failed if the reader is not aware of the complexity of making value judgments, the information costs involved, and the variations between localities of cost and outcome parameters. On the other hand, in the determination of health priorities, everyone's point of view ought to matter, especially the viewpoint of those treating patients, and it seems obvious that an understanding of how economics works should clarify its expression.

What is it that reasonable people ought to expect from a health care system's prioritization process? There is no rational basis for determining the health budget of the UK's NHS. It results from in-fighting between government departments, in a process which is unavoidably closed and unaccountable. The tax total voted by the elected representatives (which is then divided between the departments) determines the health budget indirectly; again, it is not, and probably cannot, be based on any rational formula, other than the need to convince the electorate in the electoral cycle. The key feature, in my view, is that the health budget, once determined, must be managed to deliver the greatest possible impact on health care. Costs and outcomes must both be taken into account.

Also, it has to be recognized that "reasonable people" are not all the same, and we do not live behind Rawls' "veil of ignorance" (Rawls, 1971). We all have different interests in what the health service delivers, and different reasons therefore to favor particular spending patterns. No-one at all represents the public interest; there is no-one in the health service or the electorate who has a direct self-interest in the maximizing of the common good. Economists, too, have a bias, in that they naturally seek solutions which fit the tools they have to offer, in the health sector as it is currently structured, and this focuses their work in particular directions. The expression of interests in the current political system is haphazard and often ineffectual; people start charities because of personal tragedies (and why not?), rather than to meet a need in the wider society.

Governments have attempted (in the UK, since about 1979) to resolve many of these issues through competition, in one form or another. The underlying assumption is that consumers of healthcare, assisted by their doctors, can be relied upon to select the best care, and to increase its delivery, by patronizing the best doctors, surgeons, or consultants. Even the student beginning economics knows that you need many suppliers if competition is to work to reduce costs, and that (amongst other things) the service or good produced must be identical between all of the producers. Also, competition cannot work if large producers can reduce costs simply by being large; unscrupulous firms will undercut rivals to become large .... in short, there are many reasons, even in principle, why competition between suppliers of medical services will not achieve maximum consumer satisfaction or minimize costs. The introduction of specific targets, and requiring medical institutions to meet them, is not an adequate solution either, as Bevan and Hood (2006) show.

No health delivery system is perfect; however, some imperfections might be eliminated by a different form of democratic control, in the form of a local health assembly, in which the medical professions, health lobby groups, and the general public were represented. Given charge of the health budget (e.g., of Wales, Northern Ireland, Cornwall, or Scotland), local control could include adapting to local circumstances, in specific ways, bringing local cultural influences to bear on local health issues. The whole dimension of public health tends to get overlooked in the national determination of priorities; local assemblies would have more purchase also on the processes of cultural change, which can alter lifestyles and deliver health improvements. There is an important incentive to improve public health if this reduces the demands on the budget under local control.

Conclusion

It is quite likely that people die because known possible interventions went unfunded; they are and will remain invisible. In the population at large, people do seem to understand the nature of scarcity, choice, and the inevitability of queuing. We and they, whatever our particular circumstances, deserve to have some access to the process of health prioritization, in some kind of political forum. It is remarkable how seldom the politics of health is discussed (but see the website www.pohg.org.uk); this may be explained by the lack of interest in state-based solutions on the right of the political spectrum, and the reluctance of all political parties in the European countries to raise the issues posed by social entrepreneurship (see www.sse.org.uk).

The fact remains that the daily functioning of our society depends on the health of each one of us; providing health care cannot but be a community effort, since its implications are so very pervasive, in terms of the quality of life, individuals' economic performance, and their adherence to the rule of law. The post-world war II dream (in the North Atlantic and European countries particularly) of providing for all what only the well-off had previously should be abandoned, and a truly social approach to health should be adopted. Whether the developing community-based approach to politics (in the UK, the "Big Society") will deliver such results remains to be seen; a "social" rather than a "socialist" approach to health may prove to be the way forward.

Let me end with an anecdote: a patient was being surveyed to assess his hrqol. He was very ill with cardiac disease, and stated at the first interview that he might as well use his medication to end his life. At the second interview, he was just as miserable, and made the same statement; his hrqol on both occasions registered zero. The researcher brought the case to the attention of the chief surgeon, and the patient had his operation three weeks later. Such lobbying is inevitable in health services which lack clear prioritization mechanisms; whether it was the right thing to do will never be known, and it is a good example of a decision being taken in the absence of information about the choice. Biometric assessment of patients, plus hrqol surveys, could enable the assessment of priorities on a scientific basis, taking into account changes in patient conditions which currently remain undetected by physicians. Whether or not such a resource allocation would be fair is an unanswerable question, but at least some of the value judgments involved would be known and could be argued over.

References

Bevan, G., & Hood, C. (2006). Have targets improved performance in the English NHS? *British Medical Journal, 332*, 419–422.

Drummon, M., Mohide, E. A., Tew, M., Streiner, D. L., Pringle, D. M., & Gilbert, J. R., Jr. (1991). Economic evaluation of a support program for caregivers of demented elderly. *International Journal of Technological Assessment in Health Care, 7*, 209–219.

Gold, R. M., Stevenson, D., & Frynack, D. G. (2002). HALYs and QALYs and DALYs OH MY: Similarities and differences in summary measures of population health. *Annual Review of Public Health, 23*, 115–134.

Hirst, M. (1990). Multidimensional representation of disablement. In S. Baldwin, C. Godfrey, & C. Propper (Eds.), *Quality of life – Perspectives and policies* (pp. 72–83). London, UK: Routledge.

Knaus, W. A., Wagner, D. P., Harrell, F. E., & Draper, E. A. (1994). What determines prognosis in sepsis? Evidence for a comprehensive individual patient risk assessment approach to the design and analysis of clinical trials. *Theoretical Surgery, 9*, 20–27.

Nord, E., Daniels, N., & Kamlet, M. (2009). QALYs: Some challenges value in health 12 (Suppl. 1) S10–S15.

O'Brien, B., Goeree, R., Hux, M., Iskedjian, M., Blackhouse, G., Gauthier, S., & Gagnon, M. (1999). Economic evaluation of donepezil for the treatment of Alzheimer's disease in Canada. *Journal of the American Geriatric Society, 47*, 570–578.

Oliver, A., Healy, A., & Donaldson, C. (2002). Choosing the method to match the perspective: Economic assessment and its implications for health service delivery. *The Lancet, 359*, 1771–1774.

Rawls, J. (1971). *A theory of justice*. Cambridge, MA: Belknap Press.

Sassi, F. (2006). Calculating QALYs, comparing QALY and DALY calculations. *Health Policy and Planning, 21*, 402–408.

Narrative Medicine

Stories to Some Purpose

John Skelton

Primary Care Clinical Services, School of Health and Population Sciences,
University of Birmingham, UK

There are narratives everywhere in medicine. Indeed, medicine is above all a series of personal dramas told by one individual after another to the doctor at the bedside, in the clinic or in the surgery. A series of people saying: Listen doctor, this is what happened to me. Doctors tell these narratives to each other, as part of teaching, or simply talking shop. Or, in the past, they have published them as blow-by-blow accounts, in leading journals.

The narrative voice is one of the things often perceived as endangered, in contemporary medicine, and this is a pity. Reichert, Solan, Timm, and Kalishman (2008) sum up the benefits of this voice as follows (see also Charon, 2001 for an excellent summary of the discipline).

> Many medical schools are exploring the uses of narrative writing to help students develop certain aspects of their training, primarily professionalism, patient care, and practitioner wellbeing. Writing is a means for expression and communication and a tool for learning and discovery. Current medical literature demonstrates the usefulness of expressive or reflective writing for gaining self-awareness, improving patient-physician engagement through deepening physicians' understanding of the connections between their own lived and bodily experiences and those of their patients, enhancing the empathy necessary to patient-centered care, reducing practitioner stress, helping physicians integrate the personal with the professional to enhance patient care, and developing empathy and trust between patient and practitioner and between practitioner and practitioner.

(This paragraph is buttressed by half-a-dozen references in the original.) I have cited this not merely because it is an accurate summary of the consensus, but because in itself it mimics one way in which the narrative voice is lost among contemporary conventions for reporting research. These state, for example, that a paper should begin precisely as above, with a statement of the importance of the field, and a summary of previous literature (Swales, 1990). The aim of this kind of reporting is to create an atmosphere of depersonalized objectivity, to divorce the findings from such issues as are at the heart of drama: a sense of personal engagement, of adventure, of satisfying resolution (the catharsis, as Aristotle would have said). Thus the findings in a Randomized Controlled Trial (RCT), which one might once have thought of as the end of the journey, are not presented with a fanfare at the close, but anticipated in the Abstract.

In other words, the language of modern science and the language of narrative are rhetorically distinct. The essential point is that this difference in language mirrors an epistemological difference. Throughout, I would draw the reader's attention to what seems to me the most important, and most difficult, point about narratives. They force one to consider one of the biggest of all questions: What is truth?

The epistemological difference is in part well-understood. This is the central point made by, for example, Launer, one of the most interesting writers in the field (see e.g., Launer, 2002), or Greenhalgh and Hurwitz (1998).

> Narrative medicine, in other words, reasserts the importance of lived experience, and the expression of that experience, in the face of the dominant intellectual voice in modern medicine – a voice that often creates the impression that only collectivized, abstract measurements can convey truths or carry meaning.
> "Scientific evidence" is not everything. If we understand our patients' stories, we understand their lives, the backdrop against which they have their being: and thus we can understand and help them better. (p. 168)

In this sense, narrative medicine fits in very well with the increasing emphasis over the last thirty years or so on a holistic approach to patient care, and the interest in Medical Humanities which is part of this (see e.g., the New York University website). The centrality of holistic medicine (as what ought to happen, at least) is now beyond question, though at worst a "Medical Humanities" course can seem an attempt to replace the scientific observer by someone in touch with nothing but their feelings: a person, as Malcolm Muggeridge once astutely but cruelly remarked of Arthur Koestler, "all antennae and no head" (Muggeridge, 1981, p. 208). In this context, I would prefer to stress the opportunity narratives give to enable doctors in particular to think better, rather than feel more deeply. The distinction is not between rationality and irrationality.

Narrative and Education

Narratives then have the power to make us think and reflect. Let us begin in the past. The case report, as we now call it, has always been with us, and its history is well summed-up by Hurwitz (2006). He offers examples from Hippocrates' *Epidemics* (1983). This text, written in the 5th century BC, some of it possibly by Hippocrates himself, has come down to us in an untidy, often ungrammatical form. It includes observational accounts of individual patients, told chronologically but with little attempt, as the case history unfolds, to bring the patient to life as an individual. Here is an example:

> Philiscus lived near the city wall. He took to bed on the first day of his illness with high fever and sweating and passed an uneasy night.

On the second day all the symptoms became more pronounced and later in the day his bowels were well opened following the administration of an enema. He spent a quiet night.

Third day: In the early morning and until midday, he appeared to be without fever; toward evening, a high fever, with sweating, thirst, a parched tongue and he passed dark urine. Spent a restless night without sleeping and was quite out of his mind.

Fourth day: Symptoms more pronounced, urine dark; an easier night, urine a better color.

Fifth day: About mid-day a slight epistaxis of pure blood; urine not homogeneous but containing globular particles suspended in it, like semen, which did not settle. Following the giving of a suppository, passed small stools with flatulence. Night uneasy, short snatches of sleep, talking, delirium, extremities all cold and could not be warmed, passed dark urine, slept a little toward daybreak, lost his voice, cold sweating, extremities livid.

About midday on the sixth day he died.
(p. 102)

This is essentially, as all Hippocrates' case reports are, what EM Forster (Forster, 2000) would call "stories" rather than "plots." Forster's original distinction was that to say, "The king died, then the queen died" was a story, whereas "The king died, then the queen died of grief" was a plot (p. 87).

In our terms, Hippocrates is descriptive rather than interpretative because he is not concerned, during the case report itself, with the cause and effect mechanisms which wreak change in the patient. He therefore does not supply a biological rationale (a biological "plot"). The *logic* of the textual organization is in consequence purely *chronological*. It is only when Hippocrates stands back and looks at a number of cases together that he begins to search for patterns or, in narrative terms, for interpretation, for a kind of plot. Thus, he has already told us (pp. 98–99) that Philiscus falls into the pattern of those who died in the sixth day, rather than those who had a crisis at that time, and subsequently recovered.

Contrast this with Yalom (1989), one of the finest doctor narrators of recent times. Yalom's superb *Love's Executioner* opens with a direct search for explanation, as the two uses of "because" tell us: (in the manner of contemporary medicine, Yalom raises the question of the doctors' role):

I do not like to work with patients who are in love. Perhaps it is because of envy – I, too, crave enchantment. Perhaps it is because love and psychotherapy are fundamentally incompatible.
(p. 15)

Stories describe, plots interpret: stories state facts, plots link them and explain them. And all that we see is filtered through the narrator. There is a difference between "'You look lovely, darling,'" and "'You look lovely, darling' he said sarcastically." With Hippocrates, during the case report itself, there is description only – and of course one of his messages for his audience was: don't over-interpret, don't go beyond what you observe.

We can think of Hippocrates as a teacher. These days, case discussions of various sorts are part and parcel of medical training (e.g., Evans, 2004; Robinson, Stacy, Spencer, & Bhopal, 1995). It is easy to imagine Hippocrates and his contemporaries discussing the collection of cases that have come down to us in much the same way. Easy, that is, to imagine them reflecting on the facts: Asking themselves – what do these descriptions mean? We are driven to make sense of things, and in part it is curiosity that drives us. And in fact, simple curiosity – or, to put it another way, the presentation of medical curiosities – is one of the hallmarks of the narratives that doctors have presented and reflected on. Consider this, from the mid-19th century, the story of "a labourer's daughter, aged 30 years."

She visited the author, Dr Best, in April 1869, with symptoms of some years' standing. On examination, there was a palpable mass in her abdomen, which he could not account for. Then:

On September 7th, when stooping to glean in a harvest-field, she was seized with violent pain in the abdomen, and became so faint that she was obliged to be carried home. Peritonitis immediately set in …. and after much suffering, she died on October 25th, 1869 ….

On October 27th, a "limited examination of the body" was undertaken:

The peritoneal coverings of the stomach and intestines were glued together by recent lymph. The peritoneum contained about ten ounces, of dark colored fluid, composed probably in part of brandy. On lifting the stomach to discover the tumor, it was found that this lay within the stomach …. A black tumor covered with hair was removed from the stomach and esophagus. It formed an accurate mould of these organs, and somewhat resembled a very small black swan. On section, it was found to consist almost entirely of hair …..
(pp. 630–631)

(The original has a photograph of the mass of hair). What the story *means* is hard to pin down, but it has resonance beyond what clinical relevance it has, or ever had. Look, the author is saying: How peculiar people are, and how odd the life of the doctor, who deals with such strange and fatal follies.

This tale of human oddity is what Stern and Papadakis (2006) call a "parable," even if Dr Best's moral remains implicit:

Parables are a powerful means of transmission of cultural values; the norms of professional behavior have been handed down through generations of doctors using stories with meaning. In medicine, parables often start with "I had this great case"

or "When I was an intern." What ensues is a story about a fascinating medical case with a moral about what it means to be a doctor.. .. – a story about how a patient survived when perhaps he should not have, a story about how you would have missed the diagnosis had you not stopped to ask one more question, a story about an observation from a nurse that alerted you to an unexpected problem. These stories not only serve to transmit professional values but also reveal the struggle of how we try (and sometimes fail) to meet the highest standards of professional conduct.
(p. 1796)

This way of putting it brings us directly into contact with contemporary dialog in Medical Education, and a great deal of this storytelling is acknowledged in the typical medical curriculum, through such concepts as "role-modeling" and "apprentice-style learning." The Medical Ethics courses which most contemporary medical schools have will also tend to be narrative-based, because they are naturally case-based, and the use of role-play in courses on clinical communication has the potential to fulfil much the same function through the dramatization of a narrative.

Typically, such courses will use a role-player to focus on a specific issue. Breaking bad news is the locus classicus: The medical student or doctor has to tell a patient they have a terminal illness, for example. This is very easy to use to demonstrate the contemporary emphasis on the holistic nature of illness. The role-player brief is therefore likely to have a substantial amount of detailed information about the patient's circumstances (he's male, married and sole breadwinner for a family where there are two young children, say): in acting terms, there is a detailed backstory, some of which may not surface in the consultation, some of which almost certainly will.

In this respect, both ethics and clinical communication echo another of the main contemporary themes in education, the switch from a lecture-based, top-down approach to one which invites students to accumulate examples (i.e., cases) and reflect on their similarities and differences. Robinson et al. loc. cit. exemplifies aspects of this, though the case-based tradition, in its modern form, dates back to Balint in the 1950s (see Balint, 1957, and the website of the Balint Society). This type of teaching is particularly easy to do in medicine, since the basic rhythm of the profession is the arrival and departure of patients (and their narratives) into the surgery or clinic, or into and out of the doctor's purview if they are on the ward.

What is at stake here is the conceptualization of the patient, at this moment, being at the heart of a complex web: their illness and the life which surrounds it – their family, their friends, their colleagues at work, and their own thoughts. And at the heart of another web is the doctor – representing and in contact with colleagues, systems, lines of management, the repository of clinical knowledge, the source of clinical support, and so on. And, at the point of contact, these webs touch each other. The patient's "lifeworld" to use Mishler's famous term (Mishler, 1984) and the doctor's, come together. (Mishler, incidentally, offers an excellent account of the use of narrative in research: see Mishler, 1986.) And, to change the metaphor to one in increasingly common use, the role of the doctor and the health care services is to shepherd the patient along the "illness pathway." This metaphor, of illness perceived as a journey which we take, is a common way of representing the life-narratives we tell ourselves as we seek to make sense of what we have done and will do (Skelton, 2009).

Understanding the workings of this complex nexus is the context which Stern and Papadakis (2006) are referring to when they talk of the use of narrative for learning professional values. Narratives of good professional attitudes with patients and also with colleagues, individual stories told, amount to lessons which can help one to be a doctor: and to understand what it is to be so. This doctor (quoted in O'Riordan, Skelton, & de la Croix, 2008: What follows is slightly expanded) tells the story of a patient with multiple problems, including heart disease and cancer, yet, he says, "she can see fun in the midst of calamity y'know." She is "fiery," "indomitable". . . . And what has he learned as a doctor?

> I've learned really that it's a very privileged situation . . . and there's magic moments in the career of a doctor meeting her was one of them y'know it's a very privileged situation to be there . . . and to see the courage . . . really phenomenal courage to see that in action y'know . . . and I'm interested to see her wit and her humour her character and that y'know.
> So I think that that's real privilege . . . part of the secret of surviving as a family doctor I think is to . . . well it's to treasure those moments y'know I think it's a wealth of treasure y'know unfortunately . . . there is a tendency in our job to quantify in terms of policy and expense when in actual fact it's not like that y'know it's a way of life. . ..

Narrative and Patient Care

Charon (2004) gives us this telling account of a patient narrative:

> A 36-year-old Dominican man with a chief symptom of back pain comes to see me for the first time. As his new internist, I tell him, I have to learn as much as I can about his health. Could he tell me whatever he thinks I should know about his situation? And then I do my best not to say a word, not to write in his chart, but to absorb all that he emits about his life and his health. I listen not only for the content of his narrative, but for its form – its temporal course, its images, its associated subplots, its silences, where he chooses to begin in telling of himself, how he sequences symptoms with other life events. I pay attention to the narrative's performance – the patient's gestures, expressions, body positions, tones of voice. After a few minutes, he stops talking and begins to weep. I ask him why he cries. He says, "No one has ever let me do this before."
> (p. 862)

At the level of clinical communication what this demonstrates is the virtue of good listening skills. Charon's principal achievement here is to say nothing at length. And also, as the patient talks, he presents himself in ways which Charon conjures vividly, but which we can reduce to the more formal term "holistic." The person he offers his doctor is a version of all aspects of "his life and health," his "lifeworld," as Mishler would say. And, in narrative terms, what we are looking at here is the chance for the patient to give the plot, not just the story of his life: to interpret rather than describe the hinterland in which he has his being.

By not interrupting, then, the patient is encouraged to tell his story, and this is a narrative which involves patient choice. The patient presents a version of himself and his illness – but as soon as you make the point in this way, stressing the patient-centered nature of offering freedom to mean – you draw attention to the selectivity and ambivalence of all narratives. In moving from story to plot, from description to interpretation, from the RCT to the narrative, we are moving (with the normal caveats about the nature of scientific "truth") from a truth discovered to a truth created – by the narrator as speaker, by ourselves as listeners.

Complexity is true of most kinds of story, but not all. The kinds of story one gets in crime fiction, for example, differ. The rule of the whodunnit is that there is a single, irreducible truth (Miss Scarlett, library, dagger) to which all else in the book is subservient. The dialog in whodunnits necessarily echoes less than that of Jane Austen. By letting her characters mean a dozen different things at once, on several different levels, Austen can give them a sense of reality which allows the reader to invest in them, to believe in them. In a whodunnit ambivalence gets in the way: It does not help the reader to solve the puzzle. Sherlock Holmes may have wondered what the truth was, but he never had any doubt that there was a single truth to be found, and that competing theories could be eliminated as untruths. He asks Watson (Conan Doyle gives a version of this thought to Holmes several times):

> How often have I said to you that when you have eliminated the impossible, whatever remains, *however improbable*, must be the truth?
> (p. 122)

The Holmes stories were, of course, written by one Victorian doctor, and Holmes himself was modeled on another. The role of the detective and clinician alike was perceived as paring ambiguity away, until the truth, unvarnished, stood before us. It is worth reflecting on this in the context of another locus classicus, this time from Greenhalgh (1999), who is a leading figure on narrative medicine in UK. She expands a "comment" from a GP into this account, which she calls "hypothetical." The doctor tells the story:

> I got a call from a mother who said her little girl had had diarrhoea and was behaving strangely. I knew the family well, and was sufficiently concerned to break off my Monday morning surgery and visit immediately.
> (p. 323)

The child had meningococcal meningitis. Why did the doctor pick up on this? Greenhalgh speculates it was:

> ... the potential significance of the word "strangely" and his personal knowledge about this family (their uncomplaining track record, the mother's good sense, and

the memory of the child as one whose premorbid behaviour had been nothing out of the ordinary).
(pp. 324–325)

This too, interestingly, is the doctor in Holmesian mode, forensically grasping the facts from the obscurities of language. The story may be read as an illustration of how sensitivity to language use is essential if one is to be of therapeutic value. But the lesson of narrative is far more likely to be that it offers life as it is: ambivalent, messy and uncertain.

The Unreliable Narrator

Narrators cannot always be trusted. It will not have escaped the reader that in the case of both Charon and Greenhalgh what we have are their narratives about other people's narratives (and a "hypothetical" narrative, at that, in Greenhalgh's case). These are, then, retellings at one further remove from the original events. There is an important point to be made here.

The "unreliable narrator" is a favorite plaything of the novelist and literary critic alike. The phrase, coined by Booth (1961), refers to a phenomenon much used by authors for centuries – Cervantes (2000a, 2000b) is often thought of as one of the earliest examples, but many of the narrators in Chaucer's *Canterbury Tales* (Chaucer, 1951) are not to be trusted. Incidentally, Shakespeare's notorious lack of stage directions (he never asks for a line to be spoken "sarcastically," as in the example above, about the man who evidently wished to insult his partner) is one simple explanation for how varied productions of the plays are.

Sometimes, as with Charon and Greenhalgh, the unreliable narrative involves a tale-within-a-tale. This is a device which fascinated Borges, for example, in his many references to *The Arabian Nights* (2010). This collection of tales exists in many different versions but they share as a framing device the idea that Shahrazad narrates a tale each night to King Shahriyar. Some of the *Tales* themselves contain tales within them, and one version, or so Borges asserts, includes a moment (Night 602) when Shahrazad begins to tell the king the story of themselves. He makes several references to this, for example (my translation):

The book is within the Book. Without knowing it
The queen tells to the king the now forgotten story
Of the two of them.
(Metáforas de las mil y una noches: p. 170)

Why does this matter? Because, for all the rather precious Borgesian whimsy, the extrapolation of narrative complexity to the point of circularity makes a serious point. Narratives can lose touch with the world, can travel solipsistically round and round in their own ambits. We have all I suspect listened to people and thought: well, how poorly they know themselves. We have all, frankly, used narratives to put our own actions in a better light, and in telling the story again and again have found it easier and easier to suppose it true.

Narrative Therapy

The relationship between story and truth is at the heart of discussions of Narrative Therapy. This is a technique for working with patients which was developed principally by White and Epston in the 1980s, and is centered on the Dulwich Center in Adelaide (http://www.dulwichcentre.com.au/).

The reasoning behind this kind of approach is straightforward. A "post-modern" understanding helps us to recognize that the truth is not "out there," but is a construct. (Roberts 2000). Thus:

> Some grow up with life-denying meanings and are hostage to toxic stories that adversely define and constrain their identity and self-image. They are caught in a story, and the task is first to understand this and then to find ways of modifying (reauthoring) these myths-people-live-by to promote a more constructive, effective and adaptive context for living.
> (p. 435)

People's lives and relationships, then, are shaped by the narratives they tell about themselves as a way of giving meaning to their lives and experiences. These stories become the basis of the self. If I lack a sense of self-worth, then the stories I tell myself will tend to confirm this self-perception. The aim of narrative therapy is to separate the "problem" from the "person." As and when this is done there is the opportunity for new stories to emerge: There is, that is to say, the opportunity for (part of the title of a well-known text on the subject) "the social construction of preferred realities" (Freedman & Combs, 1996). In particular, narrative therapy aims to see problems as being individual – of course – but also as existing in a particular society, a particular framework which consists of a socioeconomic context, a set of cultural preconceptions, for example, about sexuality, or the expectations of social class and so on. If this sounds like Foucault, well, it is. The originators of narrative therapy looked to Foucault for a substantial amount of their rationale. Thus White opens the classic text (White & Epston, 1990, p. 1) by saying "we believe his work to be of great importance."

Reality is, within common-sense limits, something we make for ourselves. Epston, White, and Murray (1992) (in McNamee and Gergen) mention a wide range of "social scientists" who are linked because they are "oriented" by an "interpretive method" (i.e., rather than, as the traditional scientist does, attempting to describe) and:

> ...propose that the 'story' or 'narrative' provides the dominant frame for live [sic] experience and for the organization and patterning of lived experience.

It is through these stories that lived experience is interpreted. We enter into stories; we are entered into stories by others; and we live our lives through these stories. (p. 97)

Charon's patient, we saw, had choice in what he said. This is the same point elevated to a principle. And, rather than the moment of catharsis which Charon's patient experienced, here is a deliberate encouragement, on the grounds of the relativity of knowledge, to use narrative as, essentially, a creative force.

This is in one sense absolutely fine. The young woman suffering from anorexia – where narrative therapy has often been used – *should* have a different way of thinking about herself, and the general ambivalence of life leaves plenty of scope for new stories and new metaphors to be identified which are as plausible as the old. But equally, replacing "true" with "plausible" pinpoints the difficulty. There are many cases where it is credible to help someone recognize that they are not to blame for the sadness of their lives. But sometimes, judged by the measures we normally live by, it would be neither "true" nor ethical.

The risk for narrative therapists, in other words, is that, like everyone involved in healthcare, they are in the business of making people feel better about themselves, in their case using the concept (picking up a common term already mentioned) of "re-authoring." But they need to do so with a sense of responsibility, and by extension to ensure that the stories they help to create touch reality. In a world without absolutes, this needs to mean (Epston et al., loc cit) "setting up an audience in which forms of change can be authenticated" (p. 109).

Finally, there is the issue of whether narrative therapy works. Unsurprisingly, the evidence specifically for narrative therapy (as the word "evidence" would be understood in the EBM world) is weak and, no less unsurprisingly, defenders of the approach will point to the difficulty, even the irrelevance, of getting evidence of this kind (Larner, 2004).

The long tradition of Bibliotherapy, dating back to the work of Alice Bryan in the 1930s (Bryan, 1939), is also worth briefly mentioning here. The kind of service on offer is often delivered through libraries – see for example, the service offered by Kensington and Chelsea, who define Bibliotherapy as:

... the therapeutic use of the written word to help people in any situation in life. This may include the treatment of illness or personal problems.

There is, in other words, an understanding that by helping people to read, it is possible to help people also to understand their lives and problems better, and – for instance – to recognize that they are not the first to have experienced these problems. It has been suggested (Marrs, 1995, Den Boer, Wiersma, & van den Bosch, 2004) that versions of this kind of therapy can offer success with, as the latter put it, "clinically significant emotional disorders" (loc. cit., p. 959). They conclude with a series of challenging questions, asking in particular: "Do psychiatrists underestimate the value of the acquisition of knowledge by patients?" (loc. cit., p. 969).

It will be clear that here too there is a range of possible responses from the person offered support, from the direct advice offered by a self-help book through to opportunities to read and reflect, giving perhaps a sense of emotional comfort at not being alone, or the help that a professional writer has been able to say "just how I feel", to – in the end – a complete revisioning of the way the world and one's place in it is. In the end, therefore, bibliotherapy is just reading, but not just reading as a means of passing the time. In this sense, as the library website cited above puts it:

> Many of us use bibliotherapy without realizing it. Reading is a way of making sense of the world and our place within it.

Narratives and Archetypes

One final perspective on the relationship between narrative and truth.

The ability to deal with narrative depends on "narrative competence". This is a term used inconsistently in the literature, but refers to our ability to tell and understand narratives, particularly by bringing to bear our historical and cultural knowledge, our knowledge of stylistic conventions ("Once upon a time. ..."), our common-sense knowledge of the way the world wags, and so on. It includes therefore our ability to fill in the blanks – a description of a turkey served for dinner will make us place a story in December if we are British, earlier if we are North American, without words like "Christmas" or "Thanksgiving" necessarily being used.

This means in part, however, that narratives depend on convention: if we are told something is a "fairy-tale" we think in terms of kings and princesses, and know that the narrative will slip into timelessness with the phrase "they all lived happily ever after", and so on. Our narratives fall into familiar, stereotypical patterns.

Perhaps then, constrained as we are by our human condition, we do not actually live lives with different and unique narratives. After all, when a patient tells us their story, we may try earnestly to remember that it is unique to that patient, but privately, with a guilty pang or two, we may think: how many times have I heard this story (the battered wife, the unvalued parent, and the rejected lover), and we may wonder if this retelling is more conditioned by commonplace storylines in soap opera than the patient's own experience.

But perhaps that's fair enough. Perhaps in the end we are all pretty much the same. It is typical of narrative theory, for example, to echo versions of the old cliché that there are only a limited number of plots in existence (Seven is a number often mentioned: there is a children's book museum in Newcastle called "Seven Stories" as an echo of this suggestion: http://www.sevenstories.org.uk/home/index.php). More formally, Propp's work in the 1920s suggested a limited number of functions and characters.

To drive home the point here, Brown University has a Proppian fairy-tale generator (http://www.brown.edu/Courses/FR0133/Fairytale_Generator/theory.html) which the reader might like to have a little fun using.

Conclusion

The narrative and humanist traditions are perceived then as being under threat from EBM. But the simultaneous rise of holistic medicine has invited and encourages other ways of looking at patients and their problems, and also at the role of narratives in education. These are altogether positive developments, provided always we recognize that narratives are ambivalent and unreliable. It is, however, at this stage that the study of narrative really begins to have meaning: in representing life-as-it-is, it offers amongst other things an opportunity for healthcare professionals to reflect on and use ways of thinking and ways of understanding and to challenge the nature of truth.

However, the humanistic side of medical education has been perceived as under threat for a long time. A glance, for example, at the early volumes of *Academic Medicine* demonstrates a not dissimilar pre-occupation, as if to drive home the Proppian point, that all stories are old stories. Indeed, in the very first paper ever published in that journal Cabot (1926) argues:

> If the [premedical] course is really to fulfil its purpose it must prepare students. . . . to become the medical counsellors of the community. It would seem evident that if they are to achieve this distinction they must be educated people in the broadest sense of the word. . . .
>
> . . . .I am not prepared to admit at the present time that in the equipment of the practitioner a knowledge of science is of more real value than a knowledge of the way in which humankind has behaved in the past and how he is on the whole behaving at the present time. The problems of medicine, on the whole, are quite as likely to require sound judgment based upon a knowledge of history, philosophy, sociology and psychology as on the facts of science.
>
> (p. 2)

"Educated people in the broadest sense of the word": it is all very well to contrast, as I have sought to do, the scientific, descriptive, empirical tradition and the humanistic, interpretative, narrative tradition. But what matters is probably a range of understanding which only a very few in any age have had. Here is a section from William Osler's great essay *Aequanimitas* (Osler, 1932).

Osler has quoted Marcus Aurelius, Matthew Arnold and Plato by the end of the first paragraph, picks out a line from Wordsworth's *Intimations of Immortality* in paragraph 6, and immediately offers the context for the word "aequanimitas":

> Let me recall to your minds an incident related of that best of men and wisest of rulers, Antoninus Pius, who, as he lay dying, in his home at Loriam in Etruria, summed up the philosophy of life in the watchword, *Aequanimitas*. As for him, about to pass *flammantia moenia mundi* (the flaming rampart of the world), so for you, fresh from Clotho's spindle, a calm equanimity is the desirable attitude. How difficult to attain, yet how necessary, in success as in failure! Natural temperament has much to do with its development, but a clear knowledge of our relation to

our fellow creatures and to the work of life is also indispensable. One of the first essentials in securing a good-natured equanimity is not to expect too much of the people amongst whom you dwell. "Knowledge comes, but wisdom lingers," and in matters medical the ordinary citizen of to-day has not one whit more sense than the old Romans, whom Lucian scourged for a credulity which made them fall easy victims to the quacks of the time, such as the notorious Alexander, whose exploits make one wish that his advent had been delayed some 18 centuries. Deal gently then with this deliciously credulous old human nature in which we work, and restrain your indignation, when you find your pet parson has triturates of the 1000th potentiality in his waistcoat pocket, or you discover accidentally a case of Warner's Safe Cure in the bedroom of your best patient. It must needs be that offences of this kind come, expect them, and do not be vexed.

Curious, odd compounds are these fellow-creatures, at whose mercy you will be full of fads and eccentricities,. . ..

And just what are all these references? Behind every one there is a narrative.

"Aequanimitas" is said to be the last word uttered by the great Roman Emperor, given as the watchword to the tribune of the nightwatch. He was highly effective as a ruler, and also (this is Gibbon, 2004, first published of course in the 18th century, a text much more current in Osler's time than our own) an "amiable prince", leading a "tranquil life" of "gentle repose" (p. 8–9). "Flammantia moenia mundi" is a quotation from Lucretius's defence of a rational understanding of the world, *De Rerum Naturae*. Lucretius too sought to cultivate tranquility of mind and intellectual engagement. Clotho was one of the three Fates: it was her task to spin the thread of an individual's life (the other two fates had the task of respectively measuring it and cutting it, readers of a certain age may vaguely recall). "Knowledge comes, but wisdom lingers" is a quotation from Tennyson's *Locksley Hall*, a strange poem about individual confidence and resolution in the face of the world. Lucian was a satirist, one of whose targets was one Alexander the Pahplagonian, a fraud who set up an oracle of Aesculapius, the father of medicine. And finally Hulbert Harrington Warner sold – very successfully at the time Osler was writing – a variety of so-called "Safe Cures" in bottles which were patented in 1887 and are now collectors' items.

Note how the Humanities seems to guide Osler. What he offers us is an address filled with oblique references to touchstone narratives which were part of the cultural tradition of the day. The contextualization of the students' professional life within a wider understanding is notable by being, it appears, entirely routine. And what particularly interests about Osler's references is not the display of learning, though perhaps part of it is a delight shared with his audience at a kind of florid name dropping. Rather what is of value is that the references are so apposite – they pick out the themes of superstition and science, of integrity and fraud, of self-awareness, of the need for a wide understanding and engagement with the world, for tolerance and calm in the face of the silly things people do and think. The richness and allusiveness of the text is extraordinary, in other words, and supply the context against which the doctor performs his duties.

This is the Humanities, and the narratives which they contain, at the heart of a way of thinking. "Knowledge" (putting that word in prevaricating inverted commas) is more than simply the sum of what empirical research can give us, of course. In this respect, for health care professionals, and perhaps particularly doctors who have come up through a science stream, narratives represent a new of thinking, a new way of making sense of the world professionally and personally. But beyond that, an approach to professional and personal life through which the Humanities echo, is a life which is richer.

References

Balint, M. (1957). *The doctor, his patient and the illness*. London. Pitman Medical. 2nd ed. (1964, reprinted 1986) Edinburgh. Churchill Livingstone.

Best, P. (1869). Death from accumulation of hair in the stomach of a woman. *British Medical Journal, 2*, 630–631. doi: 10.1136/bmj.2.467.630.

Booth, W. C. (1961). Distance and point of view: An essay in classification. In W. C. Booth, (Ed.), *Essays in criticism*. Oxford, UK: Oxford University Press.

Borges, J. L. (1996–1997). Metáforas de las mil y una noches. In J. L. Borges, 1996–97. *Obras completas I–IV, Tomo III* (Buenos Aires: Emecé Editores), p. 170 (Poem published, 1977).

Brown University. (2010). *Digital Propp: fairy tales and electronic culture*. Retrieved September 29, 2010, from http://www.brown.edu/Courses/FR0133/Fairytale_Generator/home.html.

Bryan, A. (1939). Can there be a science of bibliotherapy? *Library Journal, 64*, 73–776.

Cabot, H. (1926). The pre-medical course. *Bulletin of the Association of American Medical Colleges, 1*, 1–3.

Cervantes, M. S. (2000a). *Don Quixote. Motteux*, P. A Tr. Ware, Herts: Wordsworth Editions Limited. (First published 1605–1615).

Cervantes, M. S. (2000b). *The Ingenious Hidalgo Don Quixote de la Mancha*. Rutherford, J. Tr. London, UK: Penguin. (First published 1604–1605 and 1615).

Charon, R. (2001). Narrative medicine. A model for empathy, reflection, profession, and trust. *Journal of the American Medical Association, 286*, 1897–1902. Retrieved October 5, 2010, from http://jama.ama-assn.org/cgi/reprint/286/15/1897.

Charon, R. (2004). Narrative and medicine. *New England Journal of Medicine, 350*, 862–864.

Chaucer, G. (1951). *The Canterbury Tales*. Coghill, N. Tr. Harmondsworth, UK: Penguin. (Written c1387–1400).

Den Boer, P. C., Wiersma D., & van den Bosch R. J. (2004). Why is self-help neglected in the treatment of emotional disorders? A meta-analysis. *Psychological Medicine, 34*, 959–971.

Doyle, A. C. (1989). *The Sign of the Four*. In Sherlock Holmes: The Complete Stories. Ware, Hertfordshire: Wordsworth Editions Limited, pp. 97–176. (First published 1890).

Epston, D., White M. & Murray, K. D. (1992). A proposal for re-authoring therapy. In S., McNamee, & K. J., Gergen, (Eds.), *Therapy as social construction* (pp. 96–115). London, UK: Sage.

Evans, A. (2004). Helping GP trainers to improve their random case analysis teaching skills: development of a programme. *Education for Primary Care, 15*, 336–343. Retrieved October 5, 2010, from http://www.ingentaconnect.com/content/rmp/epc/2004/00000015/00000003/art00006.

Foster, E. M. (2000). *Aspects of the novel*. In O. Stallybrass (Ed.), Harmondsworth, UK: Penguin Classics. (First published 1927).

Freedman, J., & Combs, G. (1996). *Narrative therapy: The social construction of preferred realities*. New York, NY: W. W. Norton.

Gibbon, E. (2004). *The Decline and fall of the Roman Empire:* Vol. 1. In J. B. Bur (Ed.), Rockville, MD: Wildside Press. (First published 1776. Edition by John Bagnell Bury first published New York: Fred de Fau and company, 1906).

Greenhalgh, T. (1999). Narrative based medicine: Narrative based medicine in an evidence based world. *British Medical Journal, 318*, 323–325.

Greenhalgh T., & Hurwitz B., (Eds.) (1998). *Narrative based medicine: discourse and dialogue in medical practice.* London, UK: BMJ Books.

Hippocrates. (1983). Epidemics. In G. E. R. Lloyd (Ed.), *Hippocratic writings*. London, UK: Penguin Classics. (Written 5th century B.C.E.).

Hurwitz, B. (2006). Form and representation in clinical case reports. *Literature and Medicine, 25*, 216–240. doi 10.1353/lm.2007.0006.

Larner, G. (2004). Family therapy and the politics of evidence. *Journal of Family Therapy, 26*, 17–39.

Launer, J. (2002). *Narrative-based primary care: A practical guide.* Abingdon, UK: Radcliffe.

Marrs R. W. (1995). A meta-analysis of bibliotherapy studies. *American Journal of Community Psychology, 23*, 843–870.

Mishler, E. G. (1984). *The discourse of medicine: Dialectics of medical interviews.* Norwood, NJ: Ablex.

Mishler, E. G., (1986). *Research Interviewing: Context and narrative.* Harvard: Harvard University Press.

Muggeridge, M. (1981). *Like it was: the diaries of Malcolm Muggeridge.* In J. Bright-Holmes (Ed.) (p. 208), New York, NY: William Morrow.

New York University. (2008). Medical humanities. Retrieved October 12, 2010, from http://medhum.med.nyu.edu/.

O'Riordan, M., Skelton, J.R., & de la Croix, A. (2008). Heartlift patients? An interview-based study of GP trainers and the impact of 'patients they like'. *Family Practice, 25*, 349–354. doi 10.1093/fampra/cmn043.

Osler, W. (1932). Aequanimitas. In W. Osler (Ed.), Aequanimitas: *With other addresses to medical students, nurses and practitioners of medicine* (3rd ed., pp. 1–13). New York, NY: McGraw-Hill. (Talk first given 1889).

Reichert, J., Solan, B., Timm, C., & Kalishman, S. (2008). Narrative medicine and emerging clinical practice. *Literature and Medicine, 27*, 248–271. doi: 10.1353/lm.0.0028.

Roberts, G. A. (2000). Narrative and severe mental illness: What place do stories have in an evidence-based world? *Advances in Psychiatric Treatment, 6*, 432–441.

Robinson, L. A., Stacy, R., Spencer, J. A. A., & Bhopal, R. S. (1995). How to do it: Use facilitated case discussions for significant event auditing. *British Medical Journal, 311*, 315–319.

Royal Borough of Kensington and Chelsea Library Services. (2009). Retrieved October 8, 2010, from http://www.rbkc.gov.uk/leisureandlibraries/libraries/libraryservices/bibliotherapy.aspx.

Skelton, J. R. (2009). Dying in western literature In A. Kellehear (Ed.), *The study of dying from autonomy to transformation* (pp. 188–210). Cambridge, MA: Cambridge University Press.

Stern, D. T. & Papadakis, M. (2006). *Medical education: The developing physician – becoming a professional*, 355, 17, 1794–1799. Retrieved from http://www.nejm.org/toc/nejm/355/17.

Swales, J. M. (1990). *Genre analysis: English in academic and research settings.* Cambridge, MA: Cambridge University Press.

The Arabian Nights: Tales of 1001 nights (Vols. I–III). (2010). Lyons, M. C., Lyons, U. Tr. Harmondsworth, UK: Penguin.

The Balint Society. (1961). Retrieved October 12, 2010, from http://balint.co.uk/.

White, M. & Epston, D. (1990). White, M. & Epston, D. (1990). Narrative means to therapeutic ends, New York, NY: W. W. Norton.

Yalom, I. D. (1989). *Love's executioner and other tales of psychotherapy.* London, UK: Penguin Books.

Contributors

Alexander-Stamatios Antoniou, BA (Hons), MEd, MPhil, PhD, PhD, C Psychol, is a Lecturer of Psychology at the University of Athens, Greece and holds undergraduate and postgraduate degrees in psychology, philosophy, and education from universities in Greece and the UK. He also teaches in undergraduate and postgraduate programs at the School of Medicine, the National School of Public Health, and the Panteion University of Social and Political Sciences and gives seminars addressed to personnel of public and private organizations. He is the coordinator of the Division of Organisational Psychology of the Hellenic Psychological Association. He has been involved in National and European research programs and he has served, as a human resource consultant. His publications include research papers and chapters in refereed academic journals, books and edited volumes, and his work has been presented at many national and international conferences. His main research interests include occupational stress and professional burnout, leadership, work values, organisational politics, and communication networks.

Dinesh Bhugra, MA MSc MPhil MBBS PhD FRCPsych, is Professor of Mental Health and Cultural Diversity at the Institute of Psychiatry, King's College London. He is also an Honorary Consultant at the Maudsley Hospital, where he runs the sexual and couple therapy clinic. Professor Bhugra's research interests are in cultural psychiatry, sexual dysfunction and service development. He has authored/co-authored over 300 scientific papers, chapters and 20 books.

He is the Editor of the International Journal of Social Psychiatry, International Review of Psychiatry and International Journal of Culture and Mental Health.

Professor Bhugra has been instrumental in developing various training packages for health service professionals and developing strategies for psychiatric education. In conjunction with this, in 2007 the Royal College of Psychiatrists published Workplace-Based Assessments in Psychiatry, of which he was one of the editors. He has developed teaching modules and short courses for medical students and psychiatric trainees on Cultural Psychiatry and on Cinema and Psychiatry.

In 2008 he was elected President of the Royal College of Psychiatrists.

Richard J. Bogue earned his bachelor's and master's degrees from the University of South Florida. His doctoral studies at the University of Texas focused on methods of studying human behaviour. Earlier in his career, Dr. Bogue led research and demonstration projects for the American Hospital Association and its Health Research and Educational Trust. Starting in 2001, he revived the Centre for Health Futures, a strategic knowledge development unit of Florida Hospital, which is a 2100-bed eight-hospital system. He has also taught at major universities in the states of Florida, Illinois and Texas, as well as in Mexico. He has edited or authored several books and numerous peer-reviewed and other publications. Currently, as President of Richard

Bogue and Affiliates he continues his research interests in healthcare communication, physician wellbeing, and nurse empowerment.

Martin Brüne graduated in medicine at the Westphalian Wilhelms University in Münster, Germany in 1988. He completed his neurology training in 1993, and his psychiatry training in 1995. His subsequent training included a Visiting Research Scientist fellowship at the Centre for the Mind, a joint venture of the Australian National University and University of Sydney. He is currently Professor of Psychiatry and Head of the Research Department of Cognitive Neuropsychiatry and Psychiatric Preventive Medicine at the LWL University-Hospital, Ruhr University of Bochum. He has also published the *Textbook of the Origins of Psychopathology* with Oxford University Press.

Caitlin L. Burnham earned her BA in Psychology from The University of California, San Diego. She also studied Spanish language and culture at The University of Granada in Spain. She is currently pursuing her MA in Counseling Psychology at Santa Clara University, with an emphasis in Health Psychology. Additionally, Caitlin is working as a research assistant in Stanford University's Clinically Applied Affective Neuroscience Lab.

Natasha Croome studied her psychology degree at the University of Southampton, UK. Recently, she completed her masters in research methods at Southampton. She currently works as a research assistant at University College of London.

Marina V. Dalla has a doctorate in social psychology from the Department of Psychology, Faculty of Philosophy, Education, and Psychology of the University of Athens, graduated with honors. From 2000 she works as a teaching and research scientist at the Department of Psychology. She teaches social psychology modules to undergraduate and graduate (Master's) students at the University of Athens. Since 2006 she works also as psychologist at the Drug Dependence Unit-State Psychiatry Hospital of Attica. Dr. Dalla has published many papers in the form of journal articles or book chapters in Greek and English and she has held different presentations in scientific events, in Greek and in English. Her current research interests focus on acculturation and adaptation of immigrants, resilience and vulnerability of immigrant adolescents, social stigma and mental health of immigrants, immigration and drug abuse.

Rachel Davis is a research fellow in the Clinical Safety Research Unit, Department of Biosurgery & Surgical Technology at Imperial College London. She has a bachelors (First Class Honours) degree in Psychology and a masters of science degree in Health Psychology as well as a PhD. Rachel is from a health psychology background and as a researcher, primarily involved in three areas of research: communications patterns of healthcare staff in accident and emergency; factors that can predict variability in patients' surgical outcomes; and patients' perspectives on their own health and illness and how this can affect their attitudes towards their health care experiences.

Michael W. Eysenck, BA, PhD, was Lecturer and then Reader at Birkbeck College University of London between 1965–1987. He then moved as Professor and Head of Department at Royal Holloway University of London (1987–2009), becoming Emeritus Professor upon his retirement. He is now Professorial Fellow at Roehampton University. He has published 42 books and approximately 170 book chapters and articles. Most of his research and book writing has been in cognitive psychology, with his main research interest being in the relationship between anxiety and cognition. His research has been cited over 6,000 times in the literature.

Brian Fisak earned his PhD in Clinical Psychology from the University of Central Florida in 2006. He completed his predoctoral training at Geisinger Medical Center and his postdoctoral training at the University of Florida, Jacksonville. Dr. Fisak is currently an assistant professor in the Department of Psychology at the University of North Florida. He also practices as a psychologist in the Department of Community Health & Family Medicine at the University of Florida, Jacksonville. His primary research and clinical interests relate to anxiety disorders, stress management, evidence-based interventions, and health psychology. He is the author of several peer-reviewed publications and maintains an active research program. Current research projects involve the study of anxiety prevention and cognitive factors related to the development and maintenance of chronic worry and stress. Further, his research and clinical endeavours often include collaboration with primary care physicians.

Adrian Furnham was educated at the London School of Economics, where he obtained a distinction in an MSc Econ, and at Oxford University, where he completed a doctorate (DPhil) in 1981. He has subsequently earned a DSc (1991) and DLitt (1995) degree. Previously a lecturer in Psychology at Pembroke College, Oxford, he is now Professor of Psychology at University College London. He has lectured widely abroad and held scholarships and visiting professorships at, amongst others, the University of New South Wales, the University of the West Indies and the University of Hong Kong. He has also been a Visiting Professor of Management at Henley Management College.

He has written over 700 scientific papers and 55 books including *The Protestant Work Ethic* (1990), *Culture Shock* (1994), *The New Economic Mind* (1995), *Personality at Work* (1994), *The Myths of Management* (1996), *The Psychology of Behaviour at Work* (1997), *The Psychology of Money* (1998), *The Psychology of Culture Shock* (2001), *The Psychology of Physical Attraction* (2007), *The Body Beautiful* (2007), *Personality and Intelligence at Work* (2007), *and Dim Sum Management* (2008). Professor Furnham is a Fellow of the British Psychological Society. He is on the editorial board of a number of international journals, as well as the past elected President of the *International Society for the Study of Individual Differences*. He is also a founder director of Applied Behavioural Research Associates (ABRA), a psychological consultancy. Furthermore, he is also a newspaper columnist. He writes regularly for the *Sunday Times* and the *Daily Telegraph* and is a regular contributor to BBC radio and television.

Gurvinder Kalra is an Assistant Professor in the Department of Psychiatry at the L.T.M. Medical College & Sion Hospital at Mumbai, India. His primary areas of interest include mood disorders, cross-cultural psychiatry, films and psychiatry, sexual minorities and alternative sexualities, migration and cross-cultural aspects of sexuality. Some of his award-winning work has been on geriatric sexuality. He has also extensively written on cross-cultural psychiatry, and on migration and sexuality. He uses films to teach psychiatry and sexuality to his trainees, through a movie club at the department, thus educating through entertainment.

Bruce Kirkcaldy has academic degrees in psychology from the Universities of Dundee and Giessen, as well as postgraduate professional training as a behavioural therapist and clinical psychologist. He is Director of the International Centre for the Study of Occupational and Mental Health, and runs his own psychotherapy practise specializing in the treatment of anxiety and depressive disorders and psychosomatic ailments. In addition, he is Visiting Professor for Psychology at the Jagiellonian University, Cracow in Poland, and Scientific Associate at the University of Jena, Germany. He has published over 200 articles including several edited books, with research and writing interests directed towards clinical and health issues and organizational and leisure psychology.

Jutta Lindert studied at the University of Kiel, Mainz, Santiago de Compostela, and the University of Ulm, focusing on the health and social impact of violence and exclusion. Jutta has authored four books, several peer-reviewed articles, and led or participated in several major national and international research projects on mental health. She is lecturer at the Institute for Peace and Reconciliation in Auschwitz/Poland. Since 2009, Jutta leads the Institute as Professor for Applied Research at the Protestant University of Applied Sciences in Ludwigsburg. The Institute develops knowledge focusing on five areas: (1) mental health, (2) violence and health, (3) health of marginalized groups, (4) mental health promotion, and (4) cultural competencies for care providers. Jutta is President of the Public Mental Health section of the European Public Health Organisation (EUPHA).

Roy Lukman earned his doctoral degree in Educational Psychology from Andrews University, Michigan. He did his clinical work for five years before being invited to join the faculty at Florida Hospital's Family Medicine Residency Program. His focus has always been on whole person care as he contributed to the training of family physicians to be successful physicians. In 2003, he was invited to be the Director of Academic Affairs which provides oversight for all Graduate Medical Education training programs at Florida Hospital. The administrative role provided greater opportunities to focus on the training and development of physicians within the various residency programs. His focus continues to be whole person care and the balanced development of physician trainees, professionally and personally.

Terrence Martin is a graduate psychologist (Ulster University) and a human factors consultant and business psychologist specializing in the fields of health, social and organizational behaviour. A professional trainer with over fifteen years of experience in designing and facilitating learning environments with a focus on personal, group, and organizational development and change. In addition to performing management consultancy in the UK and the Netherlands, Terence is an affiliate of the International Centre for the Study of Occupational Health, and has published extensively in the area of health and organizational psychology. His specialisms include learning and development and attention to intra- and interpersonal topics (behaviour, cognition and affect) within the context of corporate business.

Douglas McCulloch, School of Economics, University of Ulster, was awarded his doctorate for a thesis on the Quality-Adjusted Life Year by the University of Ulster in 1998. His main contribution to the field is "Valuing Health In Practice – Priorities, QALYs, and Choice" (published by Ashgate, 2002), based on the thesis, and including some of the policy work carried out during his post-doctoral year at the Irish Centre for Pharmacoeconomics, St James's Hospital, Dublin. The Health Technology Evaluation Guidelines developed during that year are still in use. He has been lecturing on the Jordanstown Campus at the University of Ulster since 1975 and is currently Placement Tutor for the economics degrees. He is an executive member of the (UK) Association for Sandwich Education and Training, and is also Chairman of the ASET Practice and Research Group.

Timo Partonen was born in Helsinki, Finland, 1965. MD (Licentiate in Medicine), University of Helsinki, 1990; Licensed Physician, National Board of Welfare and Health, 1991; PhD (Doctorate in Medicine), University of Helsinki, 1996; Assistant Professor of Psychiatry, University of Helsinki, 1996–1999; Specialized Psychiatrist, University of Helsinki, 1997; Adjunct Professor (Docent) of Psychiatry, University of Helsinki, 2000; Academy Research Fellow, Academy of Finland, 2004–2009; Chief Physician, working at the National Institute for Health and Welfare (former National Public Health Institute), from 2005. The second edition of his book *Seasonal Affective Disorder: Practice and Research* was published at Oxford University Press in 2009.

René Proyer studied psychology (master level) at the University of Vienna (Austria). He received his PhD from the University of Zurich in 2006 and is currently a senior teaching and research associate at the Division of Personality and Assessment at the Department of Psychology at Zurich University. His main research interests are humor research (especially in the field of dispositions towards ridicule and being laughed at and adult playfulness), positive psychology (especially positive interventions and studying character strengths), and test development.

F. Appletree Rodden earned a PhD in biochemistry in 1969 and then did four years of post-doctoral neurochemical research with the Department of Psychiatry at Stanford

University. After that time, he asked himself whether or not one could learn anything essential about human depression from studying dead rat brains, decided that one probably couldn't, tossed his scientific career plans and became a professional ballet dancer.

After dancing in Europe and Israel for several years, he studied medicine, went into a neurosurgical residency and worked as a neurosurgeon for eight years, during which he published a number of articles on biochemical aspects of brain tumours and brain oedema. After working as a village doctor in West Africa (Burkina Faso) for a year, he began doing brain-imaging research (fMRI studies of "Humor and the Brain") with the Department of Neuroradiology of the University of Tübingen with which he is still associated. Dr. Rodden now works in the Department of Psychiatry in the Christian Hospital of Quakenbrueck. He is an active Methodist preacher in Hamburg and teaches cognitive science to seminary students at the Theological Hochschule Reutlingen.

Willibald Ruch studied psychology, education and statistics at the University of Graz, Austria and Miami University, Oxford, OH, USA. He completed his doctorate (DPhil) in 1981 at the University of Graz and his habilitation at the University of Düsseldorf in 1992. He was awarded the Heisenberg-Fellowship by the German Research Council. Previously a senior lecturer at Queen's University of Belfast he is now Professor of Psychology at University of Zurich, Switzerland. He has lectured worldwide and held scholarships and visiting professorships at different universities. He was the first European President of the International Society for Humour studies (ISHS) and founded the Annual Summer School on humour and laughter. He is on the editorial board of eight scientific journals and co-edits a book series. He has written over 150 scientific papers and written or edited five books including *The Sense of Humor: Exploration of a personality characteristic* (2007) and constructed several assessment tools. Among his research interests are topics like personality and assessment, positive psychology, and humour and laughter. Professor Ruch is a founder member of ISHS and of the International Positive Psychology Association (IPPA). He serves on several executive boards of academic societies and he loves to play classical guitar.

Shauna L. Shapiro, PhD, is an sssociate professor of counseling psychology at Santa Clara University, and previously served as adjunct faculty for Andrew Weil's Center for Integrative Medicine at the University of Arizona. Dr. Shapiro's research focuses on mindfulness meditation and its applications to psychotherapy and health care. Dr. Shapiro has conducted extensive clinical research investigating the effects of mindfulness-based therapies across a wide range of populations, and published over 50 book chapters and peer-reviewed journal articles. Dr. Shapiro lectures and leads mindfulness training programs nationally and internationally for health professionals on the growing applications of mindfulness in psychology and health care and recently co-authored the text, *The Art and Science of Mindfulness: Integrating Mindfulness into Psychology and the Helping Professions* published by American Psychology Books.

Lorraine Sherr is currently Professor of Clinical and Health Psychology and Head of the Health Psychology Unit, Research Department of Infection & Population Health, Royal Free and UC Medical School, UCL, London, UK. She is editor of several journals including *Psychology, Health and Medicine; Aids Care; and Vulnerable Children and Youth Studies* – a new international journal. She is author and editor of many articles, books, and book chapters in the area of health, clinical psychology, and medicine. She sat on the World Health Organisation Strategic Advisory Committee, the WHO Disclosure working group, the WHO Afro evaluation team on psychosocial provision for pregnant women; Medical Research Council Expert Panel 2006–2011; Save the Children and Care evaluation initiative, and she is a Winston Churchill Fellow.

Georg Siefen served as the Medical Director of the Westfalia Clinic for Child and Adolescent Psychiatry for many years and is currently Head of the Department of Pediatrics at St Josef Hospital at the Ruhr University Bochum. He graduated in psychology and went on to study medicine. He is a specialist in child and adolescent psychiatry and neurology as well as a practising psychotherapist.

John Skelton is a literature graduate who spent the first part of his career teaching English language and applied linguistics in UK, Spain, Oman, and Singapore before taking up a post in medical education at the University of Birmingham, where he is now Professor of Clinical Communication, and Head of Educational Development for the College of Medical and Dental Sciences. He also runs the Interactive Studies Unit, which delivers training in non-clinical areas to several thousand health professionals and students of the health professions. He has published on linguistics, clinical communication and medical humanities in journals from *The Lancet* to *Applied Linguistics*. He maintains his interest in international education, and has been consultant on educational projects in 20 countries around the world. He was awarded an MRCGP for services to UK Primary Care in 2002. One of his most relevant recent publications: is *Language and clinical communication: This bright Babylon*, Abingdon: Radcliffe Medical Press 2008.

Rüdiger Trimpop received his Master's degree (Diplom) at the University of Bochum in Psychology, having studied Philosophy and Law as secondary subjects. He was awarded a scholarship to Queen's University, Kingston, Canada and a PhD in the area of Industrial and Organisational Psychology (Risk Theory Management). He is currently Professor of Work, Industrial and Organisational Psychology at Jena University.

Charles Vincent is currently Professor of Clinical Safety Research in the Department of Surgical Oncology and Technology at Imperial College, London. He trained as a clinical psychologist and worked in the British NHS for several years. Since 1985 he has carried out research on the causes of harm to patients, the consequences for patients and staff and methods of prevention. He established the Clinical Risk Unit at University

College in 1995, where he was Professor of Psychology, before moving to the Imperial College in 2002. He now directs the Clinical Safety Research Unit based in Department of Department of Biosurgery and Technology, Imperial College London. He is the editor of *Clinical Risk Management* (BMJ Publications, 2nd edition, 2001), author of *Patient Safety* (2nd edition, 2010), and author of many papers on risk, safety, and medical error. From 1999 to 2003 he was a commissioner on the UK Commission for Health Improvement. In 2007 he was appointed Director of the National Institute of Health Research Centre for Patient Safety & Service Quality at Imperial College Healthcare Trust. He is a fellow of the Academy of Social Sciences and of the NHS Institute for Innovation & Improvement.